McAlpine   Heart and Coronary Arteries

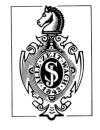

Wallace A. McAlpine

Heart and Coronary Arteries

An Anatomical Atlas for Clinical
Diagnosis, Radiological Investigation,
and Surgical Treatment

With 1098 Figures Mostly in Color

Springer-Verlag Berlin Heidelberg New York 1975

Wallace A. McAlpine, M.D.
F.A.C.S., F.R.C.S., Eng.: F.R.C.S. ED.
Cardiovascular and Thoracic Surgeon
Toledo, Ohio, USA

ISBN 3-540-06985-2
Springer-Verlag Berlin · Heidelberg · New York

ISBN 0-387-06985-2
Springer-Verlag New York · Heidelberg · Berlin

Library of Congress Cataloging in Publication Data
McAlpine, Wallace A. 1920 – Heart and coronary arteries. Biblio-
graphy: p. Includes index. 1. Heart-Atlases. 2. Coronary arteries-
Atlases. · I. Title [DNLM: 1. Biometry. 2. Coronary vessels-Atlases.
3. Heart-Atlases. WG 17 M 114 h] QM 181.M 32611′.12   74-20634

Typesetting, printing and binding:
Universitätsdruckerei H. Stürtz AG, Würzburg
Type face: Monophoto-Times
Paper: Papierfabrik Zanders
Photography: Wallace A. McAlpine
Drawings: Paul Fairchild
Reproduction of the figures: Württbg. Graph. Kunstanstalt G. Dreher
Dust cover: W. Eisenschink
Lay-out and production:
J. Tesch, H. Matthies, and H. Schwaninger

Dedicated to my wife, Shirley,

*who has sustained and encouraged
me throughout my surgical life and,
particularly, during the countless
added hours required in the preparation and photography of the
specimens seen in these pages.*

*And to my children, Kim, Fraser,
Laurel and Leigh.*

Foreword

The magnificent anatomic presentation in this book "The Heart and Coronary Arteries" has a unique importance for surgeons. It is a fundamental contribution to the anatomy of the heart and great arteries as well, because of the analytical, detailed, and imaginative anatomic approach of the author.

While surgery from time to time is influenced by the development of new physiologic principles and techniques, methods of intra- and post-operative support, and new diagnostic methodology, the excellence of its results continues to be related primarily to the precision and perfection of the operative procedure itself. The operative procedure can be precise and perfect only if it is based upon the surgeon's profound knowledge of normal anatomy, his understanding of the alterations in this normal anatomy by the pathology with which he is dealing, and his ability to use this anatomic information in organizing and effecting his surgical procedure. The cardiac surgeon, therefore, will find great rewards from intense study of this anatomic atlas. The cardiologist, the pediatric cardiologist, the anatomist, the pathologist, and students interested in cardiac disease will benefit to almost the same degree from a careful study of this work.

May 1975

JOHN W. KIRKLIN, M.D.
Professor and Chairman
Department of Surgery
University of Alabama
in Birmingham

Preface and Acknowledgements

The importance of gross anatomy in the comprehension, diagnosis, and surgical treatment of disease was impressed on me by my first teacher of anatomy, Professor Ian MacLaren Thompson at the University of Manitoba. Throughout my surgical training, in London under Lord Brock and Professor Ian Aird, in Stockholm under Professor Crafoord, and in Ann Arbor under Professors John Alexander and Cameron Haight, the role of basic sciences was always prominent in clinical considerations. To these, my teachers, this atlas is presented as a tribute.

In 1950, the surgical treatment of heart disease had entered its intracardiac phase and catheter and improved radiologic techniques had become available. In response to this challenge, I began a review of the related anatomic information. The material was limited and often not readily transferable to the clinical problems at hand. I then turned to the dissection of the normal heart. The answers to many questions were readily available; however, it was apparent that comprehension of the relations found in the operating room and the spatial anatomy seen in radiographic studies required not only a technique of fixation of the heart, which recreated the dimensions and form of the living organ, but also a technique of photography that simulated radiographic investigations.

In 1949, working in the department of surgery at Sabbatsbergs Hospital, Stockholm, I observed the pumping of fixative into lung specimens for pathologic study. I was impressed by the restoration of the form and dimension of the functioning organ. It was a natural consequence to utilize this idea and to adapt the apparatus of extracorporeal bypass in effecting the perfusion-fixation of heart-lung specimens a decade later. The importance of this type of fixation in the elucidation of the features of both normal and pathologic hearts has been attested by Dr. Maurice Lev and his colleagues.

A technique of photographic examination of the excised heart was developed to allow, first, the replication of normal in situ relationships with the implicit reference to the anatomic position, and second, inspection from any radiographic vantage point in the horizontal plane; in the text, the radiographic view of each photograph is specified. Finally, angled or elevated views may be used. These are important clinically: In the definitive arteriographic visualization of the proximal parts of the branches of the left coronary artery, the x-ray beam must be perpendicular to the axis of the vessels.

My basic aim in this work is to provide photographs of dissected, normal hearts for the study of the details and spatial disposition of anatomic structures. Photographs are the optimal medium of anatomic communication; however, if each photograph is to be a source of anatomic truth and to separate fact from opinion, it must be free of distortion. To this end, considerable time and effort were expended: Finally, incorporating recent technical advances in photography, the present technique was developed. In the photography, I attempted, first, to manipulate external lighting to demonstrate the contours, delimit the parts, and portray the relationships of the living heart and, second, to use interior lighting, not only to differentiate muscle and membrane, but also to delineate structures, such as the aortic annuli.

The physicians of this era are blessed, but also besieged, by the mass of useful new information confronting them and pressed by the need to review facts once familiar. It is hoped, therefore, that the format selected will facilitate the use of this volume. Although this format occasionally involves repetition of material, page-turning is minimized by the assignment of individual topics to two opposing pages on which the expository photographs and text appear. Although reference to valuable contributions of others is made, the format does not permit an encyclopedic account of the history of anatomic knowledge of the heart. Color-coded drawings, made from the tracings of photographs, are used to simplify orientation of the photographs. In order to avoid reduction in the scale of the photographs and expedite their examination, abbreviations are used; these provide orientation and direct attention to structures being studied. The instructions to the reader should also facilitate the study of the material.

In this presentation an anatomic method of long-standing is used. A dominating structure is first identified and studied; to it the remaining parts are then applied sequentially. In this instance, the dominating structure is composed of the aortic bulb, left ventricle, and the membrane connecting the two. This simple but eductive method clarifies relationships often deemed complex, illumines the logic inherent in cardiac design, and facilitates the acquisition of a detailed spatial knowledge of cardiac anatomy. Although the index is planned to lessen the task of a random study of its parts, review of the whole is recommended in the initial use of this volume. This instruction may be inconsistent with the subtitle of this work: The word atlas was selected to indicate both its pictorial nature and its nonencyclopedic aspect.

"In the description of the human body, all terms are used in relation to the anatomic position". The descriptions of cardiac anatomy are often unique in their disregard for this cardinal principle. The spatial examination of the heart evinces the inaptness of some currently used terms; these have been altered to effect their congruence with the anatomic position—a necessity in their clinical use. In some instances, terms familiar to workers in a narrow segment of cardiology, but not deducible by all physicians, have been changed. For example, when a branch of the left coronary artery supplies the anterolateral or the lateral sector of the left ventricular wall, the spatially correct terms, anterolateral and lateral, replace the ambiguous terms in current use—the first and second diagonal branches. In other instances, alteration is found in terms that have unfortunate connotations: For example, the traditional terms, left anterior descending and circumflex branches of the left coronary artery, are replaced by anterior and posterior divisions of the left coronary artery. This may be deemed quixotic or a mere attempt at innovation. The suggested terms—eschewing the simplistic relegation of the arteries to the sulci—invite the elicitation of the prime characteristics of an artery: its origin, its termination, its course and relations and the arterial subdivision de-

rived therefrom, its mode of branching and the precise area of supply of each of its branches. This elicitory exercise is salutary in the study of obliterative disease. The arrangement of the section on the coronary arteries effects concordance with this fundamental anatomic method. In any event, the primary purpose of this work is to present photographs of hearts for study and I have attempted to ensure that conceptual details and nomenclative changes clarify this study.

A complete knowledge of cardiac anatomy is derived from many investigative and clinical techniques—gross dissection of normal hearts is one of these. This volume is presented as a broad survey of this aspect. Gross dissection and, for example, the injection-corrosion technique exemplified by the works of James and Baroldi are not competitive—each has its own contribution to make. I have made no attempt to repeat the work of others. The location and relations of the conduction system are indicated in many figures in this volume. These inferences stem largely from the works of Hudson, James, Lev, Rosenbaum, and Titus. All 1098 photographs and drawings are original. As I have done the photography and made the tracings for the drawings, the responsibility for the illustrative material and its design is mine. In the belief that material is best studied in its complete and original form, the figures of others are not reproduced; rather, I have directed the reader to contributions that I have found helpful.

A definitive account of anatomy includes the statistical study of each structure examined. In some areas, this statistical study has been accomplished: Presenting this unpublished data, I express my thanks to two former colleagues, Dr. Axel Ehman, Michigan State University, and Dr. Toshiaki Kawakami, University of Hokkaido, for their efforts in this attainment. This has been largely a prospective study and many workers and a multitude of specimens would be needed to gain the desired statistical goal. In the discussion of specimens, features that are important but peripheral to the primary topic, are often described; This results in repetition which may prove irksome to the reader; however, it is intended to compensate, in part, for the limited statistical data. Specimens used in the demonstrations of anatomic features have been selected carefully—the exceptional specimen is not adduced in the depiction of the normal.

The index is intended to serve, not only as an aid when structures are seen in a dissection prior to their formal presentation, but also to enable the reader to examine most anatomic features in many specimens. The index also represents a second approach to the study of the material of this volume. This approach, antithetical to the format designed to minimize page-turning, affords a systematized review of each anatomic structure.

The hearts seen in this work were from individuals who exhibited no clinical or gross evidence of cardiac disease. During the past fifteen years, over 1 000 human hearts, obtained from hospitals over a wide area, have been studied. Over 300 hearts of domestic and wild animals have been used in the study of the comparative anatomy; a few will be seen in these pages.

Dr. Morris W. Selman and Dr. Hugh M. Foster, Jr., my associates in the practice of cardiovascular and thoracic surgery, have assumed an increased clinical burden without complaint. This work would have been impossible without them. Likewise, four of the nurses in our office, Patricia Sheedy, Betty Nicolen, Dorothy Fisher, and Janet Reynolds have added to their travail, sharing in the typing of the manuscript. Mr. Angus MacArthur of Kings College Hospital, London, and Dr. Donald Woodson of the Medical College of Ohio at Toledo, both surgeons, Dr. Donnan Harding, Chief of Pathology at Riverside Hospital, Toledo, and Dr. Charles Schmidt, Chief of Radiology at St. Luke's Hospital in Milwaukee, have provided help in the arrangement of the material. Without the support and encouragement of Dr. Don Nouse, Chief of Cardiology at Toledo Hospital, this work would not have been possible. During the many years of my anatomic study, the friendship and encouragement of my minister, Dr. Robert Hansen, were important. I am pleased to express my great appreciation to the medical artist, Paul Fairchild, who converted the tracings into drawings. He was engaged in this endeavor for five years; his meticulousness and his skill are evident. My late friend, Richard Jamieson, worked with me, late into the night, for many months at the inception of my studies. The importance of his contribution cannot be measured. Richard Serrick, a good engineer and fine friend, designed the mount for the heart. My friend Keith McKenney provided unwavering encouragement and a positive response to all problems. The majority of the dissections of the coronary arteries has been carried out by my daughter, Kim; the precision of her work is evident. I am grateful to Springer-Verlag for their cooperation, attention to detail and for the great efforts they have made in the production of this work. Eugen Jennewein and Kurt Söll of the Dreher Company, Stuttgart, have expended unusual effort in an attempt to capture on these pages the information contained in the photographs. Generous support has been provided by the Andersons, the Ransom Family Foundation, the Mary S. Ritter Foundation, the France Stone Foundation, Mary Stranahan, and the Institute of Medical Research of Toledo Hospital.

Toledo, June 1975

WALLACE A. MCALPINE

Contents*

* A detailed table of contents will be found at the beginning of each chapter.

Instructions to the Reader

1.

The Designation of Figures: In most instances, six figures (photographs, drawings, x-rays, or tables) appear on each page; the figures are assigned numbers in the manner depicted below: The numeration proceeds from the left to the right of the reader in each row, upper, middle and lower. This system applies when fewer or more than six figures appear. In the text, the figures are indicated by Arabic bold face numbers (**1–6**). If the figure referred to is found on the same page, the single sequence number is used (e.g. **4**); if the figure is found on a different page, both its page number and its sequence number will be used (e.g. **154—4**).

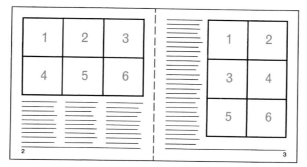

2.

The Presentation of Material: At the beginning of each chapter, the reader will find a detailed table of contents. Turn to Page 9 and note that in Chapter 2, there are four anatomic topics, A, B, C, and D. Topic C, the Aortic Sinuses and its three subtopics (designated by Roman numerals I, II, and III) comprise the **opposing pages** 20 and 21. Topic B, the Ostium of the Left Ventricle and its four subtopics occupy the two pairs of **opposing pages** 16 and 17, and 18 and 19.

3.

The Specimens: (a) **Their differentiation:** On each pair of **opposing pages,** specimens are assigned a capital letter. For example, on pages 14 and 15, six specimens (A-F) are found; one of these (Specimen E: **15—1–4**) is shown in four figures. (b) All are human unless otherwise specified. Over 200 specimens are used—19 are animal hearts—the remainder are human, only three of which show disease

(myocardial aneurysm [1] and calcification [2]).

4.

The vantage point of each figure will be noted. Usually, traditional radiographic views are used. Each of the four classic radiographic planes has two aspects which are referred to as radiographic views. With the exception of the anteroposterior plane, the terms used in this atlas, listed here, are in accord with current usage in radiology. The advantages of numerical designations are discussed on page 8.

Radiographic Views:

Abbreviations and Numerical Designations

Antero-posterior:	A.P.	0°
Postero-anterior:	P.A.	180°
Left Anterior Oblique:	L.A.O.	45°
Right Posterior Oblique:	R.P.O.	225°
Right Lateral:	R.Lat.	270°
Left Lateral:	L.Lat.	90°
Right Anterior Oblique:	R.A.O.	315°
Left Posterior Oblique:	L.P.O.	135°

When a specimen is viewed from above, detailing the spatial disposition of structures in the horizontal plane, the term **superior view** is used. When the postero-inferior aspect of the heart is seen with the interventricular sulcus disposed vertically, the term **inferior view** will be used.

5.

The mode of dissection of the specimen will be described. The heart may be separated into two segments either by a transection or an incision; the former, in contradistinction to the latter, is precisely in a single plane. An **incision** may have multiple components which are positioned to separate but still preserve the integrity of structures, e.g., the left and right aortic leaflets. **Transections** in most instances are made either in the classical radiographic planes of examination or in the planes which are customarily used in anatomic study—they will now be reviewed. The median plane is a vertical anteroposterior plane which divides the body into right and left halves. When any plane is parallel to the median plane, it is termed a sagittal plane. When any vertical plane intersects the median plane at right angles, it is termed a frontal plane. A horizontal plane intersects both the median and frontal planes at right angles.

6.

The terms medial and lateral and left and right are used in reference to the median plane of the specimen, not to the left or right of the reader. The terms anterior, posterior, superior, and inferior are used in reference to the anatomic position. To facilitate comparison with human material, when the hearts of pronograde animals are described, the above terms are retained rather than transposing to the correct counterparts, ventral, dorsal, cephalad, and caudad.

7.

The **Color Code** will be listed for reference. In the first pages, its use will be described in the text. At variance with common use, the veins are green and the right coronary artery is blue: In many drawings differentiation between the right (blue) and left (red) coronary arteries is necessary.

Red:
(a) **Left** aortic annulus.
(b) **Left** coronary artery.
(c) **Left** heart and aorta.
    Aortic valve leaflets are crosshatched.

Blue:
(a) **Right** aortic annulus.
(b) **Right** coronary artery.
(c) **Right** heart and pulmonary arteries.
    Pulmonary valve leaflets.

Green:
(a) Posterior aortic annulus.
(b) Veins.
(c) Pericardium.
(d) Muscles and valves of the right atrium.

Yellow:
The surfaces of the aorto-ventricular membrane.
(Its cut edge is white).

Purple:
Tricuspid valve leaflets.

Orange:
(a) Membranous atrial septum.
(b) Papillary muscles of right ventricle.
(c) Highlighted structures.

8.

The abbreviations are used to avoid reduction in the scale and to expedite the examination of the figures. Coincident to the presentation of the technique, in chapter 1, the reader is introduced to the color coding, abbreviations, and general features of cardiac anatomy. On many pages denotation of the abbreviations will be included in the related text, obviating turning to page 224 where they are listed in both a regional and an alphabetical manner. In a few instances, abbreviations are used for structures which are only rarely studied in this work; they will then be found only in the description of the specimen.

9.

When anatomic relations are described, the term, left ventricle, denotes the muscle part of the wall—the membranous parts of the wall are separately designated.

Section I: General Information

Chapter 1: Technique

Major Objectives

In an attempt to separate fact from opinion, only unre-touched color photographs of normal hearts or drawings made from the tracings of these photographs are used. If the photographs are to have direct clinical application, two objectives are deemed essential:

1. To fix a heart in a manner which reproduces its living appearance—the one seen daily in the operating room and in diagnostic studies. The technique used to accomplish this objective is termed **perfusion fixation.**

2. To photograph the heart in a manner which not only portrays this appearance but does so in a manner which simulates the radiographic examination of the heart in a patient—**radiographic simulation.**

Perfusion Fixation

For several years, I used the familiar technique of stuffing the washed heart with cotton and then placing it in fixative. This was not only time consuming, but failed to achieve the first objective. Since 1960, a perfusion technique, modified from the one used in open heart surgery, has been used. Heart-lung specimens are preferred. From the innominate artery and the left innominate vein, cannulae are passed into the left and right ventricles. The noncannulated entering veins and the aorta distally and its brachiocephalic branches are occluded. High-flow pumps perfuse fixative into the above chambers at pressures of 80 and 20 mm Hg, respectively. The left ventricle and aorta are distended. The excellent perfusion of the coronary and bronchial arteries results in fixation of the heart and lung. This occurs at a cellular level in four to eight hours, depending on the fixative selected. The fixative returns through the coronary sinus and veins into and distending the right atrium. The fixative pumped into the right ventricle results in its distention and perfuses the lungs, reproducing the contours, disposition, and size of the pulmo-

nary vasculature and parenchyma seen in the living patient: it returns into and distends the left atrium. All chambers are seen in their diastolic state. Formalin is used as the primary agent if the atrio-ventricular valve leaflets are to be fixed in their systolic position. In order to give rigidity to the specimen, 100% alcohol, preferably ethyl, is used either as a primary or a secondary agent following the formalin perfusion. Although only a part of the heart is examined, as a result of the rigidity, drooping or distortion is not seen; this rigidity is necessary in horizontal plane examinations and is vital when the heart is rotated in a vertical plane. The hearts are stored in alcohol. The technique has been used with equal success in the hearts of animals varying in size from a swan to a rhinoceros.

Using this technique, the coronary arteries appear normal in size and configuration. The injection into these vessels of colored plastic material has been used in conjunction with perfusion fixation and gross dissection in only a few specimens; these have been used to study the cardiac veins and the septal arteries; in larger arteries, the thickness of the wall prevents visualization of the colored substance.

The Photographic Examination of the Heart— Radiographic Simulation

In the description of the human body, all terms are used in relation to the anatomic position, which by convention is defined as one in which the body is viewed in its erect position, the head, eyes, and toes directed anteriorly, the arms by the side and supinated—the descriptions of cardiac anatomy are often unique in their disregard for this cardinal principle. Walmsley directed attention to this deficiency and stated: "Many textual descriptions and innumerable figures throughout the medical literature view the heart as it would be held in the hand, with the atria above the ventricles and the right and left hearts lying alongside each other in a sagittal plane—basic and false concepts that have caused untold confusion in the past."

In this study, the isolated heart is placed on a vertical mount, simulating its location in an upright patient during a radiographic study. The camera is located two meters from the specimen, simulating the x-ray tube. When the orientation of the heart on the mount is that seen in its living condition, **the examination is termed attitudinal.** (The heart, like a capsule in space, has a normal attitude.) This term is still applied when the specimen, like a patient, is rotated into the various radiographic planes. When a segment, or the entire heart, is viewed without regard to its anatomic position, such an examination will be designated as **nonattitudinal.** The technique used for the photographic examination of specimens appears on page 4. Examine the drawing **4—1.**

In the earliest phase of my study, **the traditional method for the photography of gross specimens was used**—the camera was placed above the specimen which was centered below two lights: the attainment of the stated objectives could not be accomplished. **The heart was then fixed to a mount,** which was designed and built to allow photographic examination in the horizontal plane. I first used a camera with a lens which was "developed for medical photography": unfortunately, its short focal length (hence, short object-film distance) resulted in distortion. I had ignored the clinical parallel—the distortion seen in a Bucky chest x-ray resulting from the short tube-film distance. The technique was obviously discarded.

In summary, **in the technique used for all the photographs in this monograph,** there are three major physical components.

1. A versatile, precision $2^1/_4$-inch by $2^1/_4$-inch-square format single lens reflex **camera** is used*. The larger size of the negative, the 45 f-stop, the built in bellows, and the ability to alter the angle of the lens are important in achieving depth of field—the critical factor in obtaining anatomic information in a multi-contoured subject, as is indeed, the heart. Also, multiple exposures are easily made—a vital necessity when a combination of interior and directional exterior lighting is used to portray the contours of the heart without loss of anatomic detail. The 250 mm f. 5.6 Carl Zeiss lens used accomplishes the radiographic simulation depicted in **4—1.** In a radiographic context this may be termed telephotography. When long bellow extensions are added magnification without distortion is possible—the Bucky effect described above is avoided.

2. The camera is firmly fixed to a stout, steel, versatile **tripod****; a level is added to ensure that the plane of examination is horizontal.

3. The heart is fixed to **the special mount,** which is sturdy and may be locked; hence, as seen on pages 6 and 7, progressive removal of parts of the heart can be carried out with a photographic recording of each stage of the dissection. Also, photographs can be taken from the opposite aspects of a plane and, if a distance of two meters or more is maintained, by viewing one as a mirror image, the two will be superimposable. The multiple photographs resulting can be projected sequentially onto drawing material and a composite tracing made which is then converted by the medical artist into an indepth drawing which demonstrates the anatomy seen in radiographic studies. A drawing placed beside only one of these photographs may contain information not seen in the photograph.

---

* Rolleiflex S.L. 66 Camera.
** Majestic Tripod.

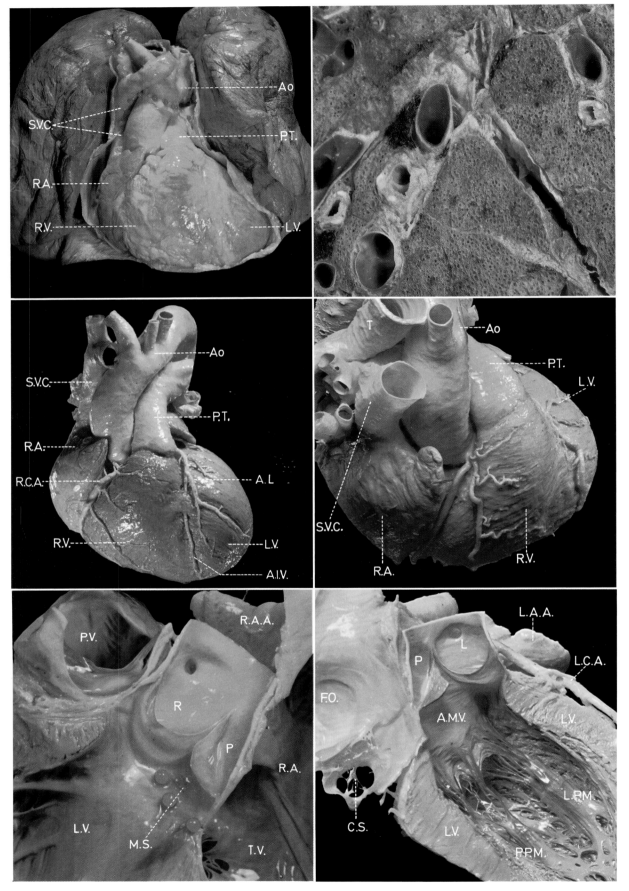

I. The Perfusion Fixation Technique— Its Advantages

Specimen A: 1–3:

1: Superior A.P. view: A heart-lung specimen resulting from this technique of fixation is seen. In order to display the heart, the lungs have been retracted and the anterior portion of the fibrous pericardium has been removed; the line of reflection of the pericardium onto the great vessel superiorly is indicated by red beads. Above, the mediastinal pleura on the right covers the superior vena cava (S.V.C.) and the right innominate vein, and on the left, the aorta (Ao). The left innominate vein is anterior to the origins of the brachiocephalic arteries. Note the fat in the anterior right atrioventricular sulcus (between the right atrium [R.A.] and right ventricle [R.V.]) and in the anterior interventricular sulcus.

2: Scale 5:1: The cross section of the lung is shown to suggest that fixation occurs at a cellular level. The parenchyma and the contour of the vessels are reproduced. Above the center and at 7:30 o'clock the pulmonary artery and vein are seen.

3: From the same vantage point as **1**, after removal of the visceral layer of pericardium and fat, observe: (a) The anterior interventricular branch (A.I.V.) of the left coronary artery runs between the right and left ventricles (R.V. and L.V.). (b) At its origin the pulmonary trunk (P.T.) is anterolateral, at its termination it is posterolateral to the ascending aorta. (Any segment of the aorta is abbreviated as Ao). The size and shape of the chambers and the vessels, large and small, seen in the living heart, are reproduced.

Specimen B: 4: Superior R.A.O. view: The shape of thin-walled vessels such as the superior vena cava is preserved as is the contour of the aorta, the innominate branch of which is seen anterior to the trachea (T).

Specimen C: 5 and **6:** The incisions pass between the following: (a) the right (R) and left (L) aortic leaflets and (b) the halves of the posterior aortic leaflet (P), (c) the membranous septum (M.S.) and the anterior leaflet of the mitral valve (A.M.V.).

5: A near P.A. view (165°) of the right anterior segment. The pulmonary sinuses have been removed. Observe: The right and the anterior half of the posterior aortic leaflets are above the membranous septum (M.S.) whose lower border is attached to the ostium of the left ventricle (which is marked by red beads).

6: R.A.O. view of the left posterior segment. Observe: (a) The adjoining halves of the left and the posterior aortic leaflets are above the anterior leaflet of the mitral valve; in this work the aortic leaflets will usually appear in their diastolic position; the mitral leaflets are fixed in either systole or diastole. The spatial disposition of structures within the chambers is also reproduced by the perfusion technique.

II. The Attitudinal Examination of the Heart— Its Definition

Specimen D: 1: A nonattitudinal examination: An incision separates the septal wall from the other walls of the right atrium. An incision passes through the aorta and the nadir of the posterior aortic annulus and leaflet (P). It is continued through the right fibrous trigone which, in the vast majority of hearts, is the junction of the two divisions of the aorto-ventricular membrane. The incision continues through the left ventricle (red), separating its posterior and the septal walls*. The A.V. membrane, which is colored yellow, is described on pages 9 and 10. With this nonattitudinal examination, two of its components, the right anterior fibrous trigone (R.A.F.T.) and the intervalvular trigone (I.V.T.), and also the left anterior fibrous trigone (L.A.F.T.) are seen between the posterior and right, the left and posterior, and the right and left aortic leaflets, respectively. In particular, we can also note that **the membranous septum**, which is divided into atrial (A.M.S.) and ventricular (V.M.S.) portions by the tricuspid valve attachment, is located between the muscular ventricular septum and the adjoining halves of the right and posterior aortic sinuses and leaflets. However, this mode of examination provides no information about the spatial disposition of any of the structures.

2: The segments resulting from a transection or other type of dissection may be examined in an attitudinal or a nonattitudinal mode. If the information gained is to be transferable to angiocardiography, the former is necessary.

Specimen E: 3–6 is examined in an attitudinal manner.

3: The right segment following a dissection similar to that just diagrammed is seen from the A.P. view. The superior vena cava (S.V.C.) and right atrium (R.A.) are on the right. The right pulmonary artery (R.P.A.), the aorta (Ao), the anterior leaflet of the mitral valve (A.M.V.), and the right and left ventricles (R.V. and L.V.) have been divided.

4, 5, and 6: Following a 45° rotation, the anatomy of the segment is seen in the L.A.O.-R.P.O. plane, first with two modes of lighting, then in a drawing. Observe: (a) The nadir of the posterior aortic annulus and leaflet (P) is above the junction (J) of the membranous septum and the anterior leaflet of the mitral valve; this is also the location of the right fibrous trigone. (b) The planes of the muscular ventricular and membranous septa meet at an obtuse angle. The latter is directed to the right, superiorly and posteriorly. It is thus apparent that the aortic valve normally overrides the muscular ventricular septum. Lack of appreciation of this anatomic fact occasioned the false concept that overriding of the aorta was a particular characteristic of the spectrum of conditions associated with defects of the membranous septum.

---

* The color (coding) may be assigned to the cross section—as seen on this page—or to the surface of a structure—as seen in **4—5** on the next page.

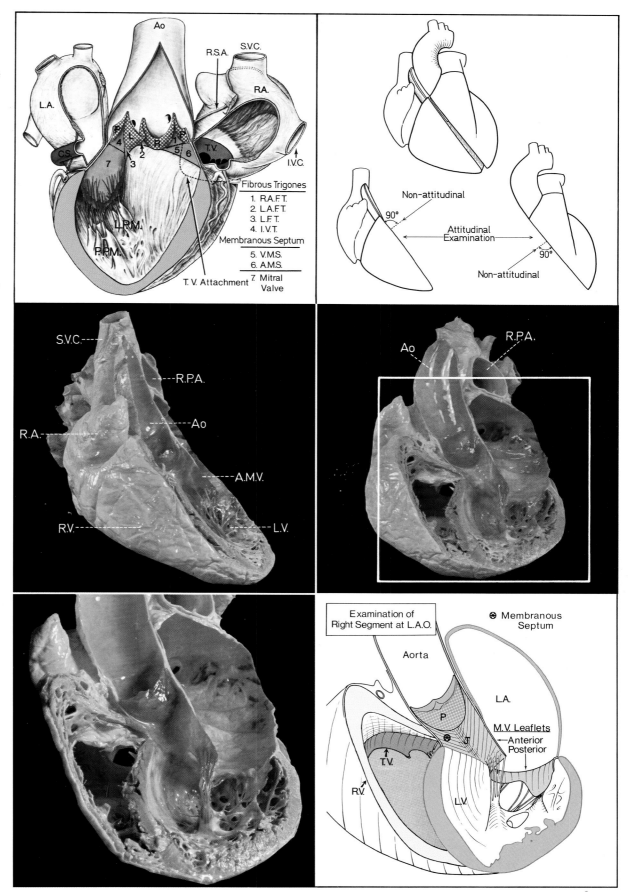

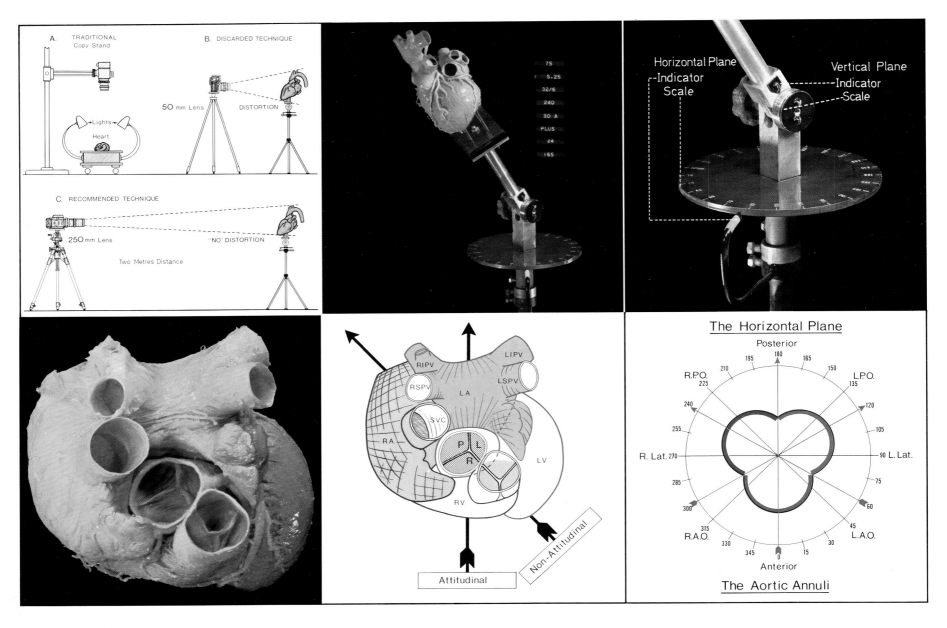

The Horizontal Plane

The Aortic Annuli

III. The Mount Used for the Photographic Examination of the Heart

1: In C is seen the technique used for the photographs shown in this work.

2: The specimen is on the special mount. The mount is fashioned to provide (a large number, if necessary, of) specially hardened, stainless steel, very sharp rods on which the heart is impaled and secured. These rods are usually masked from the photograph—in some instances they are seen as they penetrate the heart. Perforations are present in the background to allow the inclusion of eight data in the photograph. The specimen is seen rotated 20° in a vertical plane; a rotation of 90° affords examination of the specimen from **the superior view** demonstrating the disposition of anatomic structures in the horizontal plane.

3: The horizontal indicator is fixed. It marks the degree of rotation on the horizontal scale, which is attached to and rotates with the central column to which the specimen is fixed. On the upper scale, the degree of rotation in a vertical plane is measured. The heart can be rotated

in the horizontal plane into any radiographic vantage point or in a vertical plane simulating tilting of the x-ray tube or the patient.

4 and **5**: The superior view of a specimen demonstrating **the disposition of the aortic and pulmonary sinuses and leaflets in the horizontal plane.** In **5**, when the heart is viewed from the apex (a nonattitudinal examination), the aortic leaflets (color-coded red) are seen to be posterior, right and left; the pulmonary (color-coded blue) are anterior, right posterior and left posterior. When these same structures are viewed with regard to the anatomical position—an **attitudinal examination**—the aortic leaflets are seen to be anterior, right posterolateral, and left posterolateral; the pulmonary are posterior, right anterolateral, and left anterolateral; these designations will be applied to the pulmonary leaflets and sinuses. **In contradistinction to the description of all other structures in this work,** in which spatially correct terminology is employed, the widely used, but nonetheless incorrect terms, **right, posterior,** and **left**, will be applied to the aortic leaflets and sinuses. The emergence of the

right and left coronary arteries from their respective sinuses and the brevity of the designation of these structures, which are almost omnipresent in this work, can be presented to rationalize this expediency. A criticism of this nomenclative inconsistency appears on page 134.

6: (a) In all descriptions, **the point of examination** will be indicated in reference to the horizontal plane, viewed from above. The numbers increase in increments of 15° in a counterclockwise fashion; thus the L.A.O. vantage point can also be expressed as the 45° view. The abbreviations of the eight aspects of the four traditional radiographic planes of examination are listed in the "Instructions to the Reader". (b) **The disposition of the aortic annuli:** The right, left, and posterior are color-coded blue, red, and green, respectively. Each annulus occupies 120° in the horizontal plane. The three red arrows indicate the vertical planes in which the nadir of one annulus precisely underlies the commissure of the other two annuli: If a radiographic examination is carried in one of these planes, identification of the components of the aortic valve is simplified.

IV. The Use of Lighting in the Elicitation of Anatomic Information

The Aortic Annuli: Specimen A: 1: A.P. view of the left ventricle and the aorta: The aortic leaflets form the boundary between the aorta and the left ventricle. The leaflets are attached to the aortic annuli, which are tough, discrete, hemi-elliptical, thickened bands. When interior lighting is used, the annuli appear dark and form the lower boundary of the three transilluminated aortic sinuses. The coronary arteries (R.C.A. and L.C.A.) identify their sinuses of origin. The right and left annuli are attached to the ostium of the left ventricle. A membranous triangle is found between the three structures; this is called the **left anterior fibrous trigone (L.A.F.T.). The right anterior fibrous trigone (R.A.F.T.)** is between the right and the posterior annulus; below, the septal leaflet of the tricuspid valve (T.V.) is attached to the membranous septum—see its ventricular part (V.M.S.).

Specimen B: 2: Left lateral view: A frontal transection passes through the left aortic sinus. Observe: (a) **The posterior aortic leaflet (P) is suspended from its annulus.** (b) The left and posterior aortic leaflets are posterior to the right. (c) The membranous septum is between the **right and posterior aortic annuli** and the left ventricle.

The Aortic and Pulmonary Sinuses: Specimen C: 3 and 4: P.A. view:
3: A combination of lighting is used to show the following: (a) Muscle (marked by the lower arrows) is present in the two anterior pulmonary sinuses; it is between the leaflet and vessel attachments. (b) Extending bilaterally from the pulmonary annular commissure (marked by the upper arrow) are two sinus rims. (c) Surface lighting demonstrates the contour of the aortic sinuses. **4**: When interior lighting is added, (a) we can see the dark bands formed by posterior halves of the left and posterior aortic annuli, and (b) between the two we can see another membranous triangle—**the intervalvular fibrous trigone (I.V.T.)**; however, we lose the contour characteristics of the aortic sinuses. A better drawing results from a composite tracing of the sequential projection of multiple photographs, each made with lighting to elicit specific features.

The Tricuspid Valve: Specimen D: 5: A nonattitudinal view of the right segment of a transection which passes between the posterior and the left and through the middle of the right aortic leaflet. A combination of interior and exterior lighting can be used to reduce the limitations of nonstereoscopic photography; the transilluminated tricuspid valve is seen in the depth of the right ventricle and a hint of its relation to the aortic valve and membranous septum is obtained.

The Mitral Valve: Specimen E: 6: A.P. view of the posterior segment resulting from a frontal transection through the nadirs of the posterior and left aortic annuli. After removal of the posterior wall of the left ventricle, the diaphanous anterior leaflet of the mitral valve is seen and the papillary muscles are both silhouetted and illuminated.

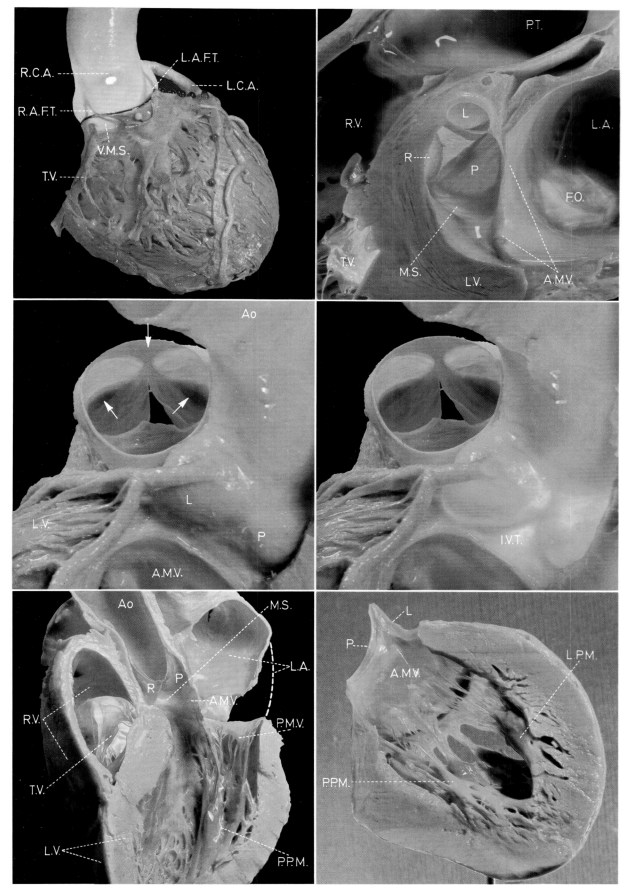

V. Progressive Dissection on the Mount

The Disposition of Structures in the Horizontal Plane

1: The ascending aorta and pulmonary trunk—usually termed the great vessels but better termed the great arteries—have been removed with the following exceptions: a) the sinus-bearing portion of the aorta—**the aortic bulb**—the left and right coronary arteries identify the left and right aortic sinuses—the barren sinus is the posterior; (b) the posterior and left anterolateral pulmonary sinuses. The specimen has been rotated 90° in the median plane, allowing a study of the spatial relationships seen in the horizontal plane. **I term this attitudinal examination the superior view.** The information derived therefrom is applicable to radiographic studies in all planes. In **2**, the left atrium has been removed—see the related drawing, **153—5**. In **3** and **4** the right atrium, and in **5** the right ventricle have been removed, leaving what I term the aorto-ventricular unit—its six components will be enumerated on page 9. In the insert in **6**, a major component of this unit, the left ventricle and its ostium, are shown after removal of the other five components. In **6** the lines of attachment of the left atrium and the right ventricle to the A.V. unit are indicated and can be examined after chapter 2 has been studied.

In order to demonstrate the importance of this type of dissection the relative disposition of selected anatomic features will be noted: (a) In **1** and **2**: **The three aortic sinuses** are related as follows: (1) The anterior half of the posterior—the right atrium. (2) The adjoining halves of the posterior and left—the left atrium. (3) The anterior half of the left forms the medial wall of what may be termed **the left coronary fossa,** the posterior wall and roof of which are formed by the left atrium and pulmonary trunk, respectively. The floor is formed by the left ventricle between its summit and the aorta. (4) The right and left halves of the right aortic sinus are related to the sinus and infundibulum of the right ventricle, respectively. (b) The **pulmonary ostium** is the highest structure in **4**. (c) In **3** and **4**: The pulmonary valve is essentially the reverse of the aortic, possessing posterior, left anterolateral, and right anterolateral leaflets. (d) In **4**: **The left ventricle** has a summit (S.); from the apex, the wall of the left ventricle ascends to this point, then descends to the left ventricular ostium. (e) The left ventricle is disposed essentially in the L.A.O.-R.P.O. plane. (f) The L.V. ostium is occupied by the aortic valve above and the mitral valve below. (g) The **posterolateral wall of the right ventricle** (orange in **4**) slopes inferiorly to the right and posteriorly. (h) The **combined axis of the "mitral" and tricuspid ostia** is disposed at a right angle to the muscular ventricular septum. (i) In **3**, the right coronary artery passes first in relation to the posterolateral wall of the right ventricle; then follows the tricuspid ostium to reach the posterior interventricular groove, whence it passes both posteriorly and to the left to reach the left ventricle.

Note: Orange, a highlight color, delimits the posterolateral wall of the right ventricle in **4**.

The Disposition of Structures in the Sagittal Plane

The right lateral view is seen in all but **2**, which is the mirror image of the left lateral view. In **3**, the right atrium, in **4**, the right ventricle, and in **5**, the left atrium, have been removed. In **3** and **4**, the beads identify the following: the attachment of the septal leaflet of the tricuspid valve (green); the posterior (red) and anterior (green) margins of apposition of the right atrium to the left atrium. **Observe:** (a) In **1**: At the superior and inferior **cavo-atrial junctions**, the posterior walls of the cavae merge imperceptibly with the posterior wall of the right atrium. Between the anterior walls of the cavae and the atrium, superior and inferior **cavo-atrial angles** are seen. A line between the angles demarcates the sinus venarum posteriorly and the body of the atrium anteriorly. (b) In **1** the **axes of the venae cavae** form an obtuse angle; in pronograde animals, they extend ventrally, forming an acute angle which results in an intervenous ridge in the interior of the right atrium. (c) The **superior vena cava**: (1) The entrance of the azygos vein marks the junction of **its two segments**—the upper is directed postero-inferiorly, paralleling the trachea—the lower is directed antero-inferiorly and medially. (2) **Its orifice** is anterolateral to the upper extremity of the atrial septum (see **6—2** and its drawing, **153—5**). (3) A vertical line dropped from **its anterior wall**—at the superior cavo-atrial angle—extends to the superomedial corner of the tricuspid valve; this line forms a part of the superior catheter pathway—a term which denotes the course followed by a catheter passed from the left arm to the right pulmonary artery. The anatomy of this pathway explains the simplicity of this technique. (d) The **inferior vena cava**: (1) **Its orifice** is located posteriorly in relation to both the right atrium and the superior vena cava. (2) The **axis of its terminal segment** is directed towards the atrial septum—a secundum defect of the latter is most easily transversed by a catheter passed from the femoral vein. (e) The **right ventricle:** (1) As seen in **3**, **4**, and **6**, the infundibulum extends above the left ventricle. (2) The tricuspid orifice extends anterior to the ostium of the left ventricle (see **3**, **5**, and **6**) and it extends inferior to it (see **3**)—hence, a left ventricular segment of the right coronary artery is directed posteriorly and superiorly as it proceeds to the left.* (f) The **axis of the left ventricle** extends superiorly and posteriorly at an angle of 45° (see **4** and **5**). In **4**, note that **the left atrium** continues the direction of the axis of L.V. Its summit is between the two superior pulmonary veins. (g) In **5**, **the aorto-ventricular unit** (defined on page 9), along with the thoracic aorta, is seen. The membranous septum and the mitral valve are colored yellow in **6**, a composite drawing made following the progressive dissection. (h) The **brachiocephalic branches** arise in a cluster early in the course of the aortic arch. The innominate (X), the proximal and largest branch, is seen in all; the subclavian (Y), intermediate in size, is seen in **2**. Between the two is the left common carotid artery. **The aortic isthmus**—the narrowing just beyond the origin of the subclavian—is well seen.

---

* The ostium of the left ventricle is divisible into mitral and aortic divisions—the tricuspid orifice is anterior to the entire mitral division—see **6**.

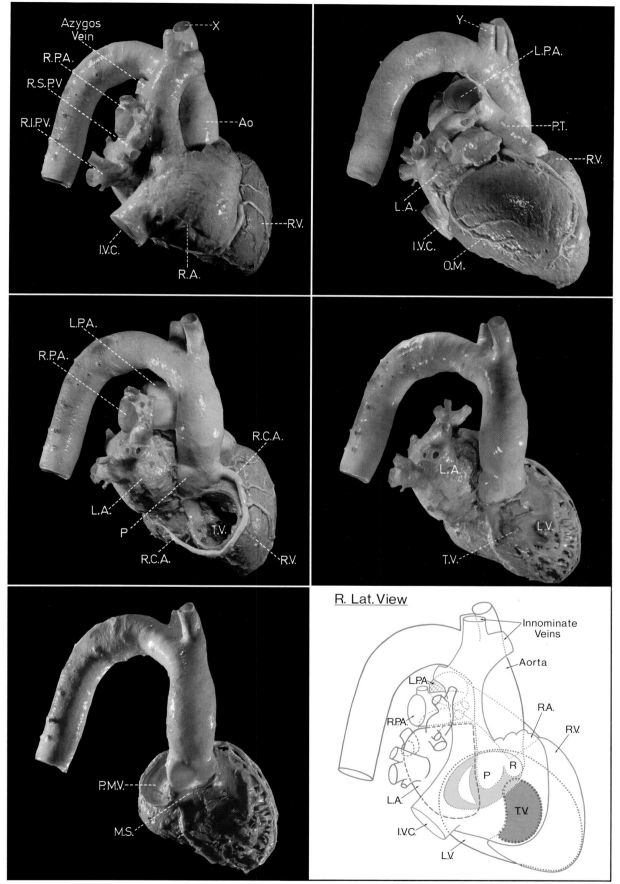

VI. Definition of Radiological Terms

The traditional radiographic planes of examination and their views are referred to in the Instructions to the Reader and on page 4. The manner of usage of these terms in this volume will be stated now.

In the study of chest x-rays, radiologic terminology has been based on the division of the chest into four quadrants by the median plane and a bisecting frontal plane. These quadrants are termed right anterior, right posterior, left anterior, and left posterior. When the x-ray beam passes parallel to the median plane or the frontal plane, **the anteroposterior and the lateral planes of examination** result. When the x-ray beam bisects the angle formed by the median and the (bisecting) frontal planes, **the oblique planes of examination** result. In order to minimize diffractive distortion—even with a teleroentgenogram—in each radiographic plane, the aspect of the chest wall closest to the area or lesion being studied is placed next to the recording device (the film cassette or the radiographic or television camera). In the oblique and lateral planes, **the designation of the view** is derived from the quadrant, or lateral aspect of the body, adjacent to the recording device. In the anteroposterior-plane examinations, when the anterior or the posterior aspect of the body is next to the recording device, the view is termed posteroanterior (P.A.) or anteroposterior (A.P.), respectively: The two designations are, therefore, derived, not from the aspect nearest the recording medium—as are the others—but from the direction of the x-ray beam. Consistence in all views would result if anterior and posterior were substituted for P.A. and A.P. The word, frontal, has been used synonymously with P.A.; however, possible confusion with the frontal plane makes this usage undesirable. Throughout this atlas, in the oblique and lateral planes, the terms used are strictly in accord with the traditional definitions; for example, R.A.O. view denotes that the plane of examination is bisecting the angle formed by the median and the bisecting frontal planes and the camera is opposite the right anterior aspect of the specimen—it occupies the 315° position—see **4**—**6**. In the anteroposterior plane, the terms A.P. and P.A. denote the 0° and 180° views, respectively. These terms indicate attitudinal examinations—anterior and posterior usually are a part of composite terms (e.g. left anterior superior) and denote nonattitudinal views.

In this atlas, a recommendation is frequently implied that the use of a numerical designation for the vantage point or radiographic view would simplify and clarify communication. Use of the anterior midline for the 0° (360°) position would not seem arguable; whether the numerical progression be clockwise or counterclockwise is immaterial if agreement is reached. In this work, the counterclockwise method is used; it has been described on page 4 and in the Instructions to the Reader. Not uncommonly, the optimal study of a structure may not be accomplished by any traditional plane of examination. The selection of the nontraditional or supplementary plane of examination may be based on anatomic knowledge. For example, it has already been indicated (page 4) that identification of the components of

the aortic valve is simplified when a 60° view is used.

Selection of the optimal view may be derived from information elicited in the patient being studied, e.g., (a) the anatomic variations present; for example, the axis of the left main branch of the left coronary artery or (b) the degree of cardiac rotation resulting from a malformation or acquired disease: Schooled in the traditional terminology, but long convinced of the salutary effect of numerical designations, I was startled on first hearing terms such as "15° R.A.O." which have developed in the era of angiocardiography. The ambiguity is apparent: is the view 15° from what is described here as the 0°—360° position in the direction of the R.A.O. vantage point or is the view 15° from the latter position? Also, is the designation of views termed "60° L.A.O." and "60° left lateral" the same? It is self-evident that terms should be simple, consistent, logical, and deducible by all physicians, not merely by a small cadre of workers in a narrow field of medicine.

The comprehension of spatial anatomy is facilitated by the use of the four traditional planes of examination, particularly in the initial examination of a patient. The anteroposterior and lateral views define structures in relation to the median and frontal planes and it is fortuitous that the long axis of the ventricular septum essentially parallels the L.A.O.-R.P.O. plane of examination, placing the jet of contrast medium from the orifice of as septal defect, in profile in this plane. As an obvious corollary, the septal wall is seen in its full expanse in the R.A.O.-L.P.O. plane. Therefore, for these reasons, these traditional planes are used in most instances in this volume. These traditional planes are, for the same reasons, useful in clinical practice in eliciting the spatial anatomy notwithstanding apparent disadvantages—for example, the vertebral column is behind the heart in the A.P. plane. To the physician, perhaps more important than the views he selects is the need for a set and repeated protocol if he is to constantly increase his spatial orientation and total comprehension of cardiac anatomy. The universal adoption of a protocol would facilitate review of the studies carried out in other centers. As knowledge and experience in the spatial anatomy grows, this desired goal may be reached.

Section II: The Normal Heart

Chapter 2: An Introduction to the Aorto-Ventricular Unit

Introduction

Aorto-Ventricular Unit—Definition

In the study of anatomy of a part, great advantage accrues from concentrating one's attention, first, on **the central structure** present. In the thigh, for example, only after the details of the femur are encompassed are the muscles added, the nerves and vessels insinuated, and the whole enveloped by fascia and skin. In the heart, there is a central dominating structure, the **Aorto-Ventricular Unit,** composed of six structures: (1) **the muscle-part of left ventricle;** (2) **the aortic sinuses;** (3) **the aortic leaflets;** (4) **the aortic annuli,** which are attached to the ostium of the ventricle either directly or through the intermediation of membrane*. The fibrous annuli, hemi-elliptical in shape, average 50 mm in length. They provide attachment to both the aortic wall and leaflets of the aortic valve. Approximately 30% of the right and 15% of the left are directly attached to the ostium of the left ventricle. The posterior annulus is a variable distance (5–25 mm) above the same ostium. Approximately the upper 10% of adjacent annuli are contiguous, forming the three annular commissures. (5) Between the left and right annuli and the ostium of the ventricle, a small triangle of membrane is present—the **left anterior fibrous trigone.** (6) From the posterior annulus and the adjoining halves of the right and left annuli, a vastly larger membrane extends to the ostium of the ventricle, and this structure will be termed the **aorto-ventricular membrane.**

The Ostium of the Left Ventricle

The opening of the ventricle is herein termed the ostium. Its margins will also be referred to as the ostium or the ostial slope. No other feature of cardiac anatomy equals it in importance. It provides attachment for the aortic annuli, the aorto-ventricular membrane, and the left anterior fibrous trigone. Its identification in radiographic studies establishes the attachment of the mitral and aortic valves and the membranous septum. Major components of the conduction system run along a segment of its upper border rendering its identification at operation of obvious importance. Its study in animals provides important insight into the anatomic variations seen in the valvular structure of human hearts.

Aorto-Ventricular Membrane

This structure moors the aortic annuli to the ostium of the left ventricle. The posterior aortic annulus is attached only by the intermediation of the membrane; in order to overcome the disruptive force of ventricular systole, it is not surprising that, between its nadir and the ostium of L.V., a thickening in the membrane may exist. This area is triangular in shape and is called the **right fibrous trigone.** The term central fibrous body has also been applied to this segment of the membrane. The attachment of the left aortic annulus to the ostium is usually meager, and it is also not remarkable that a thickening may be seen in the membrane in relation to its attachment—**the left fibrous trigone.** Cartilage may be found at the sites of these two trigones in some animal hearts, e.g., porcine. In the bovine heart, the left os cordis replaces the left fibrous trigone; the right os cordis, not only replaces the right fibrous trigone, but also the membranous septum seen in human hearts.

The Aorto-Ventricular Membrane is Continuous.

Its components, for example the right fibrous trigone and the membranous septum, are often referred to as specific entities. The drawings on the next page are used to indicate the continuity and to delimit the seven components of this membrane which result from the attachment, to it, of the atria and the right ventricle. The conjoined left and right atrial attachments between the nadir of the posterior annulus and the ostium of L.V. mark the junction of the membrane into anterior and posterior divisions. The junction point is almost always the site of the right fibrous trigone. **The anterior division** is composed of three components; (a) the right anterior fibrous trigone, (b) the ventricular, and (c) the atrial segments of the membranous septum**. **The posterior division** is divisible into four components; (a) the intervalvular trigone, (b) the left fibrous trigone, (c) the leaflets of the mitral valve, and (d) the subvalvular segment of the aorto-ventricular membrane. It is worth restating that the right fibrous trigone is a thickening in the A.V. membrane between the posterior aortic annulus and the ostium of L.V.; it is, in reality, not a separate component of the A.V. membrane but a part of both of its divisions and is therefore not synonymous with "the junction of the divisions" although the terms are often used herein interchangeably. On rare occasions the conjoined atrial attachment—the demarcator of the divisions of the A.V. membrane—may lie on one side of the right fibrous trigone.

The left and right fila of Henle (filum, L., a thread) are simply those portions of the A.V. membrane between the ostium of L.V. and the left atrial attachment that recede from the left and right fibrous trigones, respectively. (If ever justification existed for an eponymous term, this would be one, as it perpetuates the name of this worker, whose publication in 1873 remains a classic in anatomy.) The structures so designated are parts of a more extensive structure, which in this work is designated as **the subvalvular segment of the A.V. membrane.**

---

* **Annulus,** in Latin, designates a ring, i.e., a circle. In this work, the word is applied only to the fibrous attachments of aortic and pulmonary leaflets which, in reality, constitute only a segment, not of a circle, but of an ellipse. A search for a reasonable alternative term has met with failure. The term annulus, used to designate four fibrous structures to which the four valves of the heart are attached, is, in my opinion, ill-founded—no such structures are to be found.

** The left ventricular wall consists of two parts, muscular and the membranous: the fibrous trigones, the membranous septum and the subvalvular segment of the A.V. membrane comprise the membranous part. (The mitral valve forms a part of the outflow tract of L.V.) The **membranous septum** is found between the left ventricle and the two chambers of the right heart; the terms, atrial and ventricular, are applied to its divisions; the terms, atrio-ventricular and interventricular, are not used. The term membranous ventricular septum is ambiguous—it is used often in reference to what is denoted here as the membranous septum (part of which lies between the right atrium and the left ventricle).

The **atrial septum** usually has a membranous component which will be referred to as the membranous portion of the atrial septum or the valve of the foramen ovale (this term is applied when a probe patent foramen ovale exists)—it will not be referred to as the membranous septum.

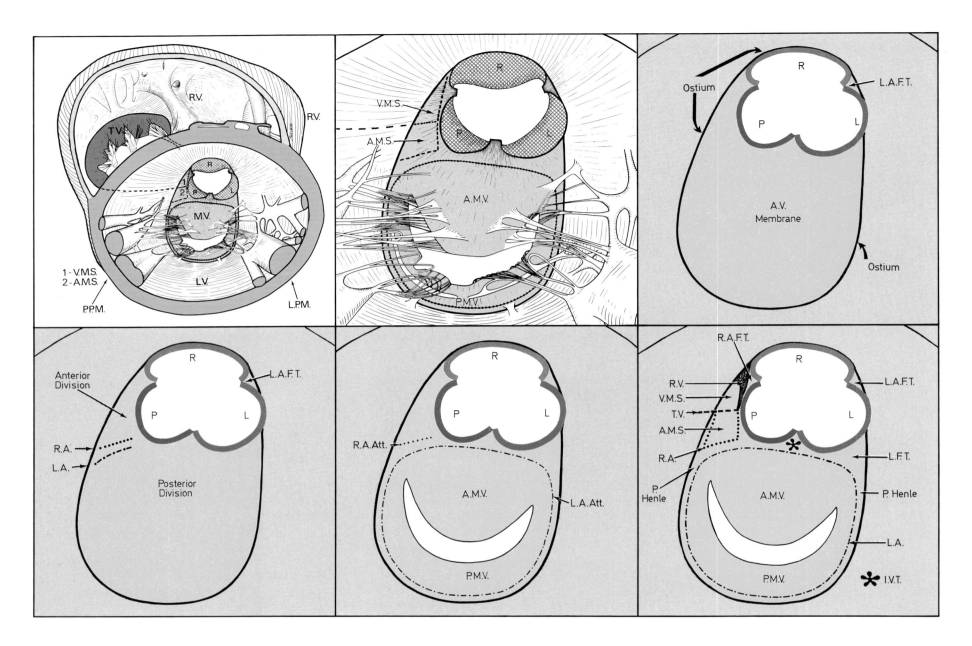

A. The Aorto-Ventricular Membrane

I. Its Design and Components

1: The heart is sectioned transversely, and we peer into the left ventricle from the apex. The walls are splayed apart to allow examination of the aortic and mitral valves simultaneously.

2: The area excerpted here provides the source for the following drawings. The three aortic leaflets, posterior (P), right (R), and left (L), are above. The anterior (A.M.V.) and the posterior (P.M.V.) leaflets of the mitral valve are below. The ventricular (V.M.S.) and atrial (A.M.S.) portions of the membranous septum are demarcated by the septal leaflet of the tricuspid valve (T.V.)—see **1**.

3: The ostium of L.V., as in all drawings and photographs in this entire work, should, when present, first be identified. The attachment of the aortic annuli to it is seen. The left anterior fibrous trigone (L.A.F.T.) is noted. The remaining structure is the A.V. membrane.

4: The right and left atria are attached on the outer surface of the membrane and are indicated here as they extend from the ostium to the nadir of the posterior annulus. The portion of the membrane at their attachment is the right fibrous trigone. Their conjoined attachment divides the membrane into **anterior and posterior divisions.** Very rarely, the conjoined atrial attachments are not attached to the right fibrous trigone—an example appears on page 25 (see the discussion on page 9).

5: The left atrial attachment is completed, the posterior division is incised, and the anterior and posterior leaflets of the mitral valve (A.M.V. and P.M.V.) result.

6: The tricuspid, the right ventricular, and right atrial attachments are added. (There is no intention to imply that the appearance depicted in **3** and **4** ever occurs during fetal development.)

The anterior division is divided into three parts by the attachments of the tricuspid valve, the right ventricle, and the right atrium to the membrane. The right anterior fibrous trigone (R.A.F.T.) is between the right and posteri-or aortic annuli and above the chamber attachments. Below the latter is the membranous septum, the ventricular (V.M.S.) and atrial portions (A.M.S.) of which are demar-cated by the attachment of the septal leaflet of the tricuspid valve to the A.V. membrane.

The posterior division is divisible into four components. (1) The **mitral valve** is, herein, by definition, that portion of the A.V. membrane which is central to the attachment of the left atrium. The orifice does not interrupt the con-tinuity of the membrane—at the commissures, it is approxi-mately, 1 cm in width. (2) The **intervalvular trigone** (I.V.T.) is that portion of the membrane between the left and pos-terior aortic annuli and above the left atrial attachment. (3) The **left fibrous trigone** (L.F.T.): Its borders are formed by (a) the ostium of L.V., (b) the left aortic annulus, and (c) the attachment of the left atrium to the membrane. The latter two structures may be contiguous; when they are separated, the left fibrous trigone and the intervalvular trigone (I.V.T.) are confluent. (4) The fila of Henle (P. Henle) are portions of the fourth component, **the subval-vular segment of the A.V. membrane.**

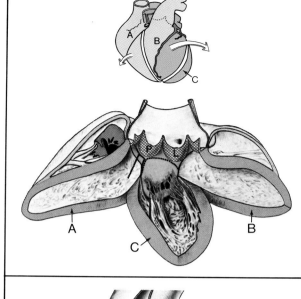

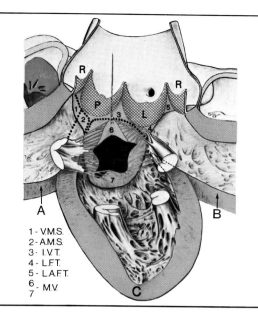

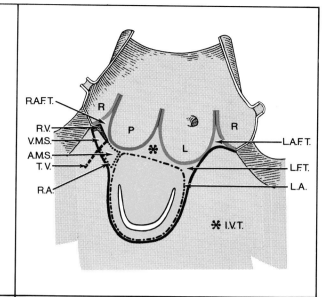

1 - V.M.S.
2 - A.M.S.
3 - I.V.T.
4 - L.F.T.
5 - L.A.F.T.
6 - M.V.
7

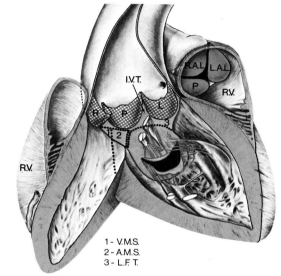

1 - V.M.S.
2 - A.M.S.
3 - L.F.T.

FIBROUS TRIGONES
100 Specimens

	Height-mm	Base-mm	Area-mm^2
Right anterior (R.A.F.T.)	11.0	20.3	17.7
Left anterior (L.A.F.T.)	6.1	4.9	8.6
Left (L.F.T.)	7.2	8.4 × 8.3	27.3
Intervalvular (I.V.T.)	12.5	23.3	59.1

AORTIC ANNULI - 100 Specimens (in mm.)

	Mean	S.D.	Range
1. Length	51.5	5.4	37 - 67.0
2. Attachment to Ostium			
Right Annulus			
To the left of the nadir	12.0	2.5	5.5 - 17.9
To the right of the nadir	4.5	3.1	1.4 - 13.0
Left Annulus	7.36	3.1	2.0 - 18.5
3. Posterior			
Height above Ostium	10.0	1.6	6.0 - 18.0

1: The intact membrane may be seen to the best advantage by the use of the incisions demonstrated here. The primary incision passes through the nadir of the right aortic annulus and is carried across the right ventricle between the segments A and B. These are distracted and two additional incisions are made to allow the interior of the specimen to be examined. The dotted line indicates the attachment of the chambers on the opposite side of the membrane.

2: A closer view is seen : Note the limited attachment of the left aortic annulus and leaflet to the ostium. Muscle is not infrequently seen in the right aortic sinus; see this specimen.

3: The components of the A.V. membrane are shown.

4: This incision passes through the left anterior fibrous trigone and across the infundibulum of the right ventricle to the apex, whence it extends to the ostium of L.V., separating the septal and posterior walls of L.V. en route. The all-important ostium of L.V. is seen after the posterior papillary muscle is divided and then elevated. The left aortic annulus is separated 3 mm from the L.V. ostium. **This represents an extreme degree of the tendency of human hearts to demonstrate a membranous type of attachment of the aortic annuli to the ostium.** The left, left anterior, and intervalvular fibrous trigones are in continuity. A heart with this type of configuration would be a prime candidate for the development of annular subvalvular left ventricular aneurysms, which are seen most often in the Bantu.

5: Here are listed the mean of the dimensions of the fibrous trigones of 100 specimens which we have studied. Each forms a portion of the wall of the left ventricle, and all are potential sites for the development of aneurysms, instances of which have been recorded in the last two and are to be anticipated in the first. The left anterior is by far the smallest; the intervalvular, much the largest. The right fibrous trigone is a thickening of the junction of the divisions of the A.V. membrane and is not delimited; hence, it is not included here.

6: The attachment of the right aortic annulus to the ostium is more extensive than the left, 16.5 : 7.36. The height of the posterior aortic annulus above the ostium is the most important determinant of the size of the membranous septum. This study was carried out in 1967: previously prosected fresh autopsy specimens were used; the specimen seen in **4** was studied later and is, therefore, not included in the data. In perfusion fixed material, the posterior annulus has been found 25 mm above the ostium.

Definitions: What forms the boundary between the left ventricle and the aorta? Certainly, no aortic ring exists, although this term remains unextinguished: During diastole, the aortic leaflets separate the aortic and ventricular cavities; during systole, the aortic annuli form three lines of demarcation between the two. What constitutes the wall of these two structures? In all instances in the human heart, the ventricular wall is divisible into two parts—one is muscle and one is membrane. When muscle is found in the right aortic sinus (see **2**), the aortic wall, then, has a muscle component, albeit small.

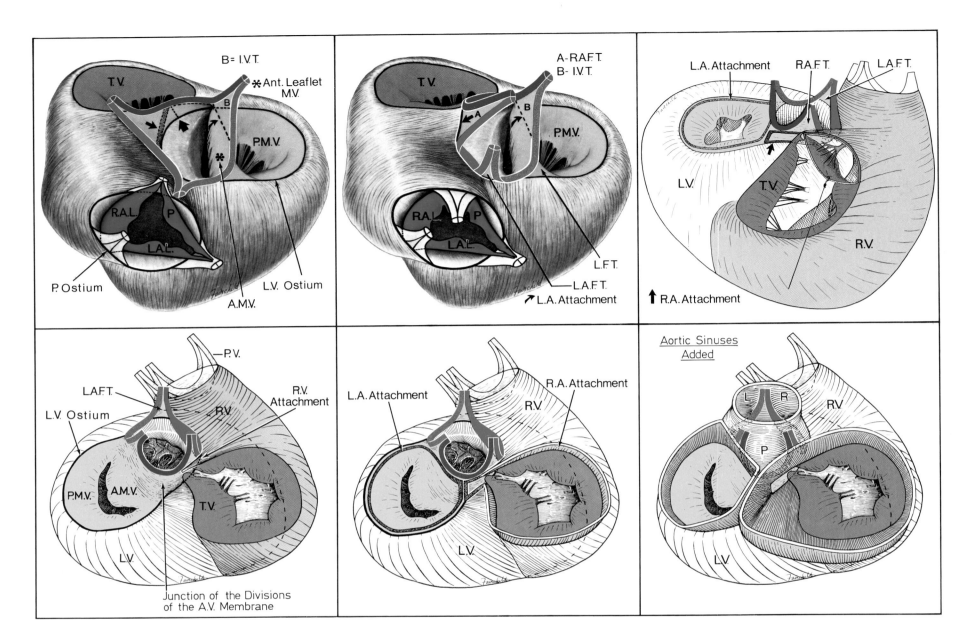

II. The Attachments of the Chambers to the Aorto-Ventricular Membrane

The Attachments of the Right Ventricle

The ventricular septum is, in this work, considered a part of the aorto-ventricular unit. The right ventricle, hence, has three walls: anterior, inferior, and posterolateral and two ostia: the pulmonary and tricuspid.

Accordingly, five lines of attachment of the right ventricle to the unit are to be described. These are: anterior, inferior, posterolateral, pulmonary or superior, and tricuspid or posterior. At this time, the posterolateral and the tricuspid attachments **to the aorto-ventricular membrane** will be examined in **1**, **2**, and **3**. The tracings were made of these specimens after the removal of the atria and the aortic and pulmonary artery walls, leaving intact the respective annuli. **1** and **2** are seen from a high L.A.O. view and **3** from 300°.

1: Identify the left ventricular ostium and note the attachment of the left (red) and right (blue) aortic annuli directly

to it. The posterior aortic annulus (green) is 8 mm above the ostial level. Where the right annulus is attached to the ostium, the posterolateral wall of the right ventricle is attached just anteriorly to the septal muscle. The attachment passes from the muscle onto the membrane at the point where the annulus leaves the ostium and the membrane begins. The upper right arrow indicates the line of attachment of the posterolateral wall of the right ventricle to the opposite side of the membrane. The stubby arrow indicates the attachment of the septal leaflet of the tricuspid valve. The curved arrow indicates the attachment of the left atrium to the opposite side of the membrane demarcating the intervalvular trigone above and the anterior leaflet of the mitral valve below. Note the circular pulmonary ostium of the right ventricle and the attachment of the pulmonary annuli to the internal surface of the ventricle and to the triangular segments of the wall of the pulmonary trunk which remain above the ostium.

2: The aortic annuli, in relation to the left (L.A.F.T.) and right (R.A.F.T.) anterior fibrous trigones, are displaced

centrally. The attachment of the posterolateral wall of the right ventricle to the outer surface of the membrane is seen.

3: A different specimen is now examined. The tricuspid and posterolateral attachments to the membrane meet beneath the commissure of the right and posterior aortic annuli.

The Attachment of the Atria to the Aorto-Ventricular Membrane

4: The atria and the great vessels down to the annuli have been removed and the specimen is examined from a high 240° view. First, identify the outline of the ostium of the left ventricle. Again note the attachments of the aortic annuli to it. Under the right and posterior aortic annuli, the posterolateral wall of the right ventricle and the septal leaflet of the tricuspid valve are seen attached to the A.V. membrane.

12–5: The attachments of the left atrium (red) and the right atrium (blue) have been added to the A.V. membrane. The left atrial attachment is central to the ostium. (Photographic demonstration of this important fact is found on pages 46–50.) The right atrial attachment to the tricuspid "membrane" and to the A.V. membrane is seen.* Note the parallel course of the two atrial attachments to the latter between the nadir of the posterior annulus (green) and the ostium of L.V.

12–6: Rims of both atria are now set in place. The inferior wall of the right atrium comes in contact with the left ventricle. The atria extend superiorly and posteriorly from their attachments. In the area where they are in apposition, the atrial septum is formed.

1–4: R.P.O. view: The atria, except for a 3 mm rim at their attachments, are removed. The aorta has been removed above the level of the aortic sinuses. In **1**, combined exterior and interior lighting is used; in **3**, only interior lighting is used; the annuli, the atrial attachments, and the posterior aortic leaflet are seen as darkened bands or areas. Between the portions of the right and left atrial attachments, which extend from the nadir of the posterior annulus to the ostium of L.V., muscle has been removed to differentiate the two attachments. Note the large intervalvular trigone between the posterior and left aortic annuli and the left atrial attachment. The coronary artery branches of this specimen will be studied on page 195 and need not concern us now.

5 and 6: The same specimen is viewed from 270°. The right atrial attachment to the aorto-ventricular membrane is relatively broad (1.2 cm); the atrial portion of the membranous septum (A.M.S.) is seen anterior to it. It is important and fundamental to realize that the membranous tissue is continuous under the site of the muscle attachment of the chambers. Between its attachments to the tricuspid membrane and the A.V. membrane, the right atrial wall extends across the posterior superior process of the left ventricle (defined on page 68). Between the right atrium (colored blue) and the left ventricle, runs the superior septal artery (this is the traditional term—as described on page 172 the spatially correct term is posterior septal artery).

Comment: The anterior division of the A.V. membrane and a large part of the anterior leaflet of the mitral valve extend superiorly from the ostium of L.V. This fact has been seen, of course, in **2—5** and **6,** and **3—5** and **6** and will be evident on page 15.

Technical note: In **1, 3,** and **5,** the transillumination was planned to differentiate muscle from membrane at the right fibrous trigone—the adjoining intervalvular trigone, membranous septum and the right two thirds of the anterior leaflet of the mitral valve are optimally illuminated and appear yellow. The red blotch just below and to the left of the center of **3** results from heat injury to this thin part of the leaflet. The remainder of the mitral valve, which is less close to the light source, appears tan colored.

---

* A description of the tricuspid membrane is found on page 94.

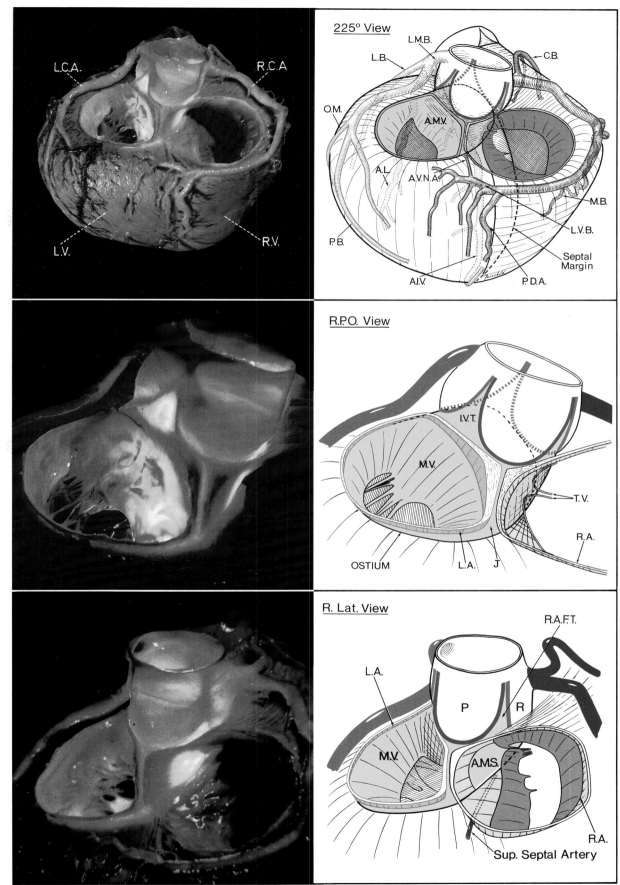

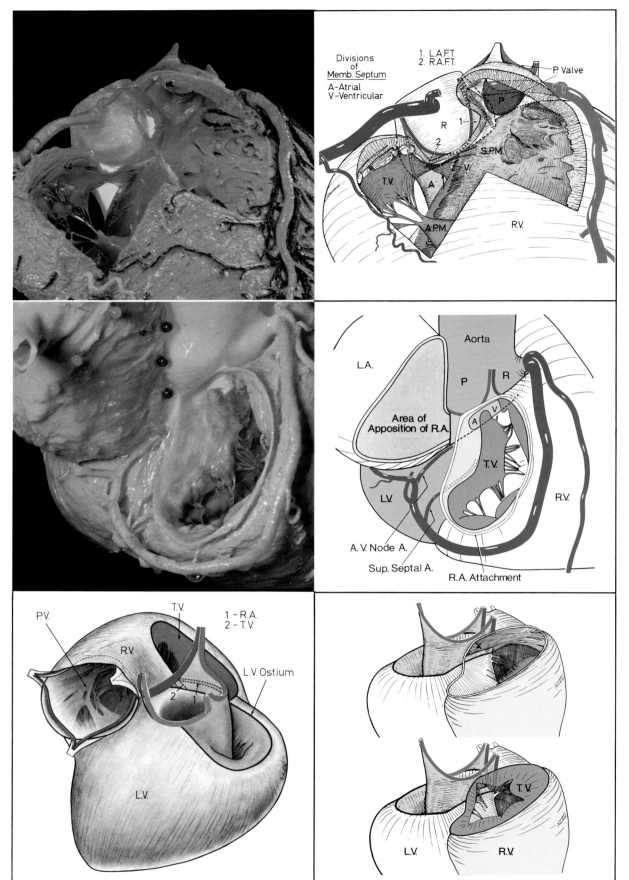

III. Variations in the Attachment of the Right Ventricle to the Aorto-Ventricular Membrane

Specimen A: 1 and **2**: An A.P. view of the specimen just seen. The cut surface of the right ventricle (R.V.) is colored blue. The ventricular septal wall is grey. A portion of the anterior wall and most of the posterolateral wall of the right ventricle have been removed, exposing the right aortic sinus (R). On either side of the latter, the left and right anterior fibrous trigones are found. The line of the attachment of the right ventricle to the A.V. membrane is seen between the right anterior fibrous trigone (R.A.F.T.) above and the membranous septum below. The atrial portion of the membranous septum in this specimen is much larger than the ventricular portion. Note the relation of the left anterior fibrous trigone (L.A.F.T.) to the posterior (P) and right anterolateral pulmonary leaflets. High ventricular septal defects occur in this area; these are best termed subpulmonic.

Specimen B: 3 and **4**: Right lateral view: The right atrium has been removed. Observe: (a) The size of the membranous septum varies directly with the height of the posterior annulus above the left ventricular ostium. In this specimen, the separation is 7 mm, in the specimen above, 16 mm. On page 25, it will be seen that on rare occasions, rotational variations of the annuli on the ostium occur, which will greatly affect the size of the membranous septum. (b) The relative size of the atrial and ventricular portions of the septum is determined by the site of attachment of the septal leaflet of the tricuspid valve to the membrane. In this specimen, in contrast to the specimen just examined in **1** and **2**, this attachment is located posteriorly on the membrane, resulting in the presence of a small atrial and a large ventricular portion.

Specimen C: 5: Superior L.P.O. view: The right ventricular and tricuspid valvular (T.V.) attachments to the membrane are located anteriorly. A very small ventricular component of the membranous septum results.

Specimen D: 6: Inferior right lateral view: An unusually broad zone of membrane is covered by the attachment of right ventricular muscle (X). Transillumination of such a specimen would suggest that the "membranous septum" is reduced to a small oval area. The important fact, however, is that the A.V. membrane is still continuous as it extends from the right and posterior annuli to the left ventricular ostium.

Technical Note:
Interior lighting has been used in **1** and **3**. In **1**, the left anterior fibrous trigone and the parts of the A.V. membrane seen in this view, viz. the right anterior fibrous trigone and the membranous septum (its small ventricular portion is obscured by covering tricuspid chordae) are well shown, placed in contrast against the less lit cavity of R.V. In **3**, with the exception of the ventricular portion of the membranous septum which is in the less lit interior of R.V., the exterior lighting largely neutralizes the transillumination effect in the aortic sinuses and A.V. membrane.

IV. The Attachment of the Left Atrium and the Mitral Valve

The mitral valve is herein defined as that portion of the A.V. membrane which is central to the attachment of the left atrium (L.A.). In **1** through **4**, this attachment is shown, and in **5** and **6**, a variation is seen.

Specimen E: 1–4:

1 and **2**: P.A. view following removal of the left atrium: The anterior and posterior margins of the area of apposition of the latter to the right atrium is indicated in the photograph by the blue and red beads. The **central red bead** is at (a) the site of the attachment of the junction of the divisions of the A.V. membrane to the ostium of L.V. and (b) the location of the A.V. node. In **1–4** note the artery to the node. The attachment of the left atrium to the A.V. membrane extends inferiorly from the left at a right angle to the axis of the aortic bulb, meeting the conjoined right and left atrial attachments to the membrane which extend between the lower adjacent red and blue beads. A posterior atrial artery passes to the right to reach the atrial septum. It is seen in **1, 3,** and **4**; in **2**, a segment of it has been removed. It is not to be confused with the attachment of the left atrium.

3 and **4**: A nonattitudinal left posterosuperior view: The muscle of the left atrium is attached to the A.V. membrane, producing the thick, dark line. The anterior leaflet of the mitral valve has appositional and nonappositional portions. There is also a nonmobile portion of the membrane which may be called the hinge of the mitral valve. This is a triangular area, the apex of which is located at the left fibrous trigone; the base is at the site of the conjoined atrial attachments extending from the posterior annulus to the ostium below. The two other sides of the triangle are formed by the left atrial attachment above and a line drawn between the central red bead and the left fibrous trigone. The height of the posterior annulus above the ostium is important in its effect on the axis of the cage of a ball-valve prosthesis: the higher the annulus, the more anteriorly directed will be the cage—an important determinant in its impingement on the septal wall of L.V.

Specimen F: 5 and 6: P.A. and superior P.A. views: The

size of the components of the A.V. membrane is determined (a) by the attachments of the chambers to it and (b) by the configuration of the ostium. In this instance, the left atrial attachment (L.A.) to the A.V. membrane is deflected posteriorly, resulting in **the enlargement of the left fibrous trigone** and its confluence with the intervalvular trigone. On page 20, a specimen will be shown where the left fibrous trigone is absent due to the presence of a large left ostial process.

Comment: The seat of a mitral valve prosthesis is round. Photographs **3** and **4** show that the mitral orifice is neither round nor in a single plane.

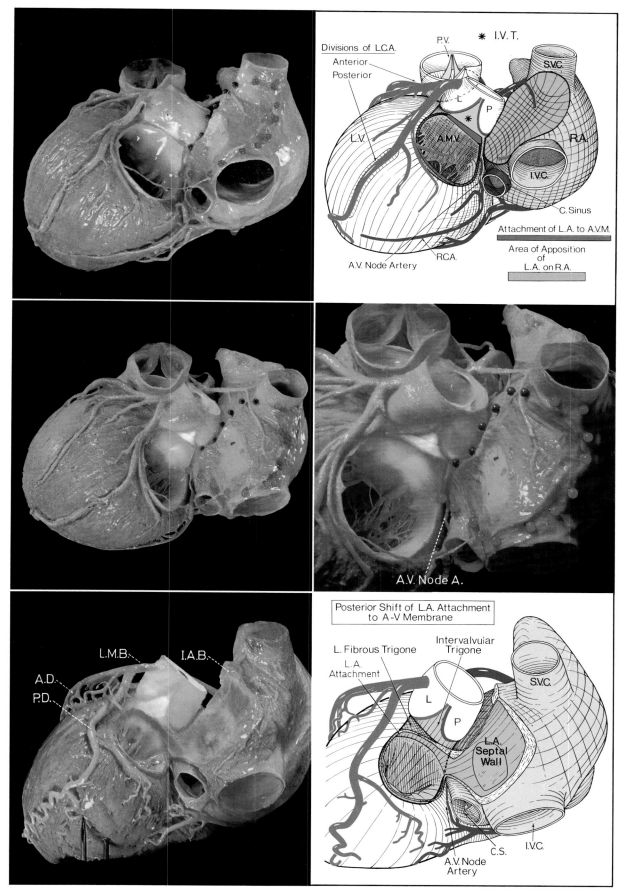

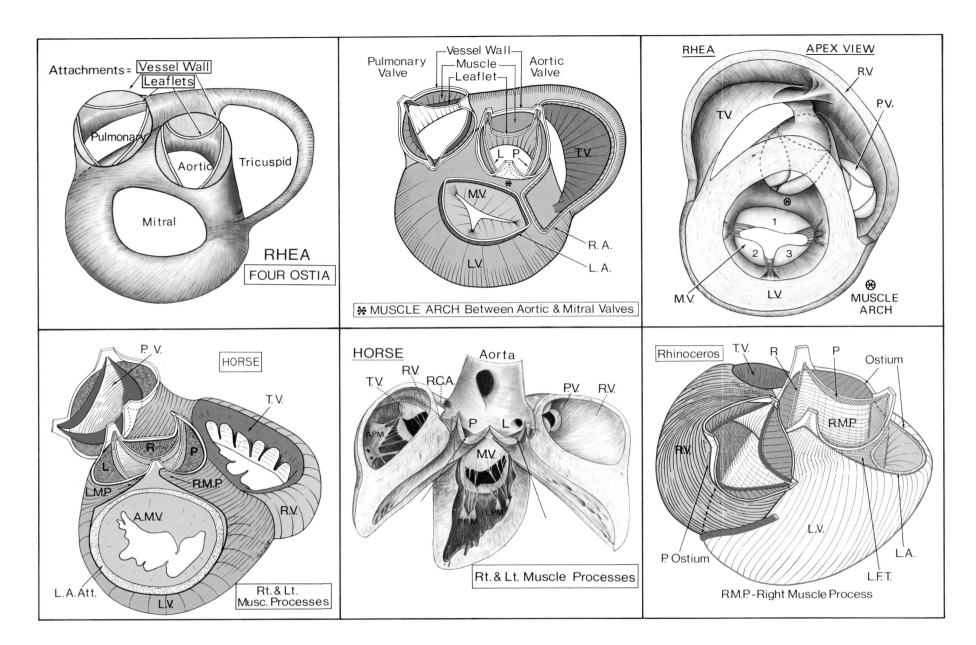

Attachments = [Vessel Wall] [Leaflets]

Pulmonary

Aortic

Tricuspid

Mitral

RHEA

[FOUR OSTIA]

Pulmonary Valve — Vessel Wall — Muscle — Leaflet — Aortic Valve

L P

T.V.

M.V.

R.A.

L.A.

L.V.

✳ MUSCLE ARCH Between Aortic & Mitral Valves

RHEA   APEX VIEW

R.V.

P.V.

T.V.

1

2 3

M.V.   L.V.   ⊛ MUSCLE ARCH

P.V.

[HORSE]

T.V.

R

P

L

L.M.P.   R.M.P.

A.M.V.

R.V.

L.A.Att.   L.V.   Rt. & Lt. Musc. Processes

HORSE   Aorta

T.V.   R.V.   R.C.A.

P.V.   R.V.

A.P.M.

P   L

M.V.

P.P.M.   L.P.M.

Rt. & Lt. Muscle Processes

[Rhinoceros]   T.V.   R   P   Ostium

R.M.P.

R.V.

P. Ostium

L.V.

L.A.

L.F.T.

R.M.P.-Right Muscle Process

B. The Ostium of the Left Ventricle

I. In Animals

Four specimens are seen on this page—in all four, the atria and great arteries have largely been removed *. In the first specimen (1, 2, and 3) and in the second (4), a large apical part of the ventricles has been removed—see the dangling chordae in 4.

1, 2, and 3: The rhea, an ostrich from Argentina: 1 and 2 are superior P.A. views, 3 is an apex view. Observe: (a) There are four distinct ostia, as the aortic and mitral valves are separated by a muscular arch. (b) The attachments of the semilunar leaflets, pulmonary and aortic, are widely separated from the pulmonary and aortic arterial attachments; hence, muscle exists in the resulting sinuses. In the pulmonary valve, this separation is found in all animal species studied and in man. (c) The right heart wraps around the left ventricle much more than it does in humans; hence, the orientation of the pulmonary valve

sinuses and leaflets is identical to that of the aortic valve, both exhibiting anterior, left posterolateral, and right posterolateral sinuses and leaflets **. (d) The mitral valve "has" three papillary muscles and three leaflets. (e) The tricuspid valve has a single anterosuperior muscular sheet. There is no septal tricuspid leaflet. [Examine features (d) and (e) in 3.]

4 and 5: The horse: 4 is a superior P.A. view. In 5, the ideal incision to examine the cardiac interior described in 11–1, passing through the midpoint of the right aortic sinus, is used. (a) Two muscle processes (L.M.P. and R.M.P.) extend across the ostium of L.V. almost separating the ostium into two orifices. This state also exists in some birds, e.g., the emu. In human hearts, vastly smaller ostial processes may be seen—on the left replacing the left fibrous trigone—and on the right at the inferior attachment of the right fibrous trigone. (b) As in the bird, the attachments of all six semilunar leaflets are widely separated from the vessel attachments by muscle. (c) The mitral valve has two leaflets and the tricuspid valve is membranous.

6: The rhinoceros: A high left lateral view: A right muscle process provides a separated attachment for the posterior aortic leaflet and the related aortic wall. The right leaflet is still widely separated from the aortic wall. The **left muscle process has disappeared,** and is replaced by membrane. A large left fibrous trigone (L.F.T.) is present. The left aortic annulus now provides attachment for both the aortic leaflet and wall. The pulmonary ostium of the right ventricle in humans, and in most animals, is circular; from within it, the pulmonary annuli extend superiorly onto the wall of the pulmonary trunk; hence, from the latter, three fibrous trigones result, each of which is bounded by the pulmonary ostium and the adjoining annuli; in the rhinoceros, however, the three interannular fibrous trigones are diminutive because the pulmonary ostium is not circular, but exhibits three triangular muscle processes which extend superiorly between the pulmonary annuli—see 74—2.

---

* In this volume, the term "great vessels", is most often used. The newer term, "great arteries", is preferable.
** The aortic valve components are labeled in the manner used in this work (R., L., and P. for right, left, and posterior).

The "ideal" incision used in **16—5** is again seen here in **1** and **2**.

1: **An ox heart**: Part of the left, and the adjoining halves of the right and posterior aortic leaflets are attached to the left ventricular ostium through the intermediation of stout bony structures (os cordis) which resemble in shape the left fibrous trigone and membranous septum of human hearts.

2: **A Poland-China pig**: The pattern **in this particular breed** is similar to that seen in humans. The difference consists in the presence of cartilage at the right and left fibrous trigone areas. The right aortic sinus has a large muscle component as is seen in some human hearts.

3 and **4**: **Spider monkey**: An R.A.O. view of the left segment following transection in the L.A.O.-R.P.O. plane. In this 30 gram heart, the posterior aortic annulus is elevated above the ostium of the ventricle. The pattern of the membrane and ostium is identical with that seen in humans. For the first time in the few animal hearts shown, the interior of the left ventricle is trabeculated. In this particular specimen, muscle is not present in the right aortic sinus (which is not shown here). At 3 o'clock in **4**, a 25 gauge hypodermic needle is partially shown to indicate the size of the heart.

II. The Ostium of the Left Ventricle and the Conduction System (Human)

5: The mitral valve and a portion of the aorta have been removed. The septal wall (red) is examined. The penetrating and branching divisions of the common A.V. bundle (H.B.) and the first division of the right bundle branch (R.B.B.) course along the ostium of the ventricle lodged at the lowest part of the A.V. membrane. The anterior and posterior divisions of the left bundle branch are directed towards the lateral and posterior papillary muscles.

6: The same specimen is viewed from R.A.O. The A.V. node is anterosuperior to the coronary sinus orifice and just posterior to the right fibrous trigone. The penetrating portion traverses the latter, and the branching portion of the His bundle runs in relation to the atrial portion of the membranous septum. The attachment of the septal leaflet of the tricuspid valve to the A.V. membrane and to the ostium of L.V. is cited as the line of demarcation between the common A.V. bundle (His) and the first division of the right bundle branch. It is pertinent, however, to consider the frequent and wide variations in location of this attachment, not only in anatomic studies, but in operations such as tricuspid-valve replacement or closure of the defects of the membranous septum. **The first division** of the right bundle courses along the ostium of L.V. **The third division** runs along the moderator band reaching the anterior papillary muscle where it terminates in the purkinje system. **The second division** is related to the septal band of the infundibulum between the two. Whenever the conduction system is indicated, either in a drawing or by the location of a bead in a photograph, the information results from the descriptions in the literature, particularly of Hudson, James, Lev, Rosenbaum and Titus.

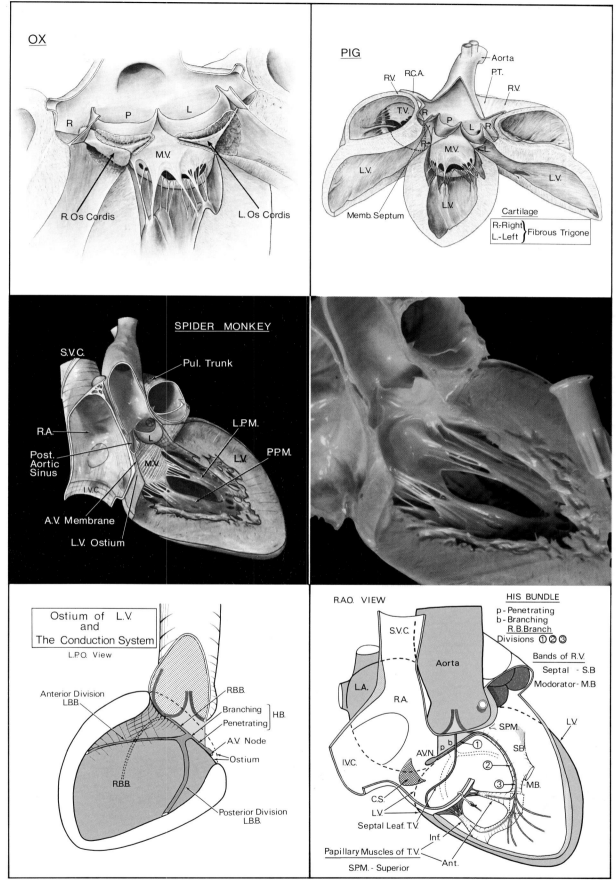

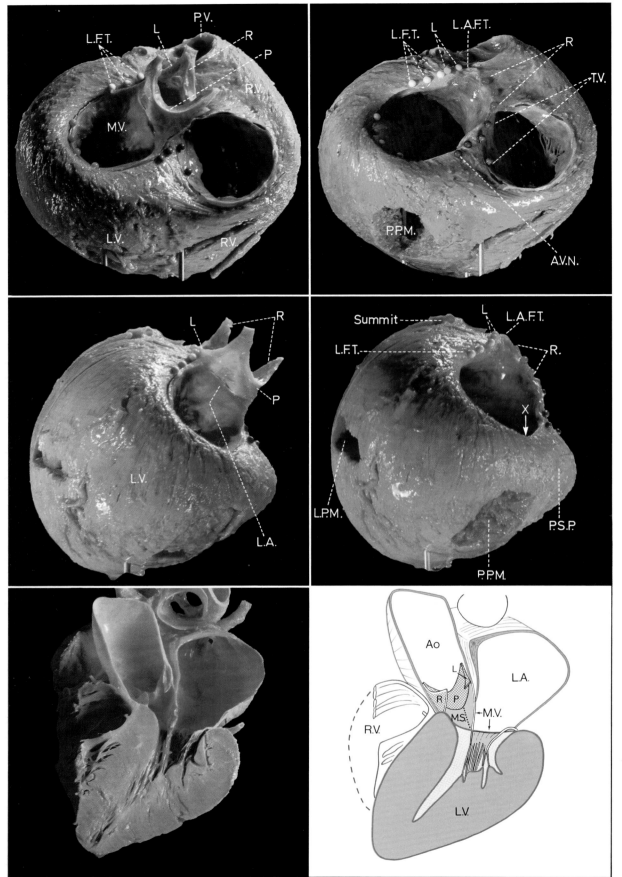

III. The Attachment of the Aorto-Ventricular Membrane and Aortic Annuli to the Ostium of the Left Ventricle

Specimen A: 1–4

1 and **2**: R.P.O. view: In this view, the ostium is most widely open (the L.V. is directed posteriorly and superiorly in the L.A.O.-R.P.O. plane). The atria and the great vessels down to the annuli have been removed. The beads mark the attachment of structures to the ostium as follows: Red—right aortic annulus; yellow—left aortic annulus. Between the two is the left anterior fibrous trigone. All three structures are attached to the outer anterior margin of the ostium. The right annular attachment is more extensive than the left (14:4 mm). The white—the left fibrous trigone; the green—the septal leaflet of the tricuspid valve. The two blue beads mark the site of the A.V. node and the right fibrous trigone. The membranous septum is attached between the red and blue beads. The left annulus is higher than the right. The A.V. membrane, peripheral to the posterior leaflet of the mitral valve (orange beads), is attached to the inner and inferior margin of the ostial slope. This is shown by the fact that the orange beads are seen with anterior lighting in **1** but are only faintly visible with posterior lighting in **2**.

3 and **4**: P.A. view, before and after removal of the aortic annuli and A.V. membrane. Observe: (a) **The left atrial attachment** (L.A.) to the A.V. membrane, extending between the nadirs of the left and posterior annuli, should be visualized in relation to **the anterior portion of the ostial slope of L.V.** The relationship of the two is critical in valve replacement, since the prosthesis is sutured to the A.V. membrane just below the atrial attachment. (b) The **lowest point of the ostium of L.V.** (X) is approximately 1.5 cm posterior to the inferior commissure of the mitral valve. (c) **The highest point** is at the site of attachment of the left anterior fibrous trigone (L.A.F.T.). (d) **The summit of the ventricle** is high above the ostium. (e) **The posterior superior process of L.V.** (P.S.P.) protrudes inferiorly and to the right. (f) The location of the base of attachment of the lateral (L.P.M.) and posterior (P.P.M.) papillary muscles is indicated.

Specimen B: 5 and 6: Nonattitudinal left lateral view:

The specimen is sectioned in the axis of the left ventricle through the midpoint of both the right aortic leaflet and the posterior leaflet of the mitral valve. The ostial slope of L.V. presents a rounded contour on cross section. Anteriorly, the A.V. membrane and right aortic annulus are attached to its upper outer margin; posteriorly, the A.V. membrane, in relation to the posterior leaflet of the mitral valve, is attached to the inner margin.

Comment: (a) The **mitral division** of the ostium of L.V. is posterior, inferior, and it extends to the left of the **aortic division.** (b) **The aortic annular axis,** marking the coplanar aortic nadirs, lies 33° below the horizontal wall (**22–2**). (c) **The posterior trigonal axis** (the axis of the left and right fibrous trigones) lies 43° below the horizontal. [See features (b) and (c) in **3** and (a) in **4**.]

IV. The Anterior Part of the Ostial Slope

Specimen C: 1 and **2**: A frontal transection: **1** is the
P.A. view of the anterior segment. **2** is provided for
orientation and to show the relation of the anterior part
of the ostial slope to the outflow tract of L.V. In **1**,
observe: (a) The maximum of the ostial slope is anterior, above the arrow; it is posterior to the right aortic
annulus, which is attached to the outer border of the
ostium. (b) The ostial slope varies throughout its course; at
the site of transection, which passes through the center
of the aortic valve, the ostial slope still intrudes prom-
inently into the cavity of L.V., and the A.V. membrane and left annulus are attached to its outer border*.

Specimen D: 3 and **4**—P.A. view. **5** and **6**—superior
views. The heart has been divided by incisions which
pass through the following: (a) the left anterior fibrous
trigone between the left and right aortic annuli; (b) the
right fibrous trigone, which is always below the nadir of
the posterior annulus and almost always the junction of
the anterior and posterior divisions of the A.V. membrane. The anterolateral segment of the specimen is seen
here; the posterolateral segment and additional views of
both segments are on page 134. Observe: (a) The right
aortic annulus and the membranous septum are attached
to the peripheral border of the ostial slope. (b) The prominence of the ostial slope is maximum under the nadir
of the right annulus; it is still marked at the lines of incision (see **6**). (c) The highest point of the ostium is at
the attachment of the left anterior fibrous trigone
(L.A.F.T.). (d) The view in **5** and **6** is similar to that
which a surgeon encounters when correction of infundibular hypertrophic subaortic stenosis is carried out
through the aortic orifice. Visualize the course of the left
bundle branch of the conduction system and its divisions. The common left bundle passes onto the ostial
slope at a point which is inferior to the commissure of
the right and posterior aortic annuli. In the above operation, the incision should not be vertical but oriented
in the axis of the ventricle, commencing under the left
half of the right aortic leaflet. The latter point is in the
center of **6**.

The anterior ostial slope is prominent in all four specimens and is maximum at 0°, decreasing towards the right
and left fibrous trigones. At the latter sites, the attachment of the A.V. membrane passes from the outer to
the inner margin of the ostial slope**. In some specimens,
the slope is less marked. This subject will be re-exam-
ined when the outflow tract of L.V. and the mitral valve
are considered in relation to the correction of subaortic
stenosis.

Goor, Lillehei and Edwards call attention to "the
variation in the contour of the left ventricular outlet" in
an article in 1969. They differentiate a prominent septum ("the sigmoid septum") from a flat ("straight septum").

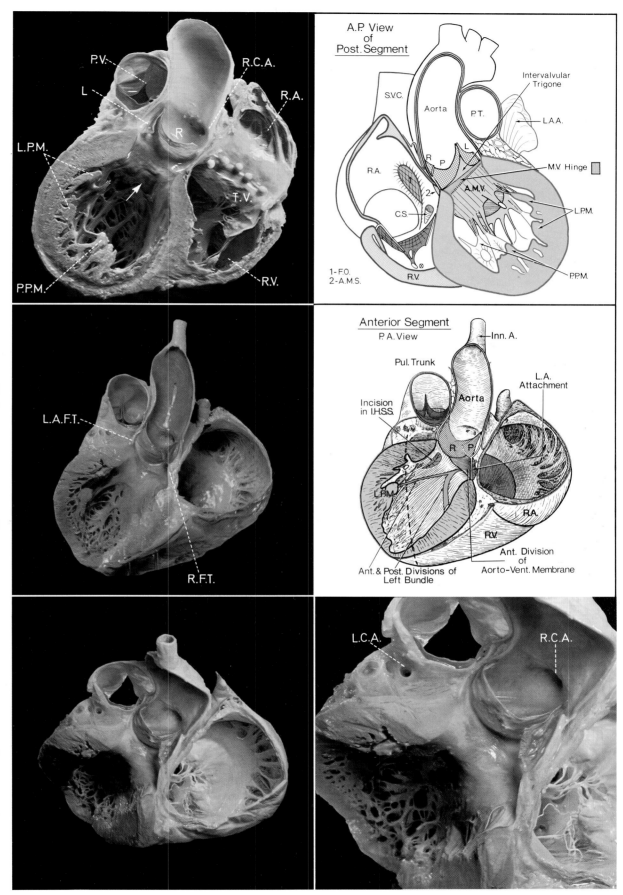

---

* This specimen appears in detail on pages 116 and 117.

** The specimens on page **53**—**1**–**4** are typical and illustrate
this point; the specimens on page 113 are atypical.

C. The Aortic Sinuses

I. An Introduction

Specimen A: 1 and **2**: A superior L.P.O. view: After removal of the atria and great vessels, all three sinuses are visualized. The left is seen in its entirety; its anterior half is in relation to the left ventricle, forming the medial wall of the left coronary fossa. The adjoining halves of the left and posterior sinuses are anterior to the left atrium (here removed) and overlie the mitral valve (M.V.) inferiorly. Note the round pulmonary ostium of the right ventricle. Note the indentation of the left ventricular ostium by the left ostial process (L.O.P.), resulting in muscular replacement of the left fibrous trigone. The shading in the ventricles is for future reference.

II. Relations to the Right Heart

Specimen B: 3, the A.P., **4,** the R.A.O., and **5** and **6,** the right lateral views: The removal of the right atrium in all, and the anterior and posterolateral walls of the right ventricle in **3, 4,** and **5,** affords inspection of the right and the adjoining half of the posterior sinus (P). The right sinus is identified by the right coronary artery. An arrow is placed above the posterior and right annular commissure.* Observe: (a) The right and left halves of the right sinus are in relation to the sinus and infundibulum of the right ventricle, respectively. In the chamber, this point of division is indicated by the superior papillary muscle (S.P.M.) (seen in **3** and **4**). (b) The anterior half of the posterior sinus bulges into the anteromedial wall of the right atrium. (c) The red and blue beads on the left atrium mark the site of the posterior and anterior margins of its apposition to the right atrium. The central red bead identifies the site of the A.V. node, whose artery is seen running to it. As described on page 26, complete heart block may, very occasionally, result from pressure of an aortic sinus aneurysm on the ostium and the A.V. bundle. (d) In **6,** the aortic sinuses and membranous septum are transilluminated, identifying the upper border of the ostium of L.V., along which runs the common A.V. bundle. (e) In **6,** a dotted line marks the attachment of the septal leaflet of the tricuspid valve to the A.V. unit. This attachment is divisible into muscular and membranous components; the latter demarcates the ventricular and the atrial (or atrio-ventricular) divisions of the membranous septum. (f) A wide gap is present between the septal and anterosuperior leaflets of the tricuspid valve. (g) As seen in **5** and **6,** the right aortic sinus bulges into the posterolateral wall of the right ventricle. **Comment:** Fistulae from posterior sinus aneurysms most often communicate with the right atrium; however, the attachment of the tricuspid valve to the A.V. membrane is variable: usually its posterior extremity underlies the commissure between the right and posterior aortic annuli; when it extends beneath the posterior sinus, the fistula may enter the right ventricle.

---

* See the drawings **115—2** and **14—4**.

III. Relations to the Left Heart

Specimen C: 1–6

1: L.P.O view: much of the left atrial wall has been removed; the superior pulmonary veins (L.S.P.V. and R.S.P.V.), the appendage (L.A.A.) and the anterior and septal walls remain. The right and left pulmonary arteries (R.P.A. and L.P.A.) are nearly at a right angle and parallel to the plane of examination.

2: An inferior 120° view following removal of the anterior left atrial wall: Note the posterior protuberance of the left (L) and posterior (P) aortic sinuses and their relation to the left atrium. The left main branch (L.M.B.) and the anterior division (A.D.) (left anterior descending) and the posterior division (P.D.) (circumflex) of the left coronary artery are seen.
3–6 are seen in the P.A. view.

3: The left atrium, except for a rim attached to the A.V. membrane, the area of the right superior pulmonary vein and its septal wall, has been removed. The left coronary artery arises from the left sinus identifying it. The adjoining "halves" of the transilluminated left and posterior sinuses are anterior to the left atrium.

4: The inferior vena cava and right atrium are retracted to the right. The pulmonary trunk and arteries have been removed, exposing the pulmonary valve (P.V.). The mitral valve and intervalvular trigone are transilluminated. The attachment of the left atrium to the A.V. membrane is the dark strip which separates the two structures. Aneurysms through the intervalvular trigone have been reported (see page 26).

5 and **6**: Note the strong, bulging contour of the aortic sinuses. The anterior "half" of the left sinus is seen in relation to the left ventricle between the pulmonary and mitral valves. Aneurysms of the left aortic sinuses are very rare. However, it can be seen that, anatomically, fistulae could develop inferiorly into the left ventricle or posteriorly into the left atrium. Fistulae into the left atrium from any sinus are very rare. **Observe:** The nadirs of the posterior and left aortic annuli are in a frontal plane. Note that the superior and inferior commissures of the mitral valve are also in a frontal plane, which is located 8 mm posterior to the plane of the annular nadirs. In the specimen shown on page 102, the frontal transection passes through the commissures, but posterior to the aortic sinuses. On page 104, a frontal transection passes through both the commissures and the two annular nadirs. The former are postero-inferior to the latter. A variable spatial relationship exists between the two sets of structures.

Comment: (a) The pulmonary sinuses are demarcated distally from the remainder of the pulmonary trunk by sinus rims (see arrows in **6**). (b) Reid noted that Valsalva (1740) was struck by the uniform presence of sinuses in a great variety of birds and animals.

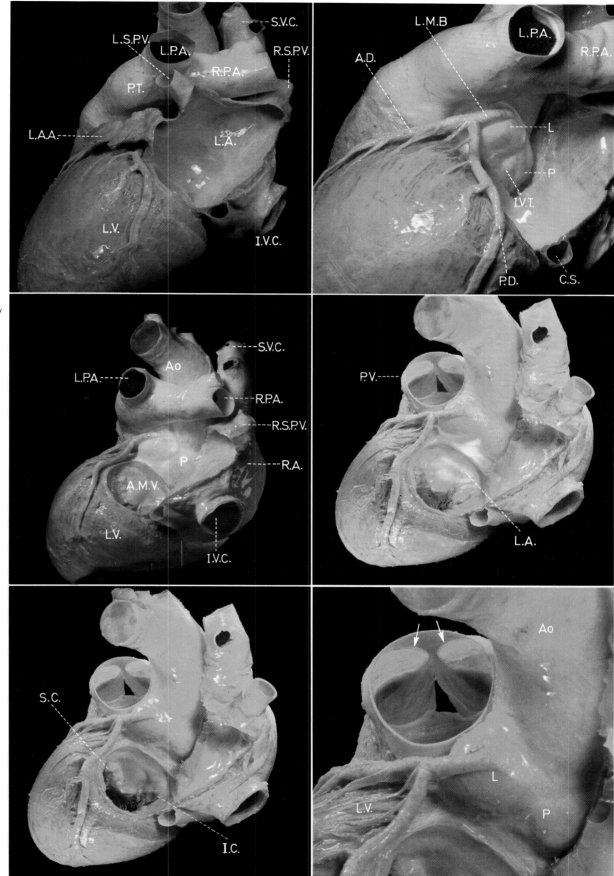

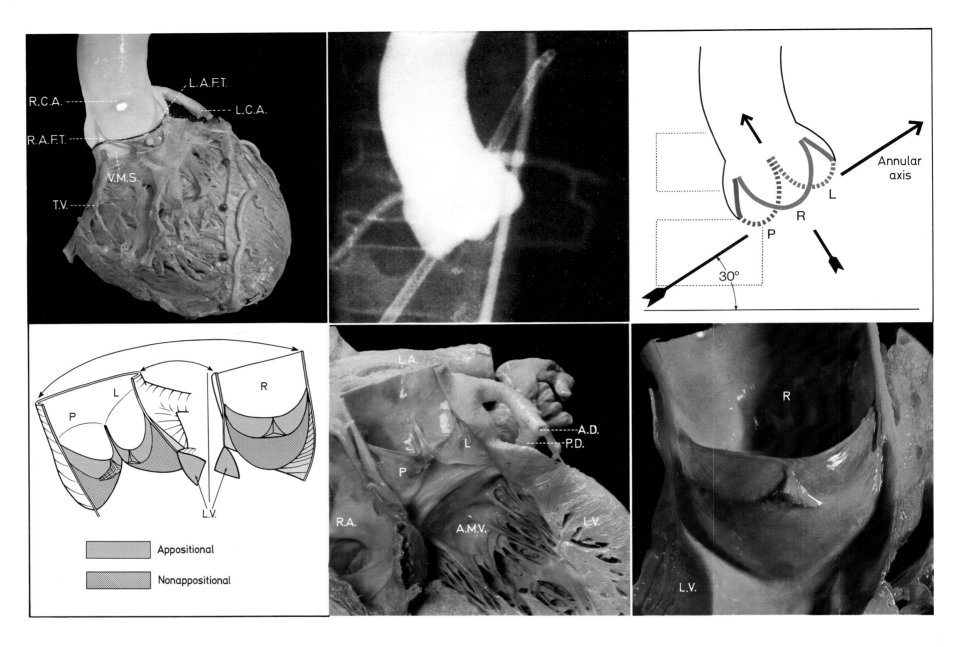

D. The Aortic Valve

I. The Spatial Disposition of the Aortic Annuli in the Anteroposterior Plane

Specimen A: 1: A.P. view: The isolated aorto-ventricular unit of a specimen, the sinuses of which were studied on page 20; the details of this dissection are on page 114. Midway between the upper ends of **the right annulus** is the right coronary orifice (the intracavitary light is seen). Below the nadir of this annulus is the yellow bead marking the site of the superior papillary muscle. The left coronary artery identifies **the left annulus.** The **posterior annulus** is seen on the right. The right anterior and the left anterior fibrous trigones are between the right and posterior, and the right and left annuli, respectively. **115—6** is the drawing of this photograph.

2: A.P. view: This aortogram provides the tracing in **3.** The aortic catheter is on the left. A second catheter crosses the field diagonally, coursing through the right ventricle, indicating the relation of the latter to the right aortic sinus.

3: The axis of the coplanar annular nadirs is 30° above the horizontal. The line passing through the nadir of the right and the commissure of the posterior and left annuli intersects the annular axis at a right angle. Characteristically, the posterior sinus is the lowest and the left the highest, as seen here. However, in a small percentage of hearts, the right sinus is at the same level and rarely below the posterior.

II. The Aortic Leaflets

1. The Mode of Suspension

Specimen B: 4, 5, and **6**

4: This drawing is intended for orientation of **5** and **6.** As shown here, the right aortic leaflet (R) and adjoining portion of L.V. has been separated from the posterior and left leaflets. The right leaflet is seen in **6**. The examination will be carried out in the A.P plane, showing the suspension of the leaflets from their annuli.

5: A.P. view: The lunules are the appositional portion of the leaflets.

6: P.A. view: The isolated right leaflet balloons into the aortic orifice in diastole. The lunule is approximately one-third of the leaflet depth. Apposition is reinforced by the nodule described by Arantius in the 16th century. In this leaflet it has four triangular surfaces—one attached to the leaflet, one ventricular, and two appositional.

Note: The equisite but simple design of the aortic valve is dependent on (a) the suspension of each leaflet and the appositional relationship of each leaflet to its **two** fellow leaflets. The ratio expressing the relationship of the leaflet surface area to the length of the suspending aortic annulus appears critical; for example, a quadricuspid valve with leaflets of equal size is usually regurgitant as the ratio is increased.

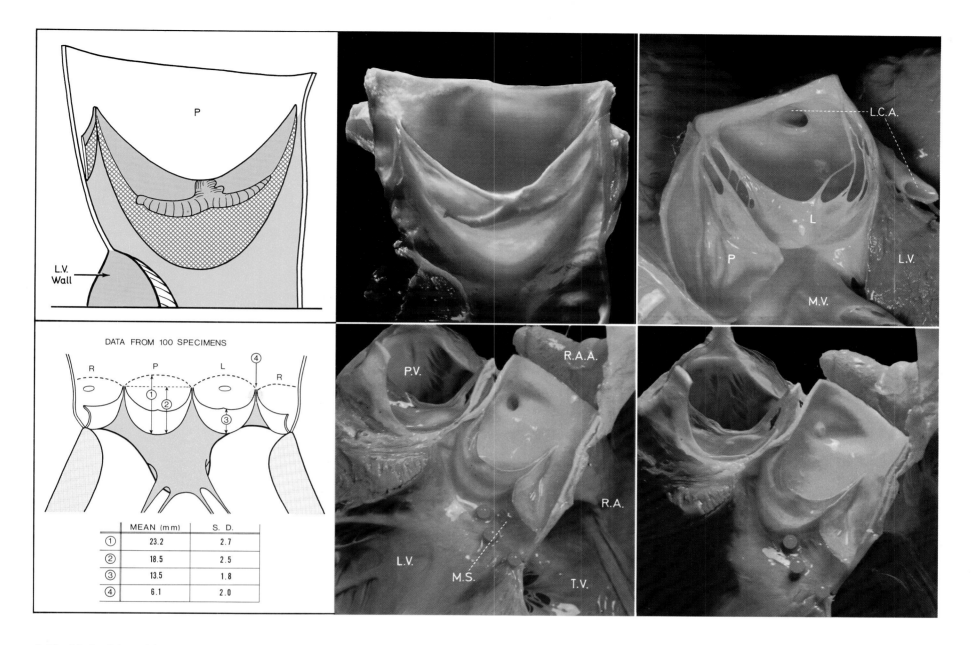

DATA FROM 100 SPECIMENS

	MEAN (mm)	S. D.
①	23.2	2.7
②	18.5	2.5
③	13.5	1.8
④	6.1	2.0

2. The Mode of Apposition

Specimen C: 1 and **2**: The posterior leaflet of another specimen: The nodule of Arantius extends along 60% of the inferior margin of the lunules. Posterior nodules are typically larger and more exuberant. The critical function of the nodules can be questioned, however, as their development may be minimal.

Specimen D: 3: The left and adjoining "half" of the posterior leaflet: The developmental abnormality, **fenestration of the semilunar leaflets,** is common (B. Friedman, and B. Hathaway). It occurs usually in the appositional portion of the leaflet in the area adjoining the commissures. In this specimen, the fenestrations are large and extend into the nonappositional area: Aortic regurgitation results. This may be of such magnitude that replacment of the valve is required.

4: Data from 100 specimens: The measurements cited here, apply equally to the right, left, and posterior com-

ponents of the valve. All were measured, and an inappreciable difference was present. The height of the sinus rim above the nadir of the annulus ① is greater than the annular height ②. The coronary orifices normally are found in a line between the upper extremities of the annuli. When the leaflet height ③ is examined, this dimension, quite apart from the lateral bulging of the sinuses, should suggest that leaflet occlusion of a coronary artery orifice would be impossible. ④ The upper extremities of adjoining aortic annuli are in contact with each other through a distance of 6 mm, forming annular commissures.

Specimen E: 5 and **6**: P.A. view: The right leaflet and adjoining "half" of the posterior leaflet are in apposition. The red beads indicate the upper border of the ventricular ostium. The membranous septum (M.S.) is seen between the leaflets and the ostium. In **5**, note the absence of a sinus rim, and the presence of an elevated orifice of the right coronary artery. In **6**, note the accessory sinus and the rim in relation to the orifice.

The sinus rim may not be recognizable in perfusion-fixed specimens. Its prominence varies directly with that of the aortic sinus itself. It is seen in the posterior aortic and the pulmonary sinuses; hence it is independent of the presence of an underlying coronary artery.

Comment: The **length of the free border of each aortic leaflet** (shown from the left ventricular aspect on this page and from the aortic aspect on the next page) equals the diameter of a circle formed by the coplanar upper extremities for the aortic annuli (see **22—3**)—the combined length for the three leaflets almost equals (3.0:3.14) the circumference of this circle, which is larger than the primary orifice at the annular nadirs. These facts, shown in **24—4** and summarized on page 26, may be adduced to show the efficiency of the aortic valve and the consequence of bicuspid and unicuspid malformations, viz., in a bicuspid valve, the combined free border lengths can, at best, double the diameter and with leaflet asymmetry, may be much less.

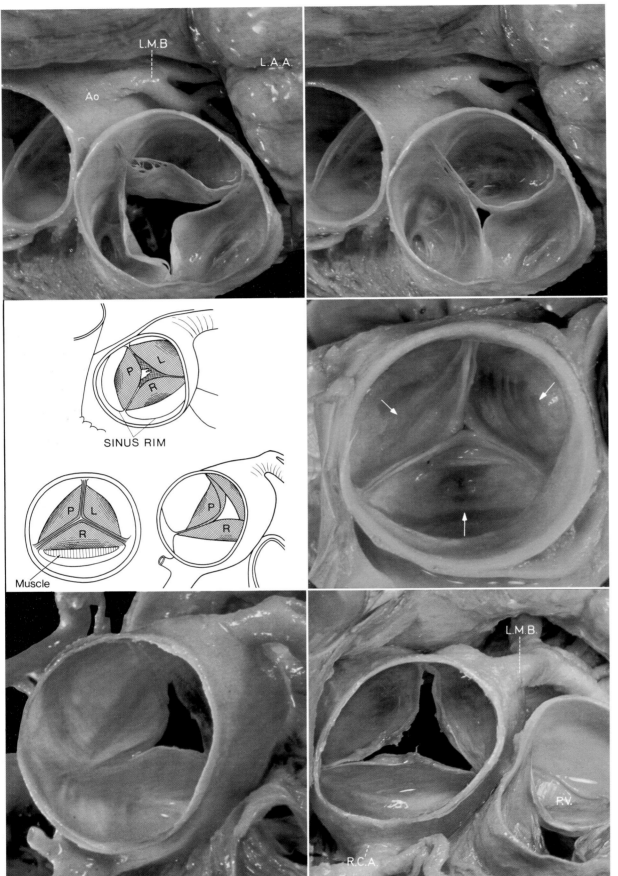

III. The Aortic Valve Orifice—Its Shape

Specimen A: 1 and **2**: A nonattitudinal view of the pulmonary valve: First note the sail-like character of the semilunar leaflets (pulmonary) and their mode of apposition. Then note that the pulmonary orifice is as triangular as the aortic. Fenestrations also occur in pulmonary leaflets. In **1,** note the fenestration in the posterior leaflet.

3: Upper drawing: The aortic orifice is roughly triangular; the sinus rims arch towards the annular commissures. Lower left and right drawings are drawings of the photographs **4** and **5**. Visualize the annuli as they extend inferiorly, affording attachment to the leaflets.

Specimen B: 4: Superior nonattitudinal view: The leaflets are seen in their normal anteroposterior relationship. The right is seen in the lower portion of the photograph. The leaflets are in apposition. The noduli are in the center of the photograph. The site of leaflet attachment at their nadir is indicated by arrows. Muscle is seen in the right sinus.

Specimen C: 5: Observe the vertical disposition of the annular attachments of the leaflets; this feature is also seen in **6**.

IV. Variations in Annular Size

Specimen D: 6: The left main branch of the left coronary artery (L.M.B.) and the right coronary artery identify the left and right aortic sinuses. A variation in size of the annuli, leaflets, and sinuses is present; the right is largest, the left is smallest.

Specimen E: 25–1: Nonattitudinal right superior view: The specimen is viewed at right angles to the plane of the aortic valve. Here and in **2**, the coronary arteries identify the right and left aortic sinuses. The posterior and left sinuses are transilluminated, indicating the site of attachment of the leaflets to the annuli and the angular disposition of the latter. Here, the disparity in annular width is marked, being 26.4, 22.9, and 21.0 mm for the right, left, and posterior annuli, respectively. The annular width was measured in 100 specimens. The arithmetic mean of the annuli, in the order noted above, was 27.6, 26.2, and 26.0, respectively; hence, a marked disparity would appear uncommon. In contrast studies of patients carried out in the R.A.O. and lateral views, the inferiorly located posterior sinus is well seen and often appears to be the largest. In 1967, Amplatz emphasized that the sinuses are not of equal size. "The posterior sinus is usually slightly larger than the right or left sinus". I have examined specimens in this regard and could not find confirmation of this statement. Also, this specimen is one of the most striking examples of the disparity in sinus size I have encountered; another example is shown on page 72.

V. Rotation of the Aortic Annuli on the Ostium of the Left Ventricle

Specimen F: 2: Superior view: The right aortic sinus faces to the right and laterally, an example of **clockwise rotation of the annuli on the ostium of L.V.** Observe: (a) The conjoined atrial attachment is shifted to the right of the midpoint of the posterior sinus. The left aortic sinus has only a minimal relationship to the left atrium. The arrow marks the posterior-left commissure. Goor and his associates show an example of marked shift in this aortic sinus-atrial relationship.

Specimen G (3–6) is an example of **counterclockwise rotation of the annuli on the ostium**

3 and **4**: R.A.O. and A.P. views of the left posterior segment:

(a) As a result of the counterclockwise rotation, the left annulus has almost lost its attachment to the ostium.
(b) In contrast to Specimen F, the conjoined atrial attachment to the A.V. membrane (A.V.M.) is normal, underlying the nadir of the posterior annulus. (c) The posterior papillary muscle (P.P.M.) is located at the apex.

In **5**, the P.A. view and in **6**, the left superior posterior nonattitudinal view, the right anterior segment of the specimen is seen. Observe: (a) As a result of the rotation, both the right and the anterior half of the posterior annulus are attached directly to the ostium of L.V. (b) The right ventricle and the right atrium (its surface is colored blue, its attachment is seen high on the sinus wall in **6**) are attached not to the A.V. membrane which normally intervenes between the ostium and the annuli but to the anterior half of the posterior aortic sinus. Accordingly the wall of the aorta is also a part of the wall of each of the two chambers (the segment between the aorta and the right ventricle is colored orange and the segment forming the wall of the right atrium is white). The tricuspid valve intervenes between the two chambers; its attachment to the aortic sinus wall is shown in **6** as an interrupted line.
This specimen demonstrates marked fenestration of the semilunar leaflets—a common variation. The aortic are seen here and in **23—3** and the pulmonary in **24—1** and **2**.

Comment: I. In radiological examination, alteration in the spatial relationships of the aortic sinuses may result from chamber enlargement; hence, the awareness of (a) the occurrence of annular rotation on the ostium as an anatomic variant and (b) variation in the size of normal aortic sinuses is important. Both features require further study in normal hearts.

II. In congenital aortic stenosis, reconstructive procedures fail to recreate **the surface area/suspension relationship of the normal three leaflet valve.** This relationship is the key to both normal function and the freedom from gradual calcification which eventuates in reformation of stenosis. The proper surgical conservatism—the inference from this relationship—reserves operation for unsustainable degrees of stenosis.

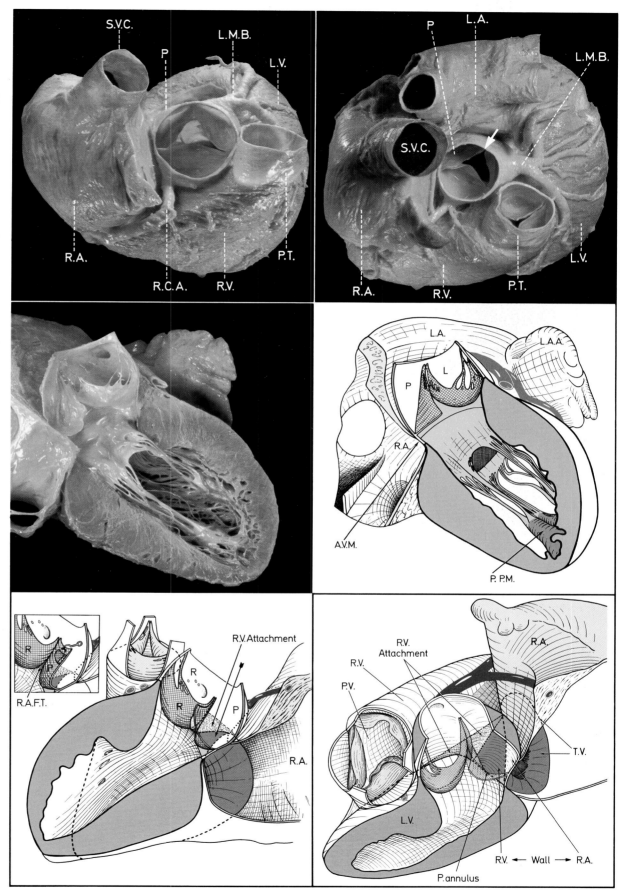

E. Clinical Comments

The aorto-ventricular membrane is continuous. The size of its components may commonly be affected by: (a) variations in the site of the chamber attachments to it, (b) variations in the height of the posterior annulus above the ostium of L.V., and less commonly, by (c) the variation in outline of the ostium, e.g., a prominent left ostial process, and rarely, by (d) rotation of the annuli on the ostium.

In this brief examination, **the aortic valve** is seen to pass from the totally muscular-based structure seen in a bird, to the one in humans which is characterized by a more membranous type of attachment of the valve to the ostium of the left ventricle. Considerable **variation in the human pattern** is seen: (1) The left annulus may have a minimal and, very rarely, no direct connection to the ostium. Conversely, in the presence of a left ostial process, the left annulus is extensively attached to muscle. The variation in the attachment of the aortic annuli to the ostium may be a factor in the development of annular subvalvular left ventricular aneurysms. (2) Very rarely, muscle is present in the left aortic sinus; however, muscle is seen not infrequently in the right aortic sinus, separating the aortic wall and the leaflet. This factor may be important in the selection of aortic valve allografts (in the search for a suitable xenograft valve, primate hearts present a membranous pattern similar to the one found in humans). The presence of muscle in the right aortic sinus is of undoubted importance during aortic valve replacement. Particular care is necessary in placing sutures in this area or paravalvular leak will result; in mitral valve replacement, this complication occurs most commonly in relation to the attachment of the posterior leaflet to the wall of the ventricle—this leaflet has been termed the mural leaflet—in this context, the right aortic leaflet might be termed the mural leaflet of the aortic valve—the greatest threat of parvalvular leak exists in relation to it. In aortic valve replacement, additional anatomic features warrant attention: (1) The aortic annuli are relatively stout structures and sutures should encircle them. (2) The coronary orifices are usually found at the level of the upper extremities of the annuli; however, they may be located at a lower level; therefore if orificial occlusion by the prosthesis is to be avoided, sutures should be confined to the lower third of the annuli. (3) Between the annuli sutures will be placed in the three fibrous trigones. The trigones are less sturdy than the annuli. This fact should be placed with two other considerations: (a) the disposition of the right annulus and leaflet referred to above; (b) the vitiation in the strength of all structures which results from the debridement of calcium. These three factors, in my opinion, demand the use of buttresses on the sutures used to secure a prosthetic valve if paravalvular leak or fistulae into the related chambers is to be avoided.

The pulmonary valve in humans displays variation in the depth of descent of the pulmonary annuli into the interior of the right ventricle; hence, this fact requires recognition in the selection of pulmonary valves if they are to be used as allografts for valve replacement. A ring is a circle, and the pulmonary muscular ostium is essentially circular in humans and in most animals. It provides attachment for the pulmonary trunk. Examination of specimens, human and animal, provides no support for the concept that a fibrous ring for valvular attachment exists (see page 74). A similar absence of a fibrous ring at the other three valve orifices may be noted.

Aneurysms of the aortic sinuses have been of interest for many years. In the era of closed heart surgery, they were of diagnostic importance; their intrusion into the right ventricle, resulting in obstruction, required differentiation from pulmonic stenosis. The development of aorto-cameral fistulae likewise required differentiation from a patent ductus arteriosus. Today, their complete correction is accomplished. Over 100 cases have now been reported, and it is of interest that over one-half of these have occurred in Japan: "Weakness" in the aortic sinus wall and "weakness" in the A.V. membrane (resulting in the annular subvalvular aneurysms of the left ventricle) occur most frequently in Japan and in Africa, respectively. Both geographic areas are relatively free of atherosclerosis. Aortic sinus aneurysms may protrude into the right atrium or ventricle and may rarely be directed against the ostium of the left ventricle; isolated cases of complete heart block and dissection into the ventricular septum have been reported (A. Onat et al.). The aortic sinus-ostial relationship is seen in **20—6**. In the 112 cases of congenital aneurysm of the sinus of Valsalva reported and collected by Taguchi and his colleagues, only one was seen in the left aortic sinus; 58 were located in the left half of the right aortic sinus and presented in the outflow tract of the right ventricle; 8 developed in the center of the right aortic sinus and presented at the junction of the divisions of the right ventricle; 26 were seen in the right half of the right aortic sinus and intruded into the sinus of the ventricle and into the right atrium in approximately equal numbers; in 15 cases, the posterior aortic sinus was the site of origin of the aneurysm. A ventricular septal defect was present in 49. Fibrosis and prolapse of an aortic leaflet may require replacement of this valve in addition to the repair of the defect in the sinus wall. Four of the 112 aneurysms were associated with a bicuspid aortic valve.

Aneurysms of the aortic sinuses must be differentiated from **aneurysms of components of the A.V. membrane;** aneurysms of the membranous septum are common. In the absence of aortic regurgitation, consecutive left ventriculography and supravalvular aortography will effect this differentiation. Aneurysms of the membranous septum have been reported presenting, not into a cavity of the right heart, but onto the surface of the heart. These may be confused with and should be carefully differentiated from aneurysms of the right anterior fibrous trigone, which would present in the right coronary fossa (the right A.V. sulcus). Killen has reported a case of spontaneous aortico-left ventricular fistula (from the right sinus) associated with myxomatous transformation. The anatomic potential for this fistula has been noted on pages 20 and 21. This very rare situation is to be differentiated also from aortic sinus aneurysms. An aneurysm of the aorto-ventricular membrane between the left atrial attachment and the adjoining left and posterior aortic annuli (the intervalvular trigone) has been reported (Waldhausen). The patient was a five year old white boy who had been kicked in the precordium by a horse. The aneurysm presented between the aorta and the anterior wall of the left atrium A false aneurysm has also been seen (Chesler) developing through the intervalvular trigone. It extended superiorly into the transverse sinus. Rupture and fatal pericardial tamponade resulted. Aneurysms through different portions of the A.V. membrane, in relation to the aortic and mitral valves, are common in Blacks.

The aortic leaflets may be compared with and contrasted to the mitral leaflets.
(1) **Their apposition: Aortic:** (a) Two appositional areas—the lunules—are present in each leaflet. A nodule may add re-inforcement at their junction. (b) Two straight lines of apposition are presented by each leaflet (**24-4**). (c) The appositional fractions of the leaflets are equal. **Mitral:** (a) One apposition area, lunular in shape (when viewed in systole), is present in each leaflet. (b) The line of apposition is lunular and serrated; therefore, multiple appositional areas occur in each leaflet (contrast **24-4** and **47-4**). (c) The appositional fractions of the leaflets are unequal, that of the posterior being larger.
(2) **Their suspension: The aortic:** Each leaflet from its own U shaped aortic annulus—**the key to the inspired design of this valve. The mitral:** Attached (indirectly) to the ostium of L.V. and confluent with the other segments of the A.V. membrane. The aortic suspension mechanism fails (a) when the aortic bulb dilates or (b) the aortic annuli are centrally dislocated due to aortic dissection. These two events most often result from Marfan's disease; as this disease process affects the entire A.V. membrane, it is added to (the many causes of) L.V. wall disease in the etiology of mitral regurgitation.
(3) **Their number: Aortic**—three—with a lesser number, the leaflet length (and orifice size) is reduced; with a greater number, the suspension is imperfect and regurgitation often results (5/11 reported quadricuspid valves were regurgitant [Hurwitz and Roberts, 1972]). **Mitral**—two—although accessory leaflets are ascribed to the valve (its posterior leaflet [Chiesi]), chordal support and leaflet apposition are unimpaired.
(4) **Their form: Aortic**—lunar and congruent: **Mitral**—the anterior—a squat pentagon, the posterior (when excised)—an elongated pentagon.
(5) **The surface area: Aortic**—usually equal (see **25—1**). **Mitral**—purportedly equal (see page 38).
(6) **Their connection: Aortic**—three units: **Mitral**—continuous at the commissures—one reason that the primary orifice is larger than the secondary orifice, which is located in the cavity of L.V. and formed by the free border of the leaflets during diastole.

Chapter 3:
The Left Ventricle—
General Considerations

Introduction

The left ventricular **apex** may be sharply angular or almost form a sector of a sphere—to it the term, apex of the heart, is usually assigned. The presence of an apex in a structure evokes definition of a **base**; the shape of the heart defies comparison to any geometric solid; nevertheless it is not unreasonable to anticipate the location of the base opposite the apex. In a horizontal plane transection neither the lateral wall of the right atrium nor the posterior wall of the left atrium subtend the apex—in spite of this fact, in most anatomic writings the term base is assigned to the latter. In an oblique A.P. transection, both the pulmonary and left ventricular ostia are opposite the apex, notwithstanding this, in clinical parlance the term base is restricted to the "origin of the great vessels". In view of the absence of a base in any geometric sense and as a result of its different denotation, the term "base of the heart" will not be used.

In this work the term **acute margin** is applied only to the right ventricle—its inferior and anterior walls do, in fact, form an acute angle. In an anteroposterior radiographic or naked eye examination, the acute margin forms the lower border, and the right atrium forms the right lateral border of the silhouette of the heart; both borders are at times combined to form the acute margin—this seems ill-advised—the former is evident on gross examination—the latter is not.

The term **obtuse margin** is usually used in a broad sense to denote the posterolateral aspect of the left ventricle and atrium. In this work it will be used to denote the junction of what will be defined as the lateral and posterior walls of the left ventricle; used in this sense, the margin is definable radiographically; it is useful in the identification of the sectors of the wall of this crucial structure in the different planes of examination used in the study of patients.

In the study of the effects of myocardial infarction, the location of the papillary muscles is important; it is helpful to create a functional separation of the left ventricular wall into papillary and nonpapillary divisions.

Since the advent of cineradiography, the clinician may daily observe the dynamic event, ventricular systole. On page 36 and 37, dissections demonstrate anatomic features which may be important in the etiology of heart block. It may be conjectured that Lenegre's disease may result from the long-continued mechanical trauma to the atrio-ventricular part of the conduction system from the distracting forces during ventricular systole, and that the fibrosis and calcification of Lev's disease results from surface trauma, which in turn is a resultant of the hemodynamic forces consequent to the anatomic configuration of the junction of the A.V. membrane. In 1935, Yater stated "... the deposition of calcium in this region is usually due to stress and strain. The main mass of the heart is really hanging from the membranous portion of the interventricular septum, and the point of junction of this part of the septum with the muscular portion of the septum and the aortic leaflet of the mitral valve is undoubtedly one of great stress and strain both in systole and in diastole". Observations made from His bundle recordings are consistent with earlier histologic evidence that lesions in the common A.V. bundle are the cause of complete heart block, albeit in a minority of instances. Lev's disease may involve varying locations of the A.V. membrane, resulting in variation in involvement of the components of the conduction system. When the calcification or fibrosis is found anteriorly, the combination of R.B.B. block and left anterior hemiblock may occur (this may be premonitory of complete heart block). Calcification in the nonmobile portion of the mitral valve is commonly seen. It may be confluent with calcification in the aortic valve and is frequently removed coincident with operations on the latter. The results of turbulence affect both divisions of the A.V. membrane; however, ordinarily only when the portion of the membrane in relation to the conduction system is involved does disease (heart block) result.

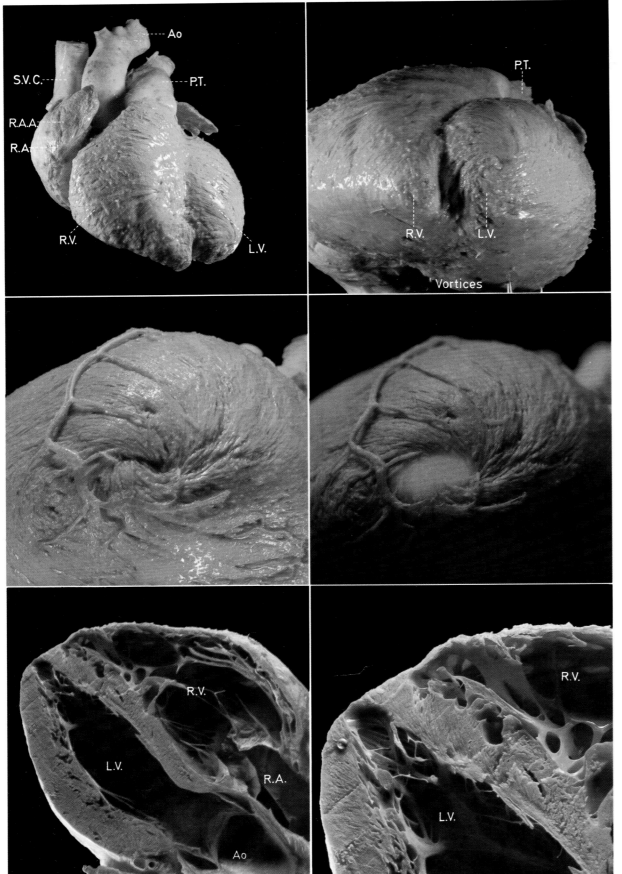

A. The Apices of the Left and Right Ventricles

Anatomic Factors in Catheterization and Perforation

Specimen A: 1 and 2

1: The apex of the left ventricle, in contrast to the right, is readily identified at fluoroscopy; in right heart catheterization and in the positioning of a pacemaker electrode, the location of the right ventricular apex, in relation to it, is important. The right is frequently inferior to the left, and the lack of consideration of this fact may cause the unnecessary concern that perforation has occurred when a catheter is seen inferior to the level of the left apex. The apex of the right ventricle may be demarcated from the left, producing an incisura; in some specimens this is marked, resulting in the sharply angular configuration of the right ventricle seen here, which results in their special vulnerability to perforation.

2: The specimen is rotated to display the apex where wide separation of the two vortices is seen.

Specimen B: 3 and **4**: The more common situation is seen in this specimen. The coronary artery demarcates the two vortices, but a fissure is not present. The left vortex is in the center of the photograph **3**. In **4**, interior lighting is used to demonstrate the thin left apex. The superficial bulbospiral muscles pass into the inner wall of the left ventricle at the apex.

Specimen C: 5 and **6**: Note the paper-thin left ventricular apex; in **6**, a common pin is shown to indicate the dimension of this feature. The angular disposition of the septal and lateral walls of L.V. would appear to direct a catheter tip against the apex making perforation a common complication which, in fact, is surprisingly uncommon in contrast to perforation of the apex of R.V., notwithstanding the greater frequency of left heart catheterizations. The complication may occur, however, and this anatomic feature provides substance for advocacy of catheters with a "pig tail" rather than a simple curved end.

For many years, the left ventricular "apex" has been the site chosen for the introduction of a decompression catheter; if used, the site should be above the thin-walled apex lest the sutures pass through it and produce a tear, the closure of which could involve encirclement of the coronary artery in the interventricular groove. The importance of the apex as a site for the development of collateral circulation militates against its use in coronary artery surgery: A relative insecurity exists when sutures are placed in this high-pressure chamber: Therefore, for these reasons, the left atrial wall, in relation to the posterior interatrial sulcus, is preferred as the cannulation site by many surgeons.

The apex of the right ventricle is selected for the engagement of a transvenous pacemaker electrode; in **6**, it is seen transilluminated, evidencing its liability to perforation regardless of its location and configuration. When a transvenous bioptome is used for myocardial biopsy, the hazard of perforation is also evident.

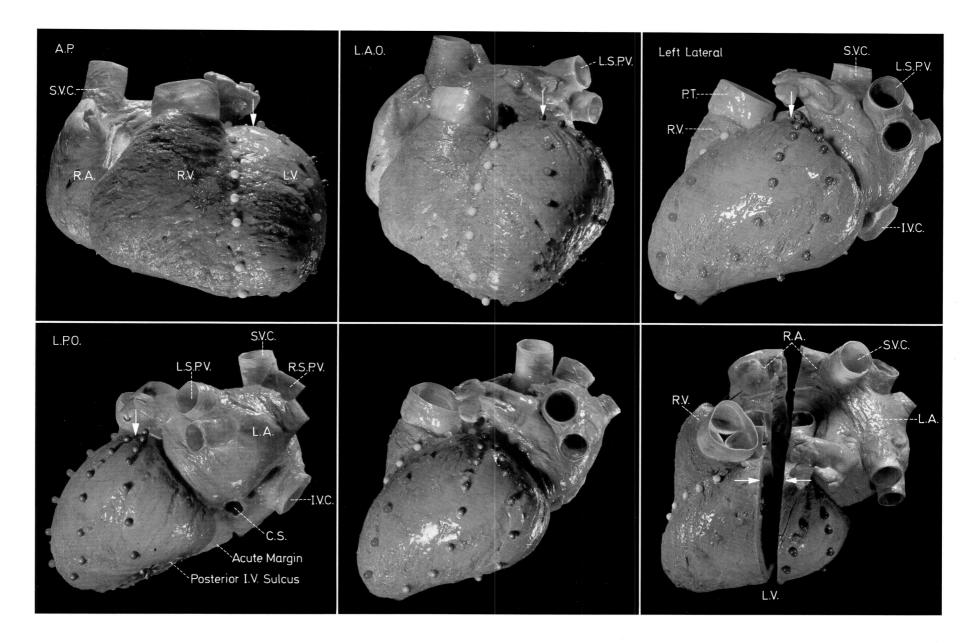

A.P.

S.V.C.

R.A. R.V. L.V.

L.A.O.

L.S.P.V.

Left Lateral S.V.C.

P.T.

R.V.

L.S.P.V.

I.V.C.

L.P.O.

L.S.P.V.

S.V.C.

R.S.P.V.

L.A.

I.V.C.

C.S.

Acute Margin

Posterior I.V. Sulcus

R.A.

S.V.C.

R.V.

L.A.

L.V.

B. The Contour of the Surface of the Lateral Wall of the Left Ventricle

Specimen D: 1–6: The summit of the ventricle is marked by vertical arrows in the following views: **1**: A.P., **2**: L.A.O., **3**: Left lateral, **4**: L.P.O. **5** is a left lateral view with 15° of elevation. In the transection in **6**, the summit is seen lateral to the left coronary fossa. The arrows are directed to the summit.

I. The Summit of the Left Ventricle and Coronary Arteriography

In this strongly muscled horizontal heart, the yellow beads mark the interventricular groove. The red, blue, and green beads, placed at intervals across the lateral wall of the ventricle, indicate its slope and simulate the anterolateral, the lateral, and the posterolateral radial branches of the left coronary artery in these radiographic views; These beads ascending the lateral wall converge toward what I term **the summit of the ventricle**, which is located above both the upper end of the anterior interventricular

sulcus and the aortic portion of the ostium of L.V. When coronary arteriography is carried out only in the horizontal plane, vessels in relation to the summit are seen end on in both the lateral and L.A.O. views and often overlapping one another in the views (A.P. and R.A.O.) when the area is placed in profile. In the left lateral view with 45° elevation (see **6**), it is apparent that the arteries traversing the summit will be well visualized.

II. An Introduction to the Radiographic Borders of the Left Ventricle

In all radiographic views, one must be familiar with **the radiographic** borders of the left ventricle and their relationship to (a) the I.V. sulci and (b) the obtuse margin and (c) the three walls of the left ventricle.

Left Border of L.V.: A.P. view (see photograph **1**): (a) The lateral branch of either division of the left coronary runs over its lower two-thirds. (b) The anterolateral branch runs along the upper $1/3$ overlapping the lateral branch. (c) The anterior I.V. sulcus is well medial to the border.

L.A.O. view (see photograph **2**): (a) The lateral branch and obtuse marginal or posterolateral radial branches run on the anterior and posterior "aspects" of the border. (b) The anterolateral branch, running midway between the left border and the anterior I.V. sulcus, can be identified in this view although its upper portion is seen end on; in the lateral and R.A.O. views, it may overlap the anterior I.V. branch. **Elevated views are needed** in arteriography.

Anterosuperior Border of L.V.: Left lateral view (see **3**): Due to the shape of the left ventricle, the anterolateral branch and the anterior I.V. sulcus (and its artery) overlap to a variable degree. **R.A.O. view** (This can be deduced from the mirror image of **4**): (a) The anterolateral branch, not the anterior I.V. branch, runs along this border. This relationship is seen better on the next two pages. (b) Note the anterior location of the lateral branch in the R.A.O. view.

Note: An anterolateral branch (usually termed diagonal) is often the highest branch in the A.P. and R.A.O. views of horizontal plane arteriograms, particularly in horizontal hearts (exemplified here).

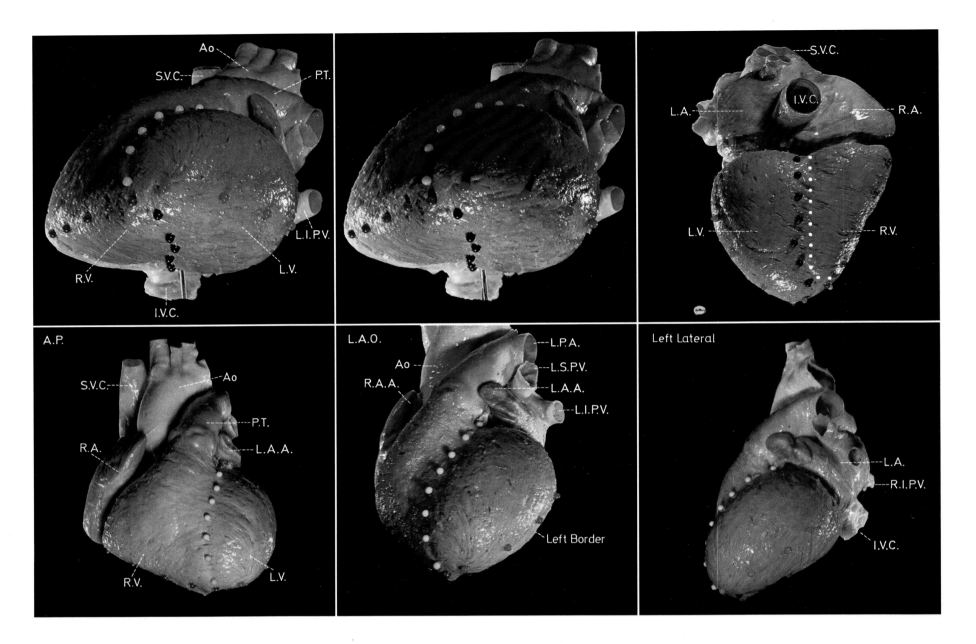

C. The Obtuse Margin

I. Its Definition

Margin is defined by Webster as "the space adjoining a bounding line or a border". The obtuse margin is a critical anatomical landmark and in many specimens a large artery courses along it. We will now attempt its photographic definition.

Specimen A: 30—1–6 and 31—1–3

1: A specimen (a vertical heart) is viewed from the apex. Yellow and black beads mark the anterior and posterior interventricular grooves; the blue, the acute margin which forms the junction of the anterior and inferior walls of the right ventricle; the red, the obtuse margin of L.V. This photograph can also be used to support the thesis that the right ventricle wraps around the left ventricle as will be later postulated.

2: The position of the red beads, that is, the obtuse margin, was selected from inspecting the specimen with inferior lighting which delimits both the posterior wall of the left ventricle and the inferior wall of the right ventricle.

3: The inferior view: Here too, the red beads, so placed, mark the lateral limit of the posterior wall of L.V. consistent with our observations in **2**. **The obtuse margin, hence, is defined as the border between the posterior and lateral walls of the left ventricle.**

Coincident with the establishment of this demarcator, we may ask what demarcates the posterior wall of L.V. and the adjoining inferior wall of R.V.? Certainly no **posterior interventricular sulcus** meeting Webster's definition (sulcus; [L., a furrow] a furrow; a groove; fissure) is to be found. As an expression of the slight degree (15°) of non-coplanarity of these two walls, a contour boundary may, with difficulty, be seen (contrast **204**—3 and **204**—6). The beads (in **3**) were the deduced boundary—none was visible—and the white dots represent the boundary established by removal of the inferior wall of R.V. Knowledge of the conformation of the crux (pages 68 and 69) is useful in plotting the boundary line—the upper white dot is below the medial end of the attachment of the inferior wall of R.V. to the A.V. unit in the crux.

II. The Spatial Disposition of the Obtuse Margin in a Vertical Heart

(a) Its location is seen in part in **4**, the A.P. view and in **5**, the L.A.O. view and in its entirety in **6**, the left lateral view.

To deduce **the location of the obtuse margin in the R.A.O. view, 31—2** and **3** can be superimposed. It lies approximately midway between the upper and lower borders of the left ventricle and demarcates the posterior wall below and the lateral wall above. (b) The anterior interventricular groove is to the right of the anterosuperior border of L.V. in the R.A.O. view. This variable relationship is determinative of the overlap of the arterial branches in the groove and on the anterolateral sector of the left ventricle. In some specimens (e.g., **196**—3), the groove forms, in large part, the border. (c) In this vertical heart, the acute margin is inferior to the posterior I.V. groove in the R.A.O. view (**31**—1 and 2). (d) Note that even in this vertical heart, a summit of the left ventricle is present.

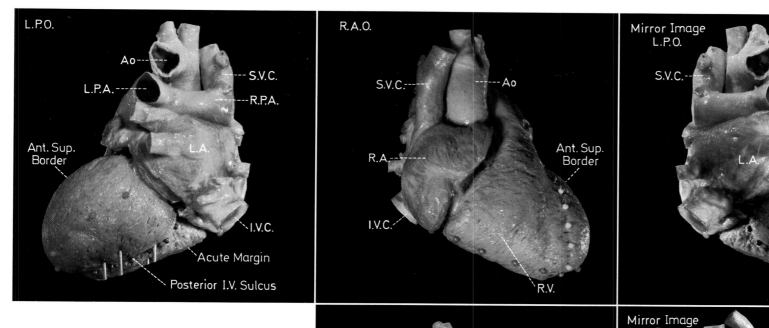

III. The Spatial Disposition of the Obtuse Margin in a Horizontal Heart

Specimen B: 4–7
4: The inferior view. **5**: The mirror image P.A. view. **6** and **7**: A.P. views—**7** results from the superimposition of **5** and **6**. The right lateral, oblique, and apex views of this horizontal heart can be seen on pages **7** and **194** and in **208—6,** respectively.

Observe: (a) The obtuse marginal artery (O.M.) identifies the border as seen in **4** and **5**. The posterior wall of L.V. is medial to this margin and passes posteriorly and superiorly in both the A.P.-P.A. and R.A.O.-L.P.O. planes.*
(b) The axis of the posterior A.V. sulcus proceeds superiorly and to the left at a 45° angle. (c) The posterior interatrial sulcus parallels, but is staggered to the left of the posterior I.V. sulcus which is identified in **5** by the posterior descending branch. In **7**, the atria and the ventricles are indicated by the dashed and dotted lines, respectively. (d) The left atrium (pink) is directed posteriorly and superiorly and to the right. (e) Note the location of the superior cavo-atrial junction (X) and the anterior right A.V. sulcus and anterior interventricular groove which are all at low level due to the poor development of both the infundibulum of the right ventricle and the right atrium.

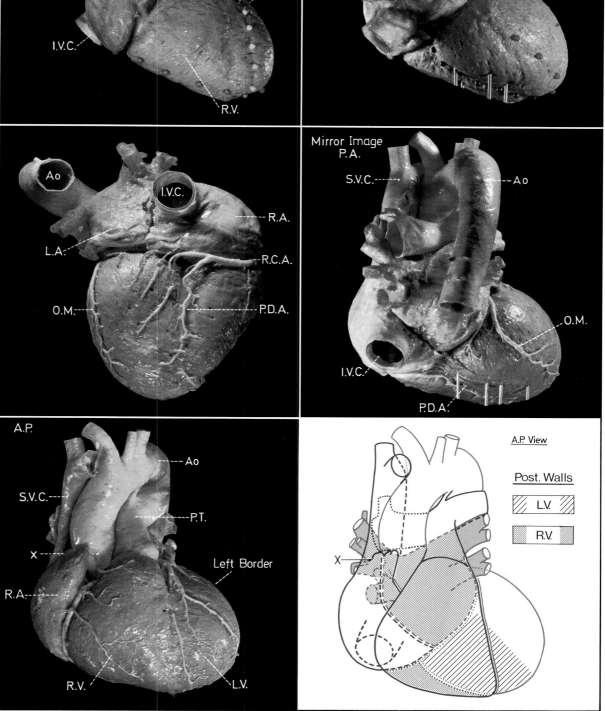

---

* See the position of the obtuse margin in a more vertical heart in **185—4**.

31

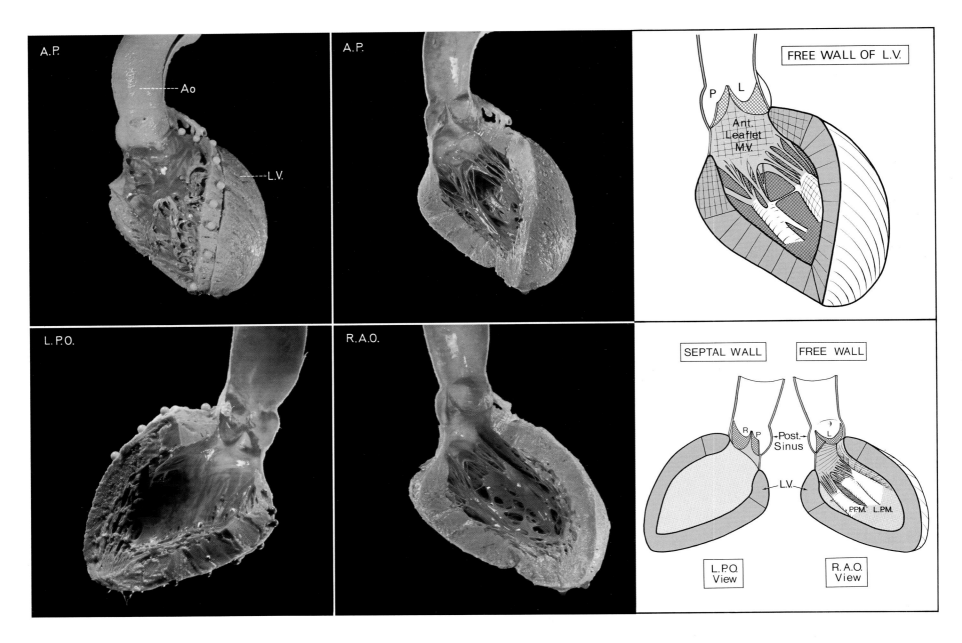

D. The Divisions of the Left Ventricular Wall

I. Anatomic

For descriptive purposes, it is obviously important to differentiate divisions in this structure. In coronary artery disease, the importance of quantitating the perfusion deficit brings the subject into an immediate practical focus. One specimen is seen in **32—1–6** and **33—1–3**.

1: The A.P. view of the isolated aorto-ventricular unit of the heart just examined on page 30. An incision is carried just to the left of the anterior interventricular groove, identified by the yellow beads, and extended upwards between the right and left aortic leaflets. A second incision is similarly directed in relation to the posterior interventricular groove and is extended up through the nadir of the posterior aortic leaflet. The left ventricle is now separated into the septal and free walls. The latter is shown in **2** and **3**.
(a) The anterior leaflet of the mitral valve is disposed at a right angle to the A.P. axis of examination. (b) As mentioned, this is a vertical heart; the axis of L.V., a

line drawn between the apex and the left and posterior aortic annular commissure measures 75° above the horizontal. This definition of the axis applies to the A.P. view—other definitions will be used in other views.

4, **5**, and **6**: The **septal and free walls** are examined at a right angle to their plane of section, simulating a right anterior oblique radiographic study. Observe: (a) The plane of the anterior leaflet of the mitral valve is now disposed at a 45° angle to the plane of examination. (b) This dissection separates the A.V. membrane into its two divisions. (c) In the R.A.O. view, the posterior papillary muscle is just above the lower border of the ventricle, and the lateral is just above the obtuse margin which, in this view, passes midway between the upper and lower borders of the ventricle. Hence, in an R.A.O. ventriculogram, the filling defect of the posterior is more commonly seen than that of the lateral. Both are attached in the intermediate third of the ventricle.
We will now transect the free wall through the obtuse margin:

Text for page 33:

33 —1, **2**, and **3**: The ventricle has been divided into septal, posterior, and lateral walls: The weight of these three divisions and the portions of aorta shown totals 254 grams. The percentages are: posterior, 30% septal, 32%; and lateral, 38%. The boundaries, especially between the septal and the posterior walls, are imprecise. However, this type of dissection is useful and does emphasize, for example, the hemodynamic importance of the septal wall. In this work, the papillary muscles are termed posterior and lateral, arising as they do from these walls. An examination of the spatial disposition of the papillary muscles in hemodynamically fixed hearts will reveal that the so-called "anterolateral" muscle is not, in reality, anterior to the "posteromedial" muscle. The blood supply to these muscles is in common with that of their respective walls.

Apart from a zone near the apex, the septal wall is atrabecular in contrast to the other two walls. Animal hearts present a sharp contrast.

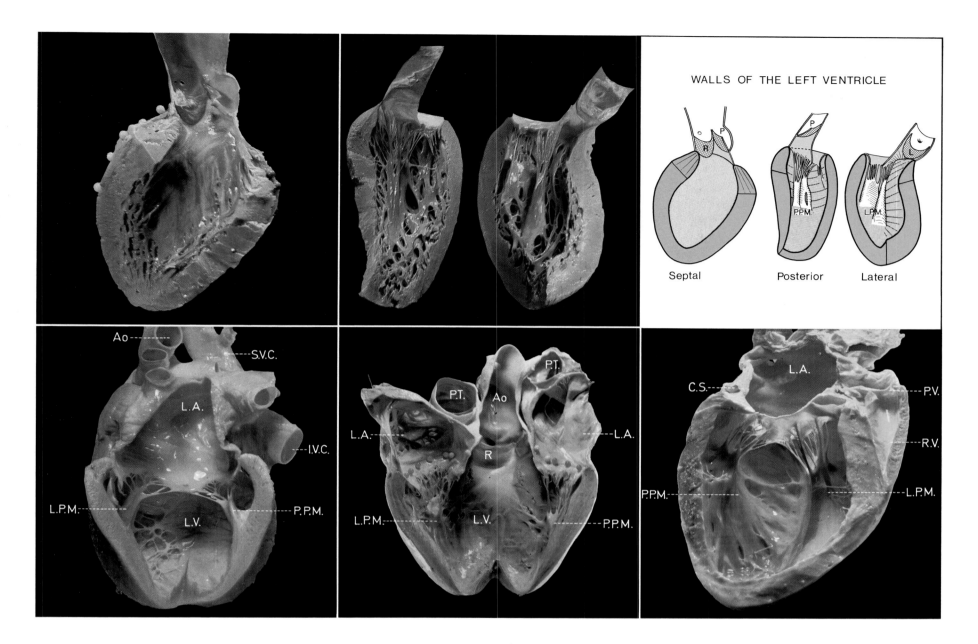

WALLS OF THE LEFT VENTRICLE

Septal   Posterior   Lateral

4: The heart of a **puma** is viewed from the postero-inferior aspect, following an incision extending from the apex through the midportion of the posterior leaflet of the mitral valve upward to the summit of the left atrium. The anterior leaflet of the mitral valve is seen in the center of the photograph. The mode of incision used here and in **5** is seen in a human heart on page 56.

5: A **pig** heart: Following the incision just described and shown in **4**, the anterior leaflet of the mitral valve was incised. The incision was then extended superiorly between the left and posterior aortic sinuses, dividing the related left atrial and aortic walls. The right aortic leaflet is in the center of the photograph. The red and yellow beads mark the site of attachment of the left atrium to the A.V. membrane in relation to the posterior and anterior leaflets of the mitral valve, respectively.

6: The heart of a **black bear**: An oblique transection extending superiorly from the apex passes through the anterior leaflet of the mitral valve. The left atrium is in the upper portion of the photograph.

With the exception of primates, mammalian hearts display atrabecular cavitary surfaces. The papillary muscles are usually short and constitute little more than a mooring for the chordae, e.g., **5** and **6**. The ratio of the unattached papillary muscle length to the apex-base length of L.V. is usually less than 0.1. This ratio is important in the separation of papillary muscle function from wall function in papillary muscle dysfunction. In the puma, the ratio is 0.17 (15:85mm). However, in other fleet animals, it may be unmeasurable (e.g., Zebra) as the papillary muscles are virtually absent.

Comments on Terminology: The publications of Walmsley, featuring photographs of cross sections of the thorax of cadavers, should be studied by all students interested in the spatial anatomy of the heart. He states—"The true posterior surface of the heart is customarily termed the base of the heart; it is formed largely by the left atrium . . .". Also, he notes—"The inferior surface of the heart is closely related to the . . . diaphragm . . . and it is unfortunate that it has become almost universally designated 'posterior'." When the heart is examined in the

operating room, the atonic diaphragm is elevated as it is in the cadaver and the walls of the ventricles under discussion largely face inferiorly. However, when the heart is viewed in an upright patient in full inspiration, these walls face postero-inferiorly; the direction in a vertical heart is more posterior, and in a horizontal heart more inferior. The designation, posteroinferior, is thus most often appropriate. In contrast studies, I have been impressed by the inferior location of the wall of the right ventricle in relation to the left ventricle, and I have used the designation, inferior, for the former. Because of the obliquity of the surfaces of the ventricles, the wall of the left faces more posteriorly than does that of the right ventricle, and its arteries in large part are seen posterior to those of the anterior or sternocostal aspect of the heart in an A.P. coronary arteriogram. Hence, I use the term, posterior, to describe the latter. In spite of these personal inclinations, the term, postero-inferior, applied to both walls, would be preferable, being less contentious regardless of the phase of respiration or the variations imposed by body habitus.

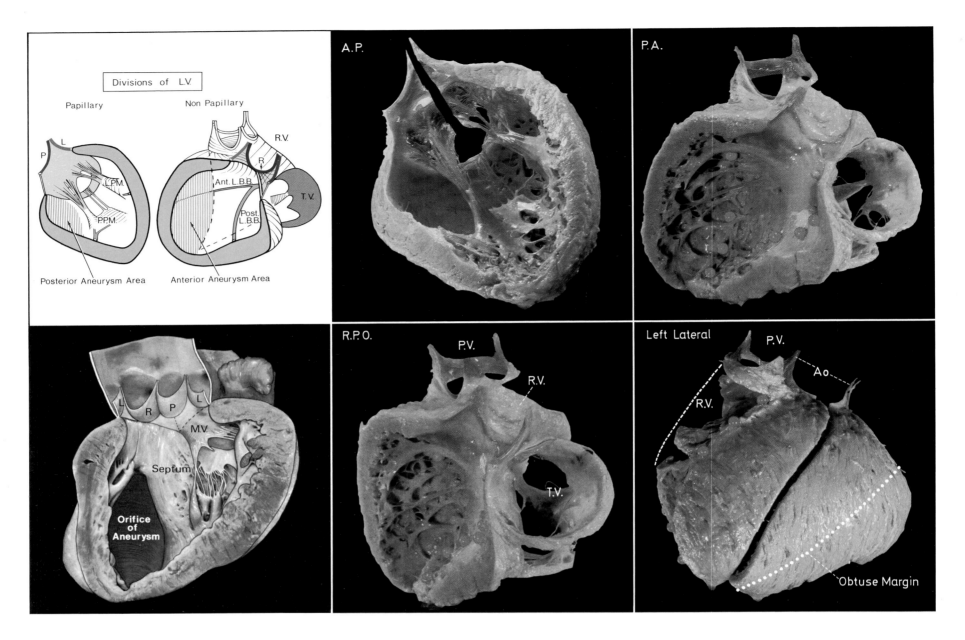

The Divisions of the Left Ventricular Wall
II. Functional —Papillary and Non-Papillary

In the specimen featured on this page, the atria, the great vessels down to the annuli, and the anterior and inferior walls of R.V. were first excised. The left ventricle was then transected as seen in **6**, the left lateral view. **1** is a drawing of the divisions which are seen in photographs **2** (A.P. view) and **3** (P.A. view). In the nonpapillary division, (**3**, **5** and **6**), the red beads delimit the septal wall anteriorly and inferiorly. **4** is the R.P.O. view of an example of an anterior aneurysm which is also seen in **35—1** with interior lighting to demonstrate the thinness of its wall.

Observe: (a) Note the large size of **the nonpapillary segment of the free wall** in **3**, **5**, and **6**. This is the anterior aneurysm area. Just above and anterior to the obtuse margin, the lateral papillary muscle is attached to the lateral wall, the remainder of which is nonpapillary, as is approximately the distal third of the posterior wall. (b) **The septal wall**, which is usually both nonpapillary and largely nontrabeculated, may be the site of a diffuse aneurysm which may

present as Bernheim's Syndrome : Septal perforation may follow. (c) The R.P.O. view of both the heart with the aneurysm and the nonpapillary segment is seen in **4** and **5**. The anterior interventricular artery normally supplies the coterminous septal wall and the anterior portion of the lateral wall. Hence, it is not surprising that a septal defect may coexist with an anterior aneurysm in ischemic heart disease. The defect is closed when the aneurysm is excised. In **4**, note the relation of the orifice of the aneurysm to the septal wall. (d) In **2** and its drawing in **1**, note the most common site for a **posterior aneurysm**. The infarcted area involves the posterior superior process of the ventricle which is below the ostium of L.V. between the right fibrous trigone and the inferior commissure of the mitral valve, an area normally free of papillary muscle attachments. It most commonly follows occlusion of a dominant right coronary artery. Variations in the dominance and distribution of this artery (see page 166) and the less common variations in the location of the posterior papillary muscle are codeterminants of associated dysfunction of the latter muscle.

Comment: (a) A large area in the lateral wall is devoid of papillary muscles, and large aneurysms may occur with a disproportionately small effect on cardiac function. For many years these have been recognized in plain x-rays of the chest. In the A.P. view, a contour—often large in size—is added to the left border of the heart.
(b) In the papillary division of the ventricle, smaller areas of wall are free of papillary muscle attachment and although aneurysms may occur through any of these areas, large aneurysms are uncommon, papillary muscle dysfunction often coexists and the physiologic effect is often disproportionate to their size. Ventriculography is today a common procedure and it has shown that posterior aneurysms, usually in the site seen in **1**, are common. A double density or calcification may be seen in an A.P. chest x-ray of a patient with a posterior aneurysm — the contour of the left heart border is usually normal ; however, alteration of this border is not confined to anterior aneurysms —on page 62 in Edwards' atlas (1961) a huge saccular posteromedial aneurysm is seen expanding and occupying the upper two-thirds of the left heart border.

E. The Shape of the Cavity of the Left Ventricle

In **2**–**6** the horizontal heart seen on page 29 has been transected.

2: A superior left lateral view demonstrates the line of section. The posterior and anterior segments are shown in **3** and **4**, with their drawings below each in **5** and **6**. Observe: (a) The line of section passes through the atrial portion of **the membranous septum**, the axis of which parallels that of the aortic bulb and is at a right angle to the annular axis; it meets the muscular ventricular septum at an obtuse angle—in a normal heart, the aorta overrides the muscular septum. In the presence of a congenital defect in the membranous septum, a catheter may be passed easily into the aorta or left ventricle from the right atrium. (b) The medial portion of the curved **inferior wall of the right atrium** is apposed to the posterior superior process of the left ventricle (P.S.P.), which is the area most often involved by a posterior ischemic aneurysm. (c) The frontal transection passes through both **papillary muscles**. Note the relation of the posterior (P.P.M.) to the septal wall (**4** and **6**) and the location of the lateral (L.P.M.) in the lateral wall. The nonpapillary portion of the free wall of the L.V. is not only anterior, but superior, to the lateral muscle. (d) Identify **the posterior wall of the left ventricle** which in this horizontal heart, largely faces inferiorly. Above, **the lateral wall extends laterally, then superiorly to reach the summit of L.V., whence it descends to the ostium of L.V.** In the area of descent, it faces superiorly and to the right. In page **29**—**1**, a segment of what is defined in this work as the lateral wall is seen to face anteriorly. As seen here, in addition, the wall also faces superiorly. **The superior convexity of the superior segment of the lateral wall is reflected in the cavity contour of L.V.; in the A.P. view, it is often above the aortic valve attachments to the ostium of L.V.**; these attachments are also obscured by the contrast material in the superior segment of the cavity in a lateral view. (e) **The ostial slope of L.V.**: In **4**, note that the anterior portion is only moderately developed; at the line of cross section, it indents the cavity, more in relation to the lateral than the septal wall. (f) **The membranous atrial septum** in the circular fossa ovalis is shown transilluminated in **3** and orange in **5**. The arrow extending through the inferior vena cava and bisecting the fossa is directed to the posterior aortic sinus. (g) The right cornu of the fenestrated **valve of the inferior vena cava** is attached to the left of, and posterior to the crista terminalis (T.B.). (h) The location of the anterior and posterior divisions of **the left branch of the conduction system** is indicated in **6** as they course towards the lateral and posterior papillary muscles. In many animals, these branches cross the cavity as free chords (see **33**—**6**) — see Edmonds *et al.* Similar transcavitary bundles may occur in the human heart — they should not be severed when the papillary muscles are excised in valve replacement. Note that the lateral papillary muscle is larger and less tethered to the ventricular wall than the posterior.

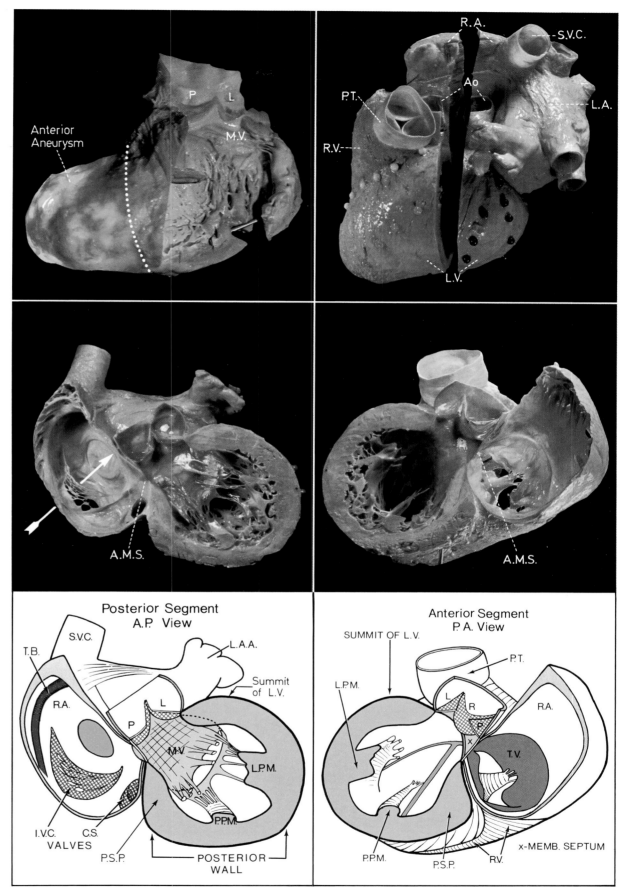

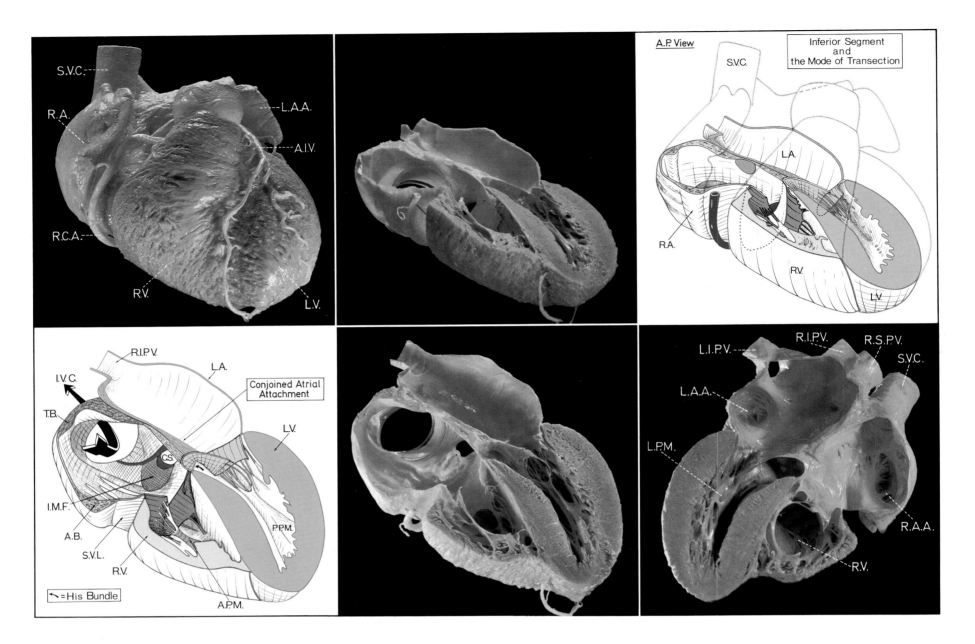

F. The Outflow Tract of the Left Ventricle in Relation to Heart Block—Lenegre's Disease

With the exception of the posterior leaflet of the mitral valve, all components of the A.V. membrane are a part of the outflow tract of the left ventricle. The junction between the anterior and posterior divisions of the membrane (the right fibrous trigone) and the membranous septum are of particular interest in this connection because the penetrating and branching portions of the His bundle run through their attachment to the ostium of L.V.: This attachment is subjected to maximal distracting forces during ventricular systole. The muscular septum moves toward the apex, exerting an inferior strain, and the blood rushing into the aorta exerts a superior distracting strain on this segment of the A.V. membrane which moors the posterior aortic annulus to the ostium of the ventricle. The membranous septum in directed, not only superiorly, but posteriorly and to the right, hence in addition to these "vertical" forces, "horizontal" strain occurs. The trauma, resulting from these distracting forces, may progressively

impair and finally destroy the function of the conduction system with the production of complete heart block; certainly the latter is not commonly the product of ischemic heart disease and gross abnormalities in affected hearts may be absent; however because of its angularity, the junction of the divisions of the A.V. membrane is also the site of maximal turbulence during ventricular systole; hence it is not surprising that fibrosis and calcification may occur on its ventricular aspect.

Specimen A : 36—1–6, and **37—1**: This transection was designed to demonstrate the anatomic features which are the basis of the above two mechanisms which may be operative in the pathogenesis of Lenegre's and Lev's disease.

1: An A.P. view of a specimen after removal of the great vessels.

2 and **3**: The lower segment is seen from an attitudinal A.P. view. The transection passes through **the angular junction of the two divisions of the A.V. membrane (the right**

fibrous trigone) just below the nadir of the posterior aortic annulus. The membranous septum extends to the right and posteriorly, intersecting a sagittal plane at an angle of 30°. During systole the anterior leaflet of the mitral valve meets this sagittal plane at a right angle, hence the two structures form an angle of 60°. The leaflet is seen here swung anteriorly in diastole which exaggerates the acuteness of the angle; perhaps this flexion is an added mechanical factor in this consideration.

In **4** and **5** the lower, and in **6** and **37—1** the upper segments are seen rotated 45° to facilitate their examination. One may visually place the upper on the lower segment and better appreciate the distracting forces during systole and the considerable possibility for trauma to the surface of the membrane where it changes direction at the right fibrous trigone, the site of entrance of the His bundle —the common atrioventricular conduction bundle (see page 17).

The line of transection passes through the upper portion of the conjoined atrial attachments to the A.V. membrane. In the upper segment, the left and right atrial attachments separate. The left atrium extends to the left along its line of attachment to the A.V. membrane, and the right atrium extends across the A.V. membrane on to the tricuspid membrane. The first division of the right bundle branch of the conduction system passes along the ostium of L.V. anterior to the tricuspid attachment and inferior to the right ventricular attachment to the A.V. membrane.* This area may be subject to distracting forces of lesser magnitude due to the lesser vertical dimension of the related segment of the A.V. membrane; however, the anatomic studies of Rosenbaum indicate that the right bundle is the thinnest; the left anterior, the left posterior, and the left main branch demonstrate a stepwise increase in calibre. This variation in calibre, Rosenbaum opines, may explain the variation in onset of function loss, the thinnest bundle being most susceptible to injury. For many years, it has been recognized that right bundle branch block is often associated with left ventricular hypertrophy. In hypertension for example, the distracting forces are increased—it is conceivable that the associated right bundle branch block results from mechanical trauma to the thin first division of the right bundle branch, lying as it does on the ostium of the left ventricle.

G. The Junction of the Divisions of the A.V. Membrane and Surface Phenomena —Lev's Disease

Two specimens will be examined, the first (Specimen B) without and the second (Specimen C) with calcification at the attachment of the right fibrous trigone to the ostium of L.V.

Specimen B: 37—2: 60° view: See pages 117 and 120 where the transection and prior dissection are seen. The posterior aortic leaflet (P) is seen almost in its entirety—fragments of the right and left (R. & L.) are present. The membranous septum (M.S.), seen in the shadow, and the well-lit anterior leaflet of the mitral valve (A.M.V.) meet at the right fibrous trigone. The septum and trigone are directed away from our vantage point, and although the angle of the junction of the divisions of the A.V. membrane cannot be accurately determined in this photograph, their angularity is apparent.

Specimen C: 3–6: Turn to page 35 for the A.P. view and the site of the frontal transection of this specimen.
3 and 4: L.A.O. (45°): A calcific mass is present at the attachment of the right fibrous trigone to the ostium—the site of penetration of the A.V. bundle into the membrane and possibly the site of maximum turbulence and distraction.

5 and 6: 345° view: The red beads indicate the A.V. node and its relation to the attachment of the right fibrous trigone to the ostium of L.V.

---

* As stated on page 10, trace the ostium of L.V. in all figures. It is shown in **37—1** as a solid line (a) for a few millimeters on the left; (b) below the left anterior fibrous trigone and (c) below the membranous septum; it appears as a dashed red line between these areas.

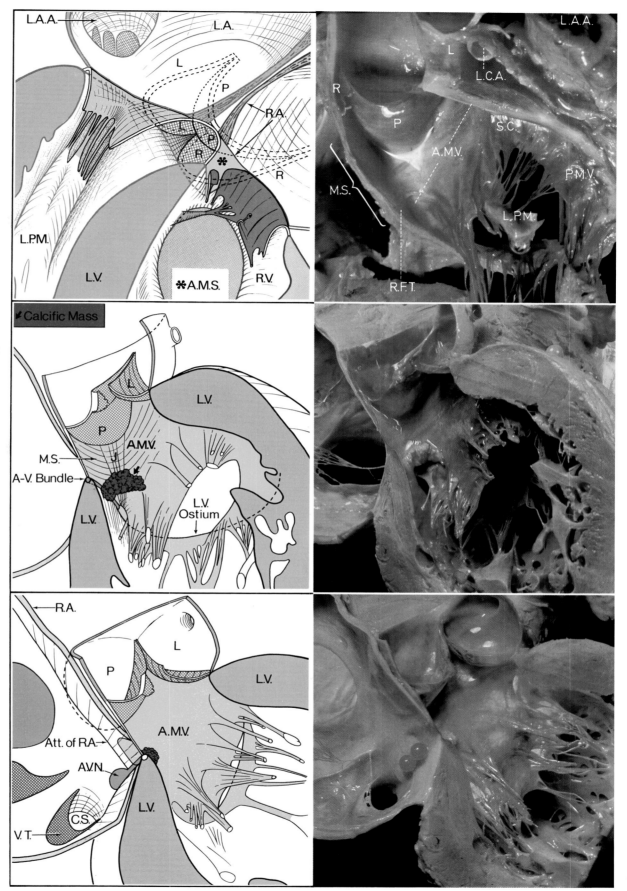

H. The Ostium of the Left Ventricle and the Mitral Valve

The ostium of L.V.—important in most anatomic considerations—provides the key to our understanding of the attachment of the aortic and mitral valves.

The borders of each of the leaflets of the mitral valve may be divided into three parts: (1) attached, (2) commissural, and (3) free. On this page we will first consider the attached border which has great practical importance in valve replacement. The dimensional interrelationships of all three borders—of interest in the biomechanics of the valve—will then be reviewed*.

The term, attached border, denotes the line of mergence of the leaflets with the other components of the A.V. membrane. **The attached border of the anterior leaflet** is divided into four parts: (1) **The intervalvular,** 2.7 cm in length, is found at the site of the anterosuperior part of the attachment of the left atrium to the A.V. membrane. It extends between the left and right fibrous trigones. (2) **The junctional,** (a)1.7 cm in length, (b) the site of the junction of the leaflet and the anterior division of the A.V. membrane and (c) the site of the conjoined atrial attachment to the right fibrous trigone. (3) and (4) **The right and left ostial:** Between the right and left fibrous trigones and the related commissures, the leaflet is attached to the ostium of L.V. through the intermediation of the subvalvular membrane; each measures approximately 1.0 cm in length. The entirety of the attached border of the anterior leaflet, therefore, measures 6.4 cm, which almost equals the attached border of the posterior leaflet (7.0 cm). However, the former forms a squat pentagon (**104—3**) and the latter forms an elongated pentagon (when excised). As the widths of the anterior and posterior leaflets in a sagittal plane are 2.7 and 1.5 cm, it is apparent that the surface area of the posterior is larger. I could find no confirmation for the statement, frequently found in medical writing, that the surface areas of the leaflets are equal. The importance of the identifying the precise attachments of the leaflets is not debatable. In mitral valve replacement, the attached border of the posterior leaflet (studied on pages 46–51) is of particular interest because of the danger of periprosthetic leak in relation to it. This complication is less common in relation to the anterior leaflet because the A.V. membrane at its attached borders is tougher and much less often involved by calcification than the posterior—the calcification also can be removed without producing serious tissue defects. During valve replacement, great care is mandatory in the placement of sutures if periprosthetic leak is to be avoided. This is of particular importance when the leaflets are in their normal state, i.e., thin and fragile, in contrast to the thickened leaflets seen following rheumatic valvulitis. Examples of the former are commonly encountered, e.g., (1) mitral regurgitation due to ruptured chordae tendinae and (2) mitral valve dysfunction due to coronary artery disease.

The term, annulus fibrosis, is still used in anatomic descriptions of the mitral valve. It is important, however, to be aware that **no ring or cordlike structure exists;** otherwise, a radiologist may be deluded in an attempt to identify the former and the surgeon may be beguiled in his concept

that the latter provides a secure site for the placement of sutures in valve replacement. Examination of the work of Henle (1873) and Zimmerman (1966) affirms the inaptness of the simplistic annular concept; nevertheless, the commonly accepted physiologic theory explaining the transmission of the cardiac impulse implies the presence of a nonconductive fibrous structure between the left atrium and left ventricle and, indeed, one exists which is described herein as the subvalvular segment of the A.V. membrane. Awareness of this is important in the comprehension of the anatomy of the so-called "annular" subvalvular aneurysms of the left ventricle (deletion of the word, annular, would seem appropriate) and is critical in the excision of the mitral valve prior to its replacement. Calcification of the mitral "annulus" is a well recognized pathologic state; however, it should be emphasized that (1) the subvalvular segment of the A.V. membrane, and the adjoining parts of both (2) the ostium of the ventricle, and (3) the posterior leaflet of the mitral valve are, in most instances, all involved; hence, this pathologic condition cannot be presented as evidence for the existence of an annulus. It is suggested on page 51 that the calcification results from hemodynamic rather than metabolic factors; it is interesting that in the single report of similar tricuspid valve calcification (Arnold et al.), pulmonary hypertension reached systemic level (R.V. pressures were 160/10 and 122/11 in the two patients studied).

The systolic reduction in the length of the ostium of the left ventricle warrants consideration in valve function: (a) Davis and Kimmonth found a reduction of the mitral division of 20–50° in dogs. (b) In a dilated, diseased left ventricle, not only may the mitral division be enlarged in diastole, but its reduction in systole may be incomplete; as a consequence, the appositional tolerance of the mitral leaflets may be exceeded, resulting in, or contributing to regurgitation. (c) As we saw above, the mitral valve attachment in relation to the ostium comprises 2/3 of its perimeter (9.0/13.4 cm); therefore, the systolic reduction of its dimension may result in a shearing strain on the sutures used to secure a prosthesis.

The ostium of L.V., consisting of aortic and mitral divisions, forms and important part of the primary orifices of the aortic and mitral valves. The longest length is 5.9 cm. **The greatest width (2.7 cm) of the aortic division,** its transverse bisector, and the width of the junction of the divisions (3.0 cm), measured between the left and right fibrous trigones, are less than **the greatest width of the mitral division** (3.6 cm) (found 1.0 cm posterior to the mitral commissures)—it is thus apparent that the ostium is oval; although when the left ostial process is prominent, the shape is pyriform (see **20—1** and **2**). The ostial perimeter is 16.1 cm—the aortic and mitral divisions measure 7.1 and 9.0 cm. The combined length of the attached borders of the mitral valve leaflets measures 13.4 cm. The lengths of the free borders of the leaflets are: anterior = 4.8; posterior = 6.2; therefore, their combined length is less than the leaflet perimeter. The orifice size is determined by the intercommissural length, 2.7 cm, and flexibility of the leaflets. A cross-sectional area of 5.0 cm^2 is common in a 70 kilo male (this measurement cannot be ascertained by the methods

employed herein). Comparison of these dimensions provides some indication of the relative inefficiency of the leaflet design and the (a) effect of loss of leaflet flexibility and (b) reduction in intercommissural length**. The secondary mitral orifice, located in the cavity of L.V. is smaller than the leaflet perimeter. In the aortic orifice, the relationship is reversed, the triangular primary orifice at the annular nadirs is less than the area at the commissures. The annular axis and its perpendicular (**22—3**) are an expression of the geometry of this uniplanar valve. On either side of the highest point of the ostium are the left and right aortic annular attachments. The inferior commissure of the mitral valve is 1.5 cm anterior to the lowest point of the ostium. The ostium of the left ventricle provides attachment for the A.V. membrane, the main components of the anterior and posterior divisions of which are the membranous septum and the mitral valve. The junction of the divisions extends above the ostium of L.V. (**3—5** and **6**), as do the confluent membranous septum and anterior leaflet of the mitral valve (**2—5** and **6**). In systole, the posterior leaflet lies in the plane of the ostium of L.V. while a large part of the anterior leaflet lies in the plane of the posterior wall of the aortic bulb (**15—1-4**)—the two meet at an obtuse angle.

---

* The dimensions are derived from a representative specimen.
** Rheumatic fever affects the leaflets—it reduces their flexibility and it results in their progressive adherence at the commissures—a progressive reduction in intercommissural length results.

Chapter 4: The Mitral Valve

Introduction

The terms used in this volume will be reviewed. The leaflets are best termed anterior (A.M.V.) and posterior (P.M.V.). The corresponding terms aortic and mural are not in common use; the objection to both will be evident. The papillary muscles are termed lateral (L.M.P.) and posterior (P.P.M.) rather than anterolateral and posteromedial. The commissures are termed superior (S.C.) and inferior (I.C.).

In any consideration of the mitral valve the following eight elements require scrutiny—they may be arranged in two groups. The first is composed of (a) the leaflets, (b) the subvalvular membrane, (c) the chordae, and (d) the left atrium whose attachment demarcates (a) and (b). The second relates to the left ventricle—(a) its cavity configuration and size; the status and dimensions of (b) the ostium, (c) the walls of L.V. as a whole and (d) the papillary muscles. Two of these elements will now be reviewed.

Four aspects of the papillary muscles may be considered. (a) The papillary muscles are attached as follows: (1) both—to the intermediate third of L.V.—their nonattached portions protrude into the orificial third; (2) the posterior—in varying proximity to the right border of the posterior wall; (3) the lateral to the lateral wall—above the obtuse margin (the left border of the posterior wall). The posterior location of the mitral valve is compatible with this relationship to the posterior wall. (b) The ratio of the unattached/attached lengths of the papillary muscle and the ratio of the unattached length/apex-base length of L.V. command attention in the separation of papillary muscle function from left ventricular wall function in this era when great attention is directed to papillary muscle dysfunction. In many animals the papillary muscles are so short that they are incapable of either shortening in health or elongation in disease. A similar design occurs in some human hearts, suggesting that anatomic measurements are needed in the study of papillary muscle dysfunction. (c) Their axes are perpendicular to the plane of the leaflets in systole, which, in turn. roughly lie in the plane of the ostium of L.V.—these axes are not parallel to the axis of L.V.—see 53. Alteration in this axis resulting from configurational changes in the cavity of L.V. may contribute to mitral regurgitation and to outflow obstruction in asymmetric septal hypertrophy. (d) Their form: In roughly two thirds of hearts the lateral muscle is a single structure and the posterior consists of separately based columns. The lateral muscle is usually larger, simpler in design and less tethered to the ventricular wall.

Knowledge of the variations in the location and number of the papillary muscles is useful in many clinical situations, examples of which are: (a) When surgical replacement of the valve is effected, the leaflets, chordae, and muscles are cleanly removed as a unit to, first, minimize the danger of leaving fragments which may embolize, and second, to minimize the area of raw surface in the ventricle; (b) the location of the muscles and their possible dispersion will affect the incidence and the degree of valve dysfunction which results from myocardial infarction in their area, e.g., when the posterior muscle is deviated medially, papillary muscle dysfunction may be associated with a posterior ventricular aneurysm; (c) elevation of the attachment increases the likelihood of intrusion of an unremoved papillary muscle into the orifice or the cage of a prosthetic valve. (d) In the valuable article of Roberts and Perloff (see References) Roberts states that in mitral valve replacement, "perforation of the left ventricular wall or ... severe thinning of the wall, with formation of a functioning or anatomic aneurysm or both may result if the papillary muscles are pulled too vigorously". Visualize this hazard in 42—6.

The recognition of rupture of the chordae tendinae as a common and often emergent cause of mitral regurgitation evokes interest in these slighted moorings: The wide spectrum of physiologic responses encountered cannot be explained by the adduction of the number of chordae ruptured—five observations are necessary for clinico-pathologic correlation. (1) Their composition—chordae tendinae or chordae muscularis (2) Their origin may be from the papillary muscles—papillary chordae—or from small trabeculae of the wall of L.V.—mural chordae (these are inserted into the posterior leaflet only). (3) Their insertion may be to (a) the free margin or to the ventricular surface of (b) the appositional or (c) the non-appositional divisions of the leaflets. The chordae are designated accordingly as (a) marginal, (b) appositional and (c) nonappositional. As a rule a stepwise increase in both diameter and length occurs as we pass from (a) to (c). Tandler (1913) divided chordae into three generation: 1st=(a); 2nd=(b) and (c); 3rd=mural chordae. Observe that his classification mixed origin and insertion. In the classification of Lam *et al.*, the mural chordae are termed the "basal", and the nonappositional to the anterior leaflet, the "strut chordae". The use of perfusion fixation is important in many aspects of anatomic and pathologic studies: Its use discloses the insertion of chordae to the nonappositional part of the anterior leaflet—this has often been unrecognized in the past. The work of Lev and Eckner has called attention to this important, but neglected technique. (4) Their diameter best indicates their functional role, although future studies may show that the site of insertion is of intrinsic importance. Their diameter varies from 0.25—1.75 mm. (Recall the diameter of nonabsorbable suture material: 000=0.25 mm; 1=0.50 mm; 5=0.75 mm). Their length varies from 0.25—2.25 cm. (5) Their number: The presence of 24 origins and 72 insertions—the numbers seen in the human (Lam *et al.*)—evinces the occurrence of chordal subdivision. Roberts and Perloff (1972) calling attention to this subdivision—and it is often obscured by Tandlers calssification—divide chordae into three orders as a consequence of this subdivision. For two reasons the size cannot be inferred from such a classification. (a) A cord may be large or small and pass without division from origin to insertion; contrariwise, more than three divisions may occur and from one cord as many as twenty filaments may arise—see the inferior commissural chorda in 41—2. (b) Unequal division occurs: No progressive diminution in diameter occurs between the "first" and "third order".

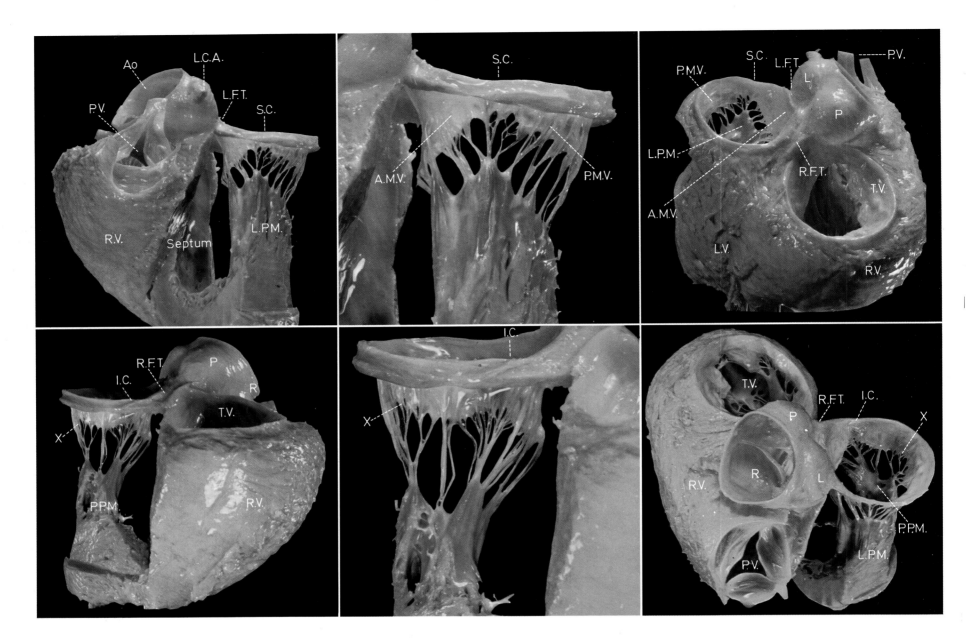

A. Plan of the Leaflet-Chordae-Papillary Muscle Complex

Specimen A: 40—1–6 and **41—1**, seen also in **20—1** and **2**, where the stippled area indicates the muscle that was removed to afford our present examination. The scale is 1.5:1.0 in **40—2** and **5** and **41—1** and 0.8:1 in the remainder.

1 and **2**: The specimen is examined in the plane of the valve orifice from a superior L.A.O. view. The **lateral papillary muscle** (L.P.M.) is attached to the middle third of the wall of the ventricle; its unattached portion is wedge-shaped. The free margins of the anterior (A.M.V.) and posterior (P.M.V.) leaflets in diastole present a reciprocal wedge-shape. From the margins of the papillary muscle, chordae pass to the leaflets; the apex of the muscle provides attachment for the commissural chordae.

3: These facts are again noted in **3**, where the **superior commissure** (S.C.) and the lateral papillary muscle are

viewed from a superior R.P.O. position. The commissure is 14 mm behind the left fibrous trigone (L.F.T.). The anterior and posterior leaflets are confluent at the commissure, the free margin of which, in this specimen, is 7 mm from the valve attachment. Rusted, in a study of fifty specimens, found a range of 5 to 13 mm in this measurement, with an average of 8 mm. Preservation of this commissural curtain is essential during a reparative operation, or serious regurgitation will result.

4 and **5**: The heart is rotated and the plane of examination is again that of the mitral valve orifice. The upper part of the posterior wall of the left ventricle has been removed, exposing the **posterior papillary muscle** (P.P.M.), which has a single base, but two heads are now present for chordal attachment. The medial head provides a stout chorda which branches into small filaments that extend to the **inferior commissure** (I.C.). The inferior commissural curtain, in this specimen, is wider than the superior, measuring 11 mm. The commissure is also 11 mm from the right fibrous trigone. Both commissures

are thus well posterior to their related fibrous trigones, a fact to remember when the terms "mural" and "aortic" are used to designate the leaflets; the "aortic", therefore, has bilateral attachments to the left ventricular wall.* A commissural scallop is seen between the inferior commissure and the indentation (X) in the posterior leaflet—it is also seen in **6**.

6: Superior left lateral view: Note the relation of the inferior commissure to (a) the right fibrous trigone and (b) to its fellow commissure—the two are usually in a frontal plane—one is not anterior to the other.
Note: The lengths of the commissural chordae (see **2** and **5**) are: superior—0.8 cm; inferior—1.4 cm; the former are usually shorter (Rusted *et al*). (Lam *et al* found average lengths of 1.2 and 1.4 in 50 hearts). The lateral papillary muscle not only protrudes more into the cavity of L.V., but—if unremoved—more into a valve prosthesis.

---

* The anterior leaflet has been termed the aortic and the posterior leaflet, the mural.

Specimen A: 1: Inferior view: The plane of examination is that of the orifice of the valve. Chordae, either appositional or non-appositional, are attached to the entire ventricular aspect of the posterior leaflet. Chordae pass from the posterior muscle to supply a portion of the left half of this leaflet. The two papillary muscles are frequently connected by cord-like bands, as seen in this specimen.

Specimen B: 2: From the same perspective as **40 —4**, the inferior commissure is viewed in a different specimen. Note the absence of a commissural scallop and the presence of a large posterior leaflet. The greatest dimension of the widths of the posterior and anterior leaflets are 2.0 and 2.7 cm, respectively. These measurements are usually approximately 1.5 and 2.5 cm.

Specimen C: 3–6

3: Superior P.A. view: The atria and great vessels have been removed. The leaflets are in their diastolic position. The relation of the commissures to the left and right fibrous trigones is evident but can be confirmed in **4**. The two arrows are directed toward the anterior and posterior interventricular grooves.

4: The mitral leaflets have, in large part, been excised. The yellow and red beads mark the sites of the trigones and commissures, respectively. The apices of the papillary muscles are directed to the commissures.

5 and 6:

The internal surface of the lateral papillary muscle displays a separate commissural component (X), which is located below the red bead that marks the superior commissure. Black cloth is present between the commissural head and the remaining muscle which has papillae in tiers which supply the related portions of the leaflets.

The posterior muscle is concave and has a triangular shape; the chordae are attached to the margins.

Comments: (a) Wide variations are found in the papillary muscles. In the simplest form, seen in **40—1** and **2**, the chordae are attached to the margins of the wedge-shaped terminal part of the papillary muscle—a single column attached through much of its outer aspect to the wall of L.V. The posterior papillary muscle (**40 —4** and **5**) has a single base and two heads. In **41 —6**, muscle bands join the two heads. When two heads or two separately based muscles are side by side, the anterior of the two usually supplies the commissure in addition to the anterior leaflet. In **41 —5**, two separate muscles are present—one above the other—the upper supplies the commissure—a common arrangement.

(b) The papillary muscles are often convex-concave; however, they also may be globular, conical, fusiform, or quadrangular.

(c) The order and approximation of the chordae lengths are: commissural—1.25 cm; appositional—1.5 cm; nonappositional—1.75 cm.

(d) From the commissural chorda in **2**, twenty small filamentous insertions result—see comments on page 39.

(e) The right and left fibrous trigones lie in a frontal plane as do the commissures—the planes are 10 mm apart (**3** and **4**).

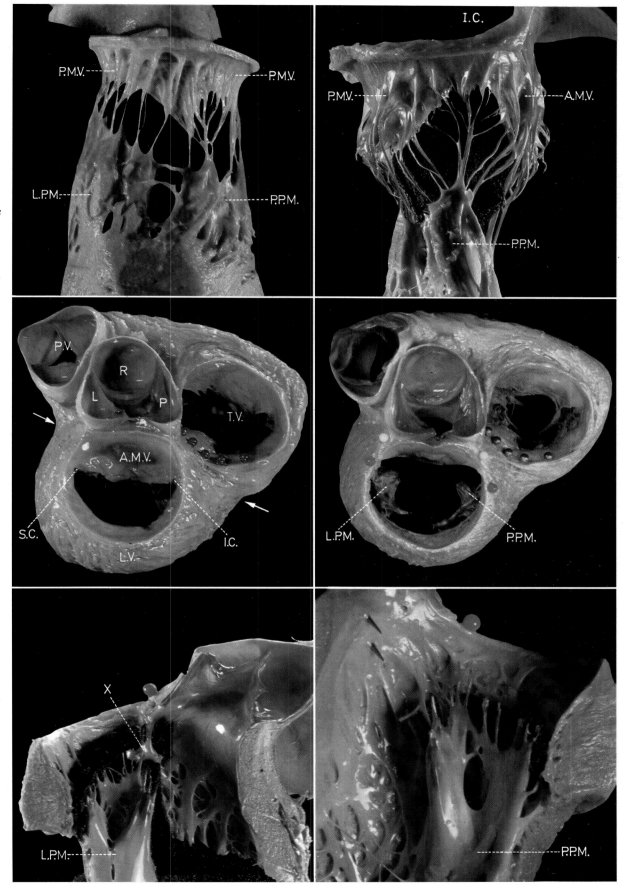

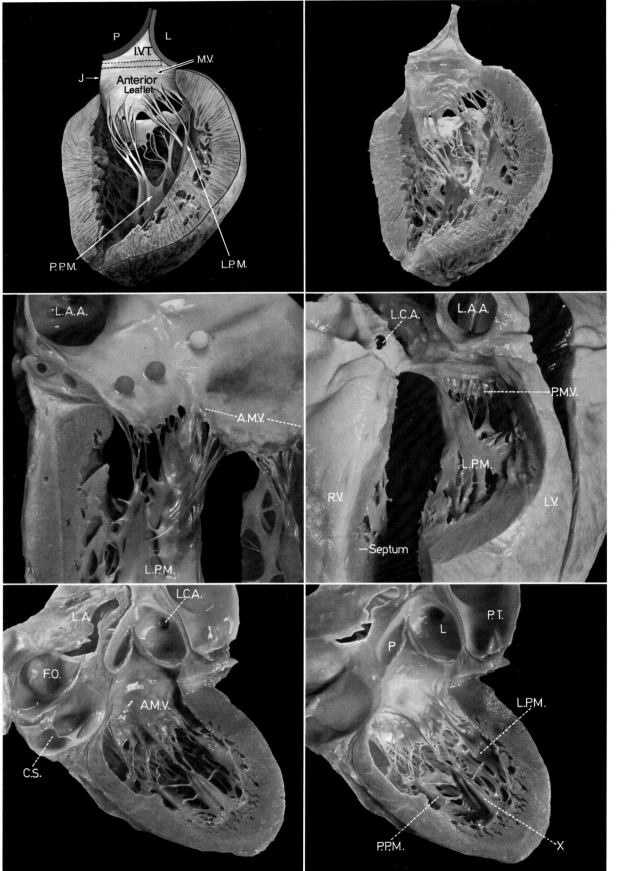

B. The Papillary Muscles

I. Variation in Location

Lateral Translocation of the Posterior Papillary Muscle
Specimen A: 1 and **2**: In a nonattitudinal A.P. view, one incision separates the septal and posterior walls and is carried up through the junction (J) of the divisions of the A.V. membrane. The second incision passes through the junction of the papillary and nonpapillary divisions of the free wall of L.V. The posterior papillary muscle arises with the lateral, a situation recalling the condition of the parachute mitral valve, wherein all chordae arise from a single papillary muscle. This specimen exhibited local prolapse of the posterior leaflet, and one can wonder if any relationship exist between this pathologic finding and the anatomic variation present.

Superior Translocation of the Lateral Papillary Muscle
Specimen B, 3 and **4**, is shown also on page 94. The scale is 1.3 : 1.0
3: The line of transection is through the obtuse margin. The red and yellow beads identify, in turn, the ostium of L.V. and the left fibrous trigone. The papillary muscle extends to the commissure. This papillary muscle, if unremoved in valve replacement—and at one time this was recommended—would intrude into the valve prosthesis. Note the wedge-shaped left atrioventricular sulcus, with the coronary artery above and the great vein below.

In **4**, an L.A.O. nonattitudinal view, a window has been made in the lateral wall of the ventricle. The incision through the obtuse margin is on the left. The incision on the right identifies the septal margin, adjacent to which is the attachment of the papillary muscle to the superior segment of the lateral wall of L.V. This is also an example of virtual muscularization of chordae, which is shown on page 45 in its complete form.

The Inferior Location
of an Anterior Accessory Papillary Muscle
Specimen C: 5 and **6**: An A.P. view of the left posterior segment of a specimen which has been transected in the L.A.O.—R.P.O. plane. In **6**, interior lighting is added. The accessory papillary muscle (X) is attached just above the apex of the ventricle. It receives chordae from the apex of the anterior leaflet of the mitral valve, an area which normally is free of chordae. This is an uncommon variation—much less common than a posterior inter-mediate papillary muscle supplying chordae to the posterior leaflet, seen on the next page in **43—4** and **5**. The non-appositional chordae insert on the anterior leaflet central to the left and right fibrous trigones—they extend to the attachment of the leaflet as shown in **6**. A surgeon, determined to ablate all papillary muscles, should realize that they may be located deep in the ventricle. A similar, inferiorly located papillary muscle is shown in **45—2**.

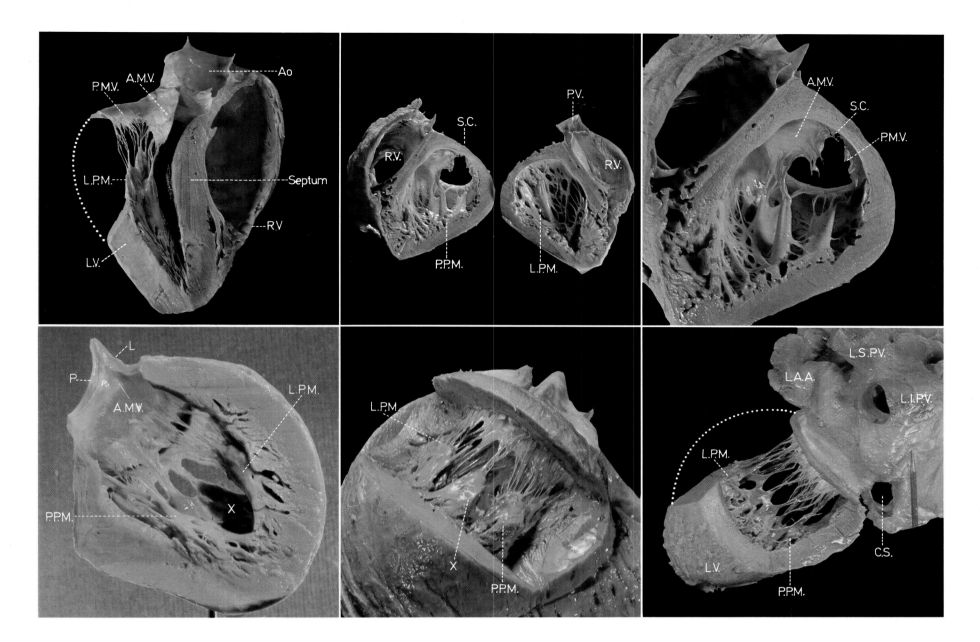

II. Variation in Number

Specimen D: 1: A nonattitudinal examination of the left segment of a specimen. The transection passes midway through both mitral leaflets. A part of the lateral wall has been removed to silhouette the **lateral papillary muscle**. Note the single base and the three heads; the upper supplies chordae to the commissural area, and the lower two supply the respective "halves" of their adjacent leaflets. A single base, with single or multiple heads, may be present. Frequently, two heads are present, each on adjacent but discrete muscle bases. The next specimen presents a contrast with these more common patterns.

Specimen E: 2 and **3**: Nonattitudinal L.A.O. view: An oblique transection, extending from above downwards towards the apex, passes through the superior commissure. Note the presence of two sets of three papillary muscles. The bases of attachment of all six muscles are unusually separated. In the left segment, which has been everted, the lateral papillary muscles are seen. The com-

missures and the adjoining portions of the two leaflets are each attached by chordae to separate papillary muscles. In the presence of this variation, the result of rupture and the effects of the complication, papillary muscle dysfunction, might be less severe.

Specimen F: 4 and 5

4: This specimen has been sectioned in a frontal plane through the nadirs of the left and posterior aortic annuli. The posterior segment is seen in an attitudinal A.P. view. **A posterior intermediate papillary muscle** (X) can be seen.

5: The posterior leaflet and the papillary muscles are viewed posteroinferiorly at an earlier state of dissection. In addition to the two normally situated muscles, the separate intermediate papillary muscle (X) is located posteriorly, a condition which is normal in birds.

Specimen G: 6: L.P.O. view: In this specimen, a row of small papillary muscles extends between the two major

papillary muscles. In the replacement of a mitral valve, the papillary muscles should be deftly removed; otherwise, partially severed fragments may necrose, become separated, and result in embolism.

Comment: (a) **The ratios of the unattached/attached lengths** of the papillary muscles are small in specimens **B**, **D**, **F**, and **G** and large in **C** and **E**. In **B**, the unattached length is seen in **42—4**; in **D** it lies above a line joining the labels L.P.M. and Septum; in **F** (**5**) the white lines to the three muscles mark the junction of their free and attached segments. The cavitary aspect of **G** appears in **99—1**. (b) **The ratio of the unattached papillary muscle length/apex-base length of L.V.** in **E** is unusually large. (c) The axis of the papillary muscles is normally angled posteriorly to the long axis of L.V. as seen in **E** and in **53—3-6** and **94—4**. The collinear axes in **C** are unusual.

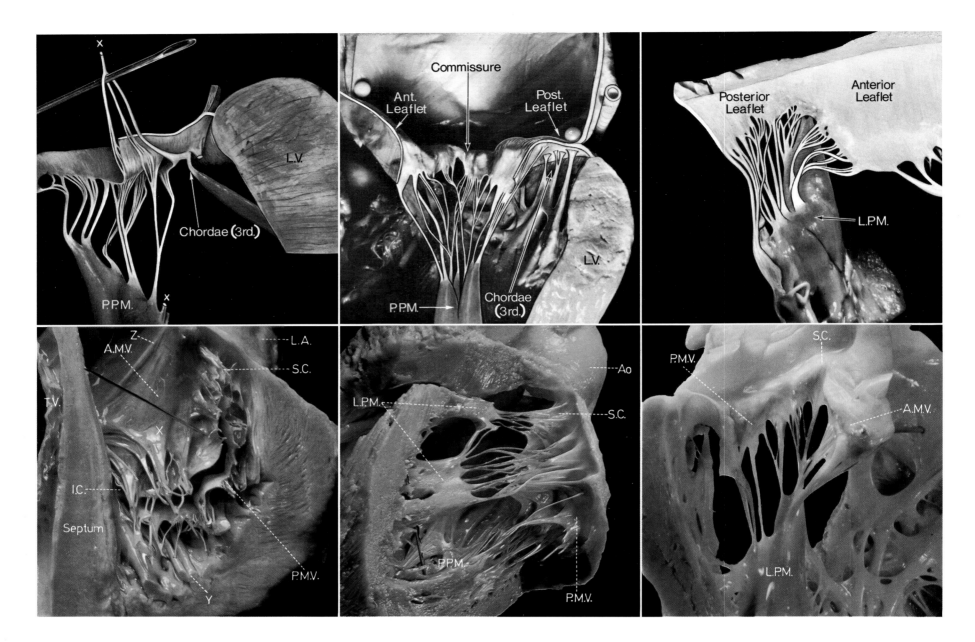

C. The Chordae of the Mitral Valve

Six specimens are examined. The upper three are shown in retouched photographs.

1: A chorda has been sectioned at point X and elevated on a Keith needle. It provides filaments to the (a) free edge of the leaflet, that is, 1st generation chordae, and also, (b) filaments to the under aspect of this posterior leaflet—2nd generation chordae. These are Tandler's terms. In the terminology suggested on page 39, these three chordae would be termed marginal, appositional, and nonappositional. The third generation chordae of Tandler are termed mural chordae.

2: From muscle trabeculae on the ventricular wall, chordae extend to the peripheral portion of the posterior leaflet—mural chordae. These chordae provide some support and substance to the posterior leaflet which presents poor material for the placement of sutures in valve replacement in mitral regurgitation associated with normal leaflets. The trabeculae of origin do not intrude into

the prosthesis. Hence, care should be taken to avoid their injury or removal.

3: When chordae arise from the margins of a wedge-shaped papillary muscle, their susceptibility to the cohesive effects of rheumatic disease may be lessened, and they are in less jeopardy at operation for the reconstruction of the mitral valve. However, as shown here, even when a wedge-shaped papillary muscle exists, the chordae may exhibit what may be referred to as **linearization**, the chordae presenting a conjoined linear attachment to the inner surface of the muscle.

4: An attitudinal L. A. O. view: On the anterior leaflet, the appositional area is the major site for chordal attachment, however, central to each commissure large nonappositional or "strut chordae" (see X) extend from the junction of the above area and the nonappositional portion of the leaflet onto the nonappositional portion and their terminal elements may reach the attached margin of the leaflet. Note the trabeculae (Y) which supply mural chordae. The valve is in a systolic state; it is held

open by a needle. Note the sickle shape of the orifice and the ridge (Z) at the junction of the mobile and nonmobile portion of the anterior leaflet.

5: The left lateral view of a mitral valve fixed in systole: In contrast to the anterior leaflet, chordae are widely attached to both the appositional and the entire nonappositional portion of the posterior leaflet. Separately based components of a "papillary muscle" are usually located in a plane at right angles to the axis of the ventricle. Here two widely based lateral papillary muscles are disposed in that axis.

6: The valve leaflets have been fixed in their systolic position. The line of transection passes through the midpoint of the two leaflets. The left half of both are seen; the leaflets are distracted. Only five chordae are attached to the lateral papillary muscle. In the presence of such **concentration of chordae**, ischemic injury to a small segment of muscle could result in significant regurgitation. The appositional area of the leaflets are thickened and dark in color.

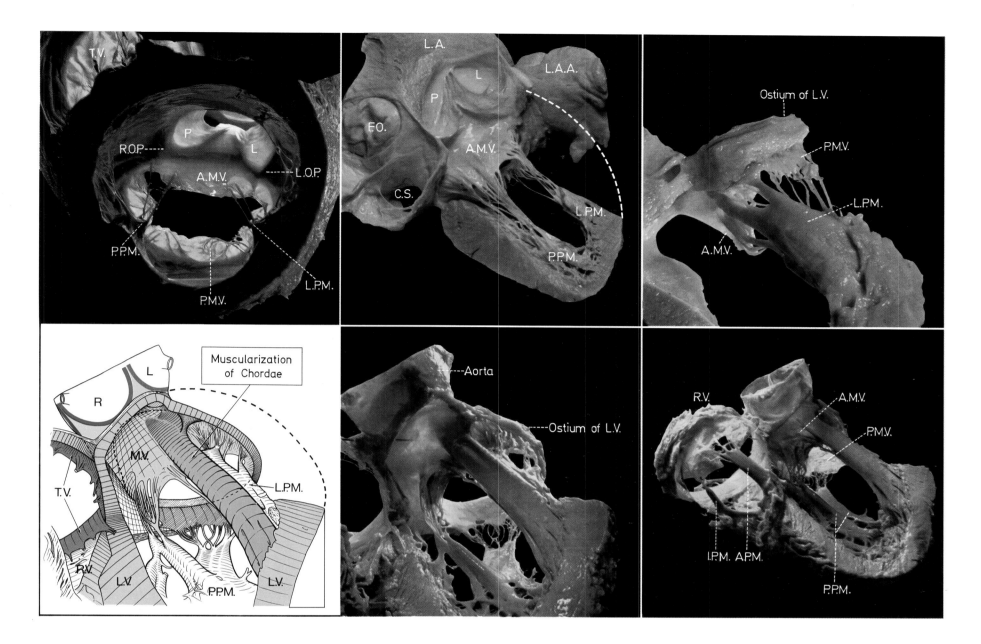

On this page four specimens are seen—they are designated with the letters A, B, C, and D.

Specimen A: 1: Black bear: Following its transverse section, we peer into the left ventricle from the apex and note the aortic valve above and the mitral valve below. A transverse darkened zone, passing between the wedge-shaped right and left ostial processes (R.O.P. and L.O.P.) is produced by the left atrial attachment on the opposite side of the A.V. membrane. In addition to atrabecular ventricular cavities, the hearts of most animals demonstrate simple wedge-shaped papillary muscles and sparse delicate chordae, in contrast to the profusion and considerable substance of the latter in the human heart (emphasized in **44—4**). We now return to human hearts.

Specimen B: 2: R.A.O. view of the left posterior segment resulting from a transection in the L.A.O.—R.P.O. plane. Both segments are seen after the transection in **25—3–6**. Here, much of the lateral and posterior

walls has been removed below and behind the interrupted line. The chordae are unusually long, passing to the inferiorly located papillary muscles.

Specimen C: 3: A.P. view of the lateral papillary muscle. Muscularization of chordae is seen. A second example is seen next.

Specimen D: 4, 5, and **6**: The scale in **4** and **5** is 0.7:1.

After removal of large segments of the walls of both ventricles, the L.A.O. view of the heart is seen in **4** and **5**, and the A.P. view in **6**. A massive column of muscle extends from the lateral wall of the left ventricle to the anterior leaflet of the mitral valve and passes up to be continuous with the muscle of the left ventricular ostium.

This degree of muscularization probably would interfere with the posterior motion of the anterior leaflet during ventricular systole; however, no clinical data relative to this specimen are available.

Lam and his colleagues (1970) found muscular chordae ("chordae muscularis") in 8 of 50 normal valves. These averaged 0.3 cm in diameter. All were attached to the anterior leaflet and "none of the eight patients had a history of systolic murmur or ... mitral insufficiency". Roberts and Perloff (1972) indicate their benignity. Regurgitation at the mitral valve results from the enlargement or reduction of the dimensions of any of its functional components (enumerated on page 39). Leaflet and chordal shortening in rheumatic fever once assumed a major mechanistic role. Today the attribution of many clinical events and manifestations to chordal rupture, papillary muscle dysfunction, leaflet prolapse, and asymmetric septal hypertrophy (see page 39) has induced consideration of each of these components.

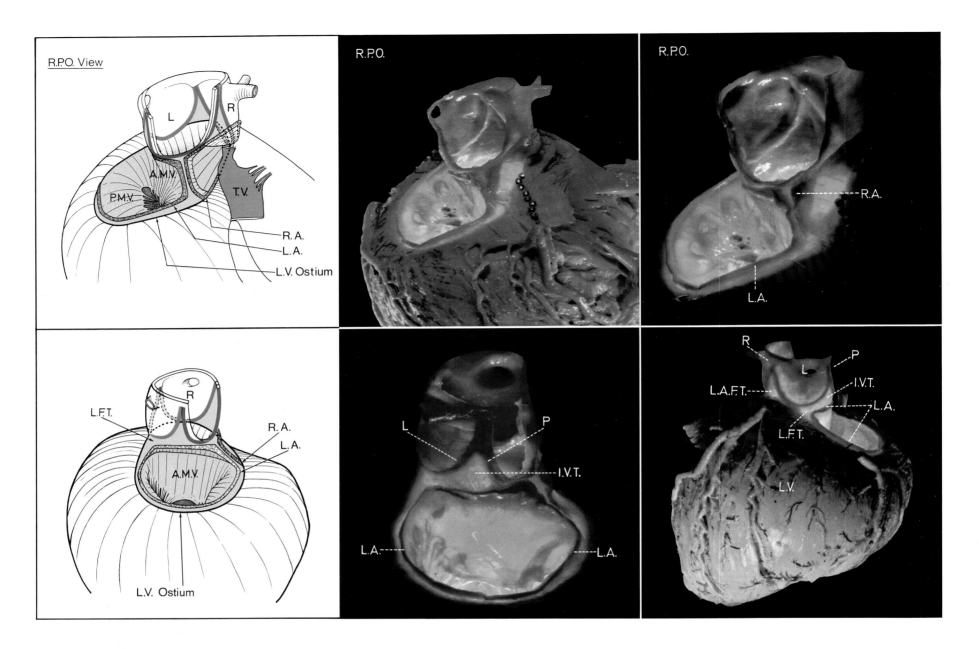

D. The Mitral Valve Leaflets and the Ostium of the Left Ventricle

I. The Disposition of the Subvalvular Segment of the Aorto-Ventricular Membrane in the Plane of the Ostium of the Left Ventricle

In the diagrams on page 12, the left atrium is shown to be attached to the aorto-ventricular membrane central to and separated from the left ventricular ostium. The mitral valve was defined as that portion of the membrane within the left atrial attachment; the latter will be seen now in photographs.

Specimen A: 1–6: The aorta has been transected above its sinuses. The posterior aortic sinus wall and the aortic leaflets have been excised. With the exception of 3 mm rims at their attachment to the A.V. membrane, the atria have been removed, as has the right ventricle.

1, 2, and **3:** R.P.O. view: **1** is a drawing of **2** in which a combination of interior and exterior lighting is used.

In **3**, only interior lighting is used and the scale is 1:1. The residual rim of the left atrial attachment appears as the dark strip, separating two of the components of the translucent A.V. membrane: The mitral valve leaflets are within the attachment and the subvalvular segment is between it and the ostium of L. V.

4 and **5:** Superior P.A. view: A combination of lighting was used for the photograph from which the tracing of **4** was made. Only interior lighting is used in **5**, which is shown in a 1:1 scale. A strip of aorto-ventricular membrane, peripheral to the left atrial attachment, its subvalvular segment, is continuous on the left with the left fibrous trigone and on the right with the right fibrous trigone. Henle described membrane extending posteriorly from the left and right fibrous trigones; these areas have been termed the "fila of Henle". The fact to be emphasized, however, is that the left atrial attachment, throughout its course, is central to the attachment of the aorto-ventricular membrane to the left ventricular ostium. Although the degree of separation is variable,

the four specimens shown on these pages (46–49) are not extreme, unusual examples of this anatomy.

6: A nonattitudinal L.P.O. view with a combination of lighting. The aortic annuli and the left atrial attachment appear as dark broad lines against the transilluminated aortic sinus walls (labeled R, L, and P) and the A.V. membrane. Observe: (a) In the next specimen to be examined on page 47, a left ostial process is present and the attachment of the left annulus is extensive; hence the left fibrous trigone (L.F.T.) is absent. In this specimen, by contrast, the left aortic annulus, which is seen in its entirety, demonstrates only a 4-mm attachment to the ostium. A large left fibrous trigone is present. (b) Due to posterior displacement of the atrial attachment to the A.V. membrane, the intervalvular (I.V.T.) and left fibrous trigones (L.F.T.) are confluent. (c) The left anterior fibrous trigone is seen between the right and left aortic annuli.

Specimen B: 1–6: The aorta and the pulmonary trunk have been transected above the sinuses (the left anterior pulmonary sinus has been excised); the atria, except a 3-mm rim at the site of their attachments to the aorto-ventricular and tricuspid membranes, have been removed. With transillumination the left atrial attachment appears as a dark strip and is marked by the letters L.A.

1: A nonattitudinal left posterior view: A combination of interior and surface lighting again demonstrates the band of the A.V. membrane—its subvalvular segment—peripheral to the left atrial attachment and central to the ostium of L.V. A strikingly large left ostial process (L.O.P.) results in the absence of a left fibrous trigone.

2: P.A. view: Observe: **The anterior leaflet:** (1) Its axis is shown by the arrow; it is parallel to the axis of the aortic bulb, extending superiorly and to the right. (2) Its free border extends between the superior (S.C.) and inferior (I.C.) commissures.

3: L.P.O. view, and **5:** 240° view: Interior lighting alone is used. Observe: (a) **The left atrial attachment is divisible into three segments:** (1) The **anterosuperior segment** extends between the nadirs of the left and posterior annuli, X and Y. (2) The **right vertical segment** descends with the right atrial attachment on the right fibrous trigone to the ostium of L.V. (3) The **posterior segment** is related to the ostium of L.V. (b) The attached border of the anterior leaflet is divisible into four parts. Two are formed by the first two segments of the left atrial attachment just noted. Two are found between the commissures and the left and right fibrous trigones. In **3**, note that 10 mm separate the superior commissure (S.C.) and the nadir of the left annulus (X). (c) At the midpoint of the posterior leaflet of the mitral valve, the subvalvular segment of the A.V. membrane is less translucent because: (1) It normally narrows here, and in a few specimens, no subvalvular segment is recognizable by naked-eye inspection in the region. (2) In the hearts from older patients, fibrosis and calcification may be present, since this is the site where calcification of the so-called mitral annulus displays its maximum development.

4: L.P.O. and **6:** 240° views: Exterior lighting alone is used. Observe: (a) The line of apposition of the two leaflets of the mitral valve seen extending between the commissures is sickle-shaped, with the concavity directed to the right and superiorly. (b) The infolding of the leaflets produces multiple appositional areas, particularly within the posterior leaflet. These result in increased thickening and loss of leaflet mobility in rheumatic valvulitis. (c) The **mobile portion** of the anterior leaflet is in the plane of the ostium of L.V.; the relatively **nonmobile portion** is in the plane of the aortic bulb—on the ventricular aspect a ridge is seen at their junction—the hinge of the mitral valve. (d) In **6**, a small atrial division of the membranous septum results from the posterior location of the membranous attachment of the septal leaflet of the tricuspid valve.

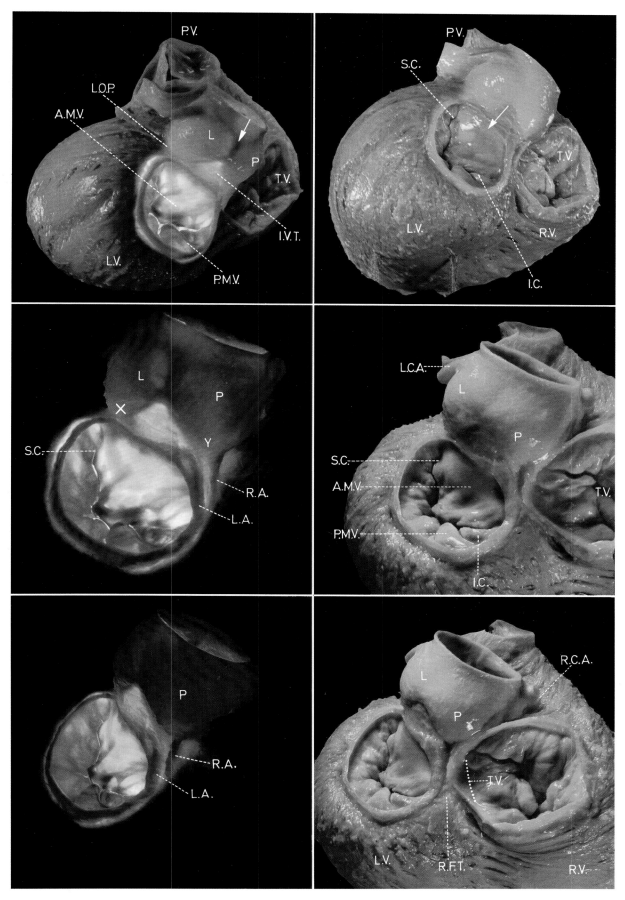

47

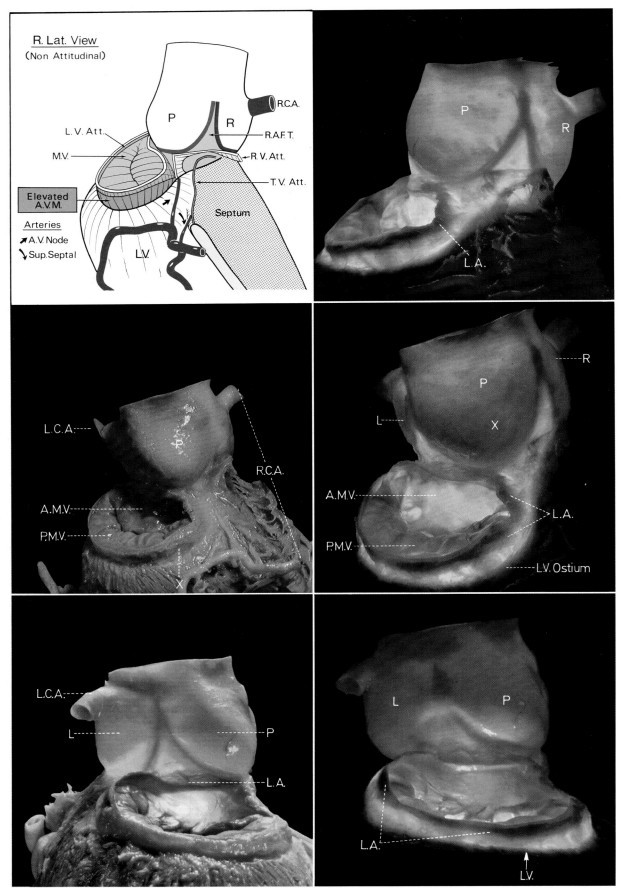

II. The Disposition of the Subvalvular Segment of the Aorto-Ventricular Membrane in the Axis of the Left Ventricle

The subvalvular segment may extend from the left ventricular ostium superiorly to the site of the left atrial attachment, where is merges at a right angle with the leaflets of the mitral valve. This arrangement is seen on these two pages, where all the photographs and drawings are from a single specimen with the exception of **49—5** and **6**. At both commissures, the subvalvular segment of the membrane extends 8 mm above the left ventricular ostium, and at the midpoint of the posterior leaflet, 3 mm.

Specimen A: 48 —1–6 and 49 —1–4

1 and 2: Right lateral nonattitudinal view: **1** is traced from photograph 147—1 and is intended to orient the reader for the photographs on this page. The subvalvular segment (or as it is less well termed, the elevated A.V. membrane) is colored orange. It is disposed in the axis of the ventricle. In the enlargement **2**, the dark aortic annuli and the left atrial attachment are seen delineated from the translucent aorta and aorto-ventricular membrane.

3 and 4: A nonattitudinal R.P.O. view: In **3** at X, surface lighting demonstrates the elevation of the subvalvular segment. In **4**, interior lighting alone shows the subvalvular segment between the ostium of L.V. and the attachment of the left atrium to the A.V. membrane. Again note the more translucent anterior and less translucent posterior leaflets. The posterior aortic leaflet creates a darkened zone (X) in the posterior aortic sinus.

5 and 6: A nonattitudinal P.A. view: Using a combination of lighting in **5** and interior lighting alone in **6**, the elevation of the subvalvular segment above the left ventricular ostium is seen. It extends from the right fibrous trigone around to the left fibrous trigone, as shown on these two pages. Note that the widths of the nonappositional portion of the anterior and posterior leaflets are almost equal (in this specimen).

When the term annulus fibrosus of the mitral valve is used, and a cordlike structure, providing attachment for both the left atrium and the mitral valve, is believed to exist, it is difficult to comprehend the development of aneurysms in this area. It is not difficult to see how aneurysms could develop through this subvalvular membrane. These aneurysms can result from infection, mesodermal abnormalities, or from surgical excision; this is a particular hazard during mitral valve replacement in the presence of calcification in this area. Annular subvalvular aneurysms of the left ventricle, seen most often in the Bantu, may involve this membrane, and it is suggested that the word annular be deleted therefrom. (It is the purpose of these dissections to show that the fibrous structure present is a flat membrane, not a cord.) See articles by Abrahams, Beck, Chesler, Cockshott, and Pocock on subvalvular aneurysms.

1: A left posterior nonattitudinal view, demonstrating the elevated subvalvular segment of the aorto-ventricular membrane. The photograph from which this drawing has been taken is **79—1**. The drawing is intended for use in the study of **2**, **3**, and **4**.

2: A closer examination of the elevated subvalvular segment is seen with a combination of lighting from essentially the same perspective as **1**.

3 and 4: The specimen has been rotated counterclockwise and is now examined from a nonattitudinal L.P.O. view. In **3**, the subvalular segment (X) between the left ventricular ostium and the left atrium may be seen with exterior lighting. In **4**, the maximum development of the elevated segment is seen in relation to the superior commissure of the mitral valve. (S.C.)

Specimen B: 5 and 6

5: This specimen has been transected through the obtuse margin. The subvalvular segment of the aorto-ventricular membrane (orange) extends 10 mm above the ostium of the left ventricle, merging with the mitral valve (yellow).

6: The photograph from which the drawing was made: The aortic leaflets have been removed. The mitral valve and the chordae tendinae are seen as dark areas against the transilluminated subvalvular segment of the aorto-ventricular membrane. A drawing of the entire lower segment of this same specimen is seen in **92—6**.
At operation for the replacement of the mitral valve, the surgeon may incorrectly assume that the mitral valve leaflet is directly attached to the left ventricular ostium—excision of the subvalvular segment might be carried out, resulting in separation of the left atrium from its moorings. Serious bleeding may occur early in the postoperative course or aneurysm development or paravalvular leak may present at a later time. Correction of these complications may be difficult and also dangerous if the posterior division of the left coronary is nearby.

Technical Note

In these four pages, interior lighting has been used to differentiate membrane from muscle. When the external surface of a specimen is examined, the presence of membrane intervening between the atrium and ventricle may not be recognized if interior lighting is not used. This material may be presented to show the information which may be garnered from gross dissection alone. It might be argued that transillumination may not differentiate thin muscle from membrane. This is not my opinion; a transilluminated membrane presents a homogenous ground-glass appearance, quite unlike the streaked appearance seen when a wall of muscle is transilluminated. It would be fractious to decry the use and value of microscopic studies of this area; however, it is apposite to state that when such a technique is applied, perfusion fixation should be used in the preparation of hearts; otherwise, the dimensions and the direction of the subvalvular membrane will not be recognized.

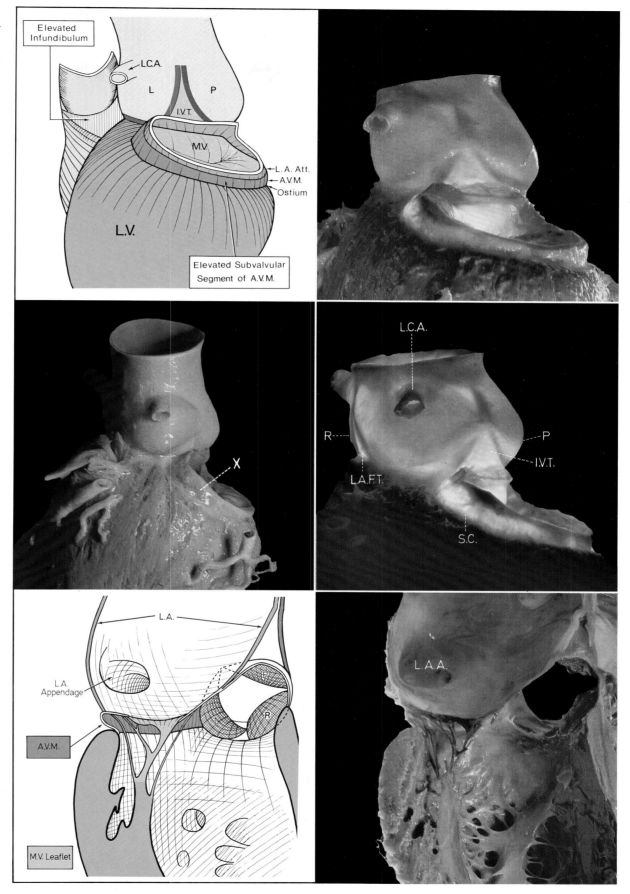

49

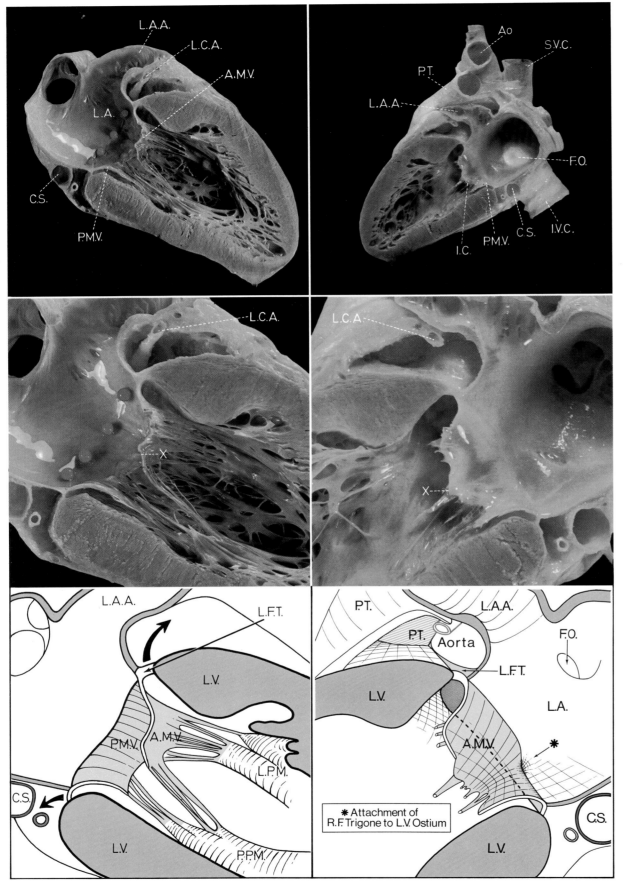

III. The Development of Aneurysms through the Subvalvular Segment of the Aorto-Ventricular Membrane

Specimen A: 1–6: The heart has been transected in a vertical plane extending from the apex posteriorly, on the left of the aorta. The left segment is seen in **1**, **3**, and **5** and is viewed from R.A.O.; the right segment is seen in **2**, **4**, and **6** and is viewed from L.P.O. The fat has been removed (leaving the pericardium intact) displaying the aortoventricular membrane and left atrial attachments thereto and, coincidentally, the left coronary artery in both the left coronary fossa and, along with the coronary sinus (C.S.), in the posterior left A.V. sulcus.

In **3**, the scale is 1:1; in **4**, 1.1:1.0. Their related drawings are **5** and **6**. The subvalvular segment is 2.2 mm in width at the mid-point of the posterior leaflet of the mitral valve; this is almost always the site where the segment is narrowest. Above, the anterior leaflet (A.M.V.) and the left fibrous trigone are continuous.

The arrows in **5** indicate where aneurysms can develop in the subvalvular segment and how excessive surgical excision can disrupt the continuity of the cardiac walls.*
In **4** and **6**, a dimple is seen at the attachment of the right fibrous trigone to the ostium of L.V. Just posterior to this point is the A.V. node, which is, as is its artery of supply, in jeopardy during mitral valve replacement.

Apart from our topic, note in **2**, that a catheter passed in the axis of I.V.C. will bisect the horseshoe-shaped (transilluminated) membranous floor of the fossa ovalis (F.O.) and traverse the small patent foramen ovale at the junction of the septal and anterior walls of the left atrium. In **4**, the muscular derivative of the septum secundum lies on the right side of the membranous derivative of the septum primum.

Before examining **Specimen B, 51—1** and **2**, study the drawings and photographs of this transected specimen in its entirety in **79—3–6**. As seen in **51—1** and **2**, a sagittal transection passes through the lateral portion of the left aortic sinus, the intervalvular trigone (I.V.T.), the anterior leaflet of the mitral valve (A.M.V.), and the subvalvular segment of the A.V. membrane, which is marked by the arrow (X) and is seen best in **2**. The attachment of the left atrium to the A.V. membrane is seen. The right ostial attachment of the anterior leaflet extends posteriorly from the right fibrous trigone. At operation, a dimple is seen at the junction of this attachment and the right fibrous trigone (also see **50—4**). The left coronary artery is in contact with the posteroinferior wall of the pulmonary trunk. Note the vertical orientation of the anterior leaflet of the mitral valve and, in particular, its relation to the anterior wall of the left ventricle. The two structures form the anterior and posterior walls of **the outflow tract of the left ventricle.** In the latter, note both the location of the membranous septum (M.S.) and its relation to the aortic leaflets (marked R., L., and P).

---

* See the articles by Roberts and Morrow and by MacVaugh, *et al.*

IV. Anatomic Factors in Calcification of the "Mitral Annulus"

Specimen C: 3 and **4**: The details of the essentially horizontal transection of this specimen are on page 105. Here, the inferior segment is examined. The lighting is planned to demonstrate the relation of the anterior and posterior leaflets to **the two "tracts" of the left ventricle**, which are differentiated in **4** (which is made from the left ventricle of **3**). During the ejection phase, the **outflow tract** is indicated by the arrow B; this tract is seen in **51—1** and **2**. There is also **an isovolumic stress area,** indicated by the arrow A, between (1) the posterior leaflet of the mitral valve, (2) the subvalvular segment of the aorto-ventricular membrane and (3) the ostial slope of L.V. Great force is directed into this region, and the resulting turbulence and stress is probably the cause of the so-called annular calcification. Commonly all three structures are involved; however, an isolated central zone of calcification may be seen which is indicated to represent specific involvement of the "annulus" of the mitral valve; this has been mooted as evidence for the existence of a mitral annulus.

Usually the calcification does not extend onto the appositional portion of the posterior leaflet and no serious functional disturbance results.

Specimen D: 5, 6, and **7**

5 and **6**: The characteristic location of the maximal development of the calcification is at the midpoint of the posterior leaflet. When full-blown, the calcification (1) presents a horseshoe shape (in standard chest x-rays) which marks the location of the mitral portion of the ostium of L.V. and (2) may interfere with the systolic reduction of the ostium of the left ventricle.

7: The left segment is viewed from the apex. The calcification (green) involves the three elements enumerated above. The severed papillary muscles are orange.

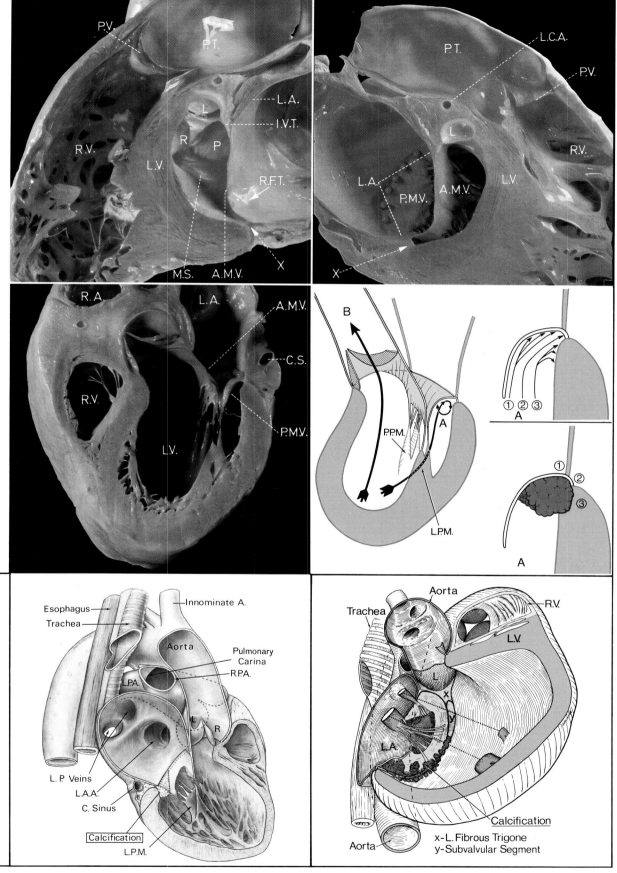

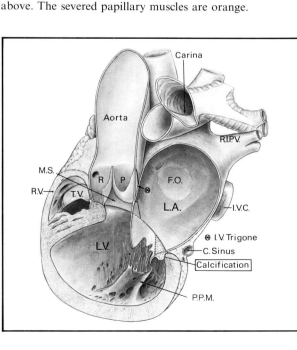

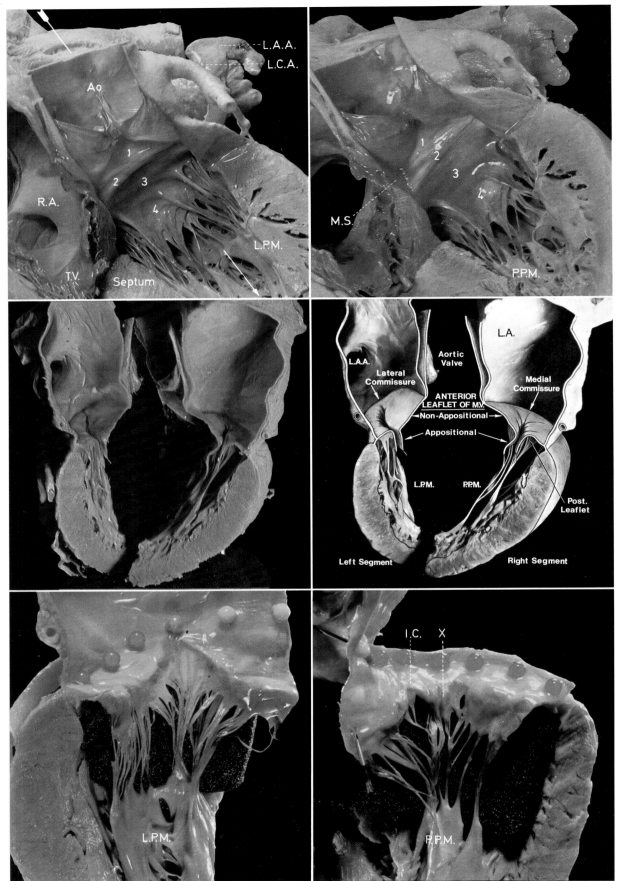

E. The Functional Anatomy of the Mitral Valve

Specimen A: 52—1–6 and 53—1 and 2.

I. The Divisions of the Anterior Leaflet

1: The A.P. view: The right aortic sinus and much of the lateral and septal walls of the left ventricle have been removed. The mitral leaflets are in their systolic position.

In **2**, the vantage point is now 15°, i.e., to the left of A.P. and we are now able to see the junction between the membranous septum (M.S.) on the right and the mitral valve on the left. Examining these photographs together, first observe that 4 planes can be noted between the commissure of the posterior and left aortic leaflets and the free edge of the anterior leaflet of the mitral valve. ① The intervalvular trigone is disposed in the axis of the aorta. ② The **mitral valve hinge**, extends between the left and right fibrous trigones, as an obtuse angled ridge between the planes or segments ① and ③. It is best seen in **2**, although its lower edge is seen in **1**. ③ The **nonappositional portion of the anterior leaflet** is disposed in the plane of the left ventricular ostium. ④ The **appositional portion of the leaflet** meets the nonappositional portion at a right angle. The junction is distal to the attachment of the strut chordae of the mitral valve. The attachment of the anterior leaflet of the mitral valve extends 10 mm behind the right and left fibrous trigones, which are disposed in a frontal plane. During diastole, the anterior leaflet moves anteriorly to lie in or just anterior to a frontal plane. During systole, as seen here, the nonappositional segment is disposed in the plane of the ostium of the ventricle, directed inferiorly from the left at an angle of approximately 45°.

An incision (see arrow in **1**) is now made in the axis of the ventricle between the left and posterior aortic leaflets and is carried through the mitral valve, left atrium, and left ventricle to the apex. The line of division passes through the midpoint of the posterior leaflet of the mitral valve.

II. The Appositional Fractions of the Leaflets

3 and **4**: The two segments resulting from the incision are everted and are examined from a posterior vantage point (180°) in a nonattitudinal fashion. The appositional fractions of the anterior and posterior leaflets are 30 and 50%, respectively.* In **4**, the commissures of the mitral valve are designated as lateral and medial, rather than superior and inferior, respectively. Both are correct; the latter are usually used in this work.

5 and **6**: The left and right portions of the mitral valve are now seen. The anterior and posterior leaflets are distracted to demonstrate their appositional surfaces. The appositional area is marked by thickening in the tissue, which increases with aging, and is the site of the excres-

---

* Appositional Fraction $= \dfrac{\text{width of appositional portion}}{\text{width of leaflet}}$

cences described by Lambl. As Magarey points out, Lambl described filiform processes on the aortic leaflet—they were later found on the mitral valve. The red and yellow beads mark the attachment of the left atrium to the A.V. membrane, in relation to the posterior and anterior leaflets, respectively. In **52—5**, note that the junction of both the nonappositional and the appositional portions of the leaflets extends to the blue bead, which marks the junction of the leaflets. The free margins of the anterior and posterior leaflets of this specimen meet 10 mm below this point. If the commissure is defined as the junction of the leaflets, it is seen that one must differentiate between their appositional and nonappositional portions, since the latter meet at the left atrial attachment while the free margin of the former meet 10 mm below. In **52—6**, a commissural scallop (X) is present, and at the primary inferior commissure, the appositional portions of the two leaflets are separated from the left atrial attachment.

III. The Anterior Leaflet of the Mitral Valve in Systole and Diastole

Its Location in Systole in a Sagittal Plane

Specimen A: In **1** and **2**: The left lateral view of the right segment of the specimen seen on the preceding page. Note the three parts of the anterior leaflet and the subvalvular segment of the A.V. membrane (X). Observe: (a) The hinge of the leaflet, lies in a frontal plane. (b) The nonappositional portion lies in the plane of the ostium of L.V. (c) The commissure is often seen in a left lateral ventriculogram as a wedge-shaped filling defect.

Its Location in Diastole in a Sagittal Plane

Specimen B: 3 and **4**: An attitudinal left lateral view of the right segment: The plane of transection is anteroposterior, in the axis of L.V., dividing the aortic valve into left and right halves. Observe: (a) The position of the hinge is constant. (b) The axis of the anterior leaflet is angled slightly anteriorly to the frontal plane. (c) The greatest dimension of the left ventricular cavity is indicated by a horizontal line extending anteriorly from the attachment of the posterior leaflet of the mitral valve.

Its Location in Diastole in the Horizontal Plane

Specimen C: 5: The drawing of this specimen is seen in **103—1**. Observe: The mobile portion billows anteriorly.

Its Location in Systole in the Horizontal Plane

Specimen D: 6: Regardless of the level of transection, the cut edge of the leaflet is perpendicular to the median plane.

Note: The relevance of the anatomy on these two pages to echocardiography is evident.

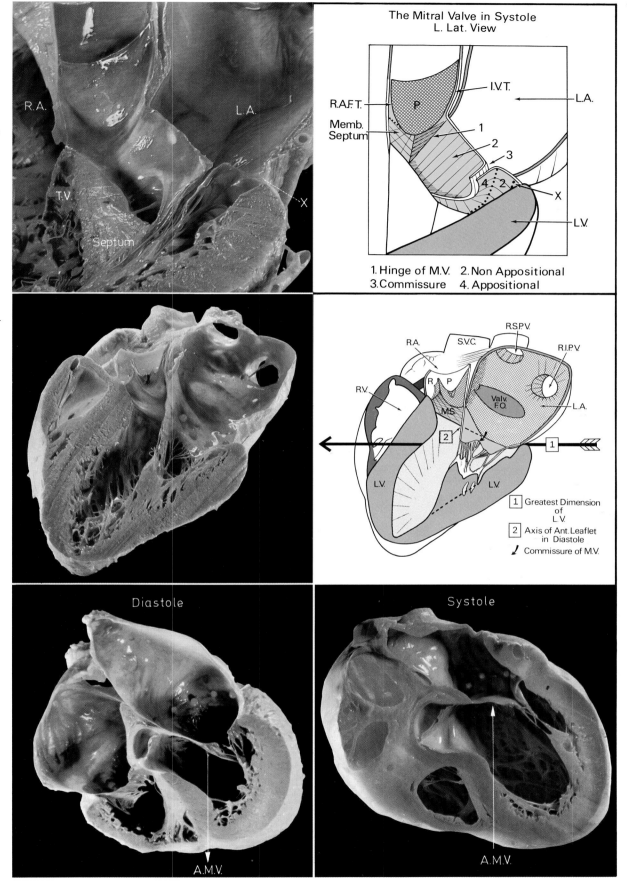

The Mitral Valve in Systole
L. Lat. View

1. Hinge of M.V.   2. Non Appositional
3. Commissure   4. Appositional

1 Greatest Dimension of L.V.
2 Axis of Ant. Leaflet in Diastole
Commissure of M.V.

Diastole

Systole

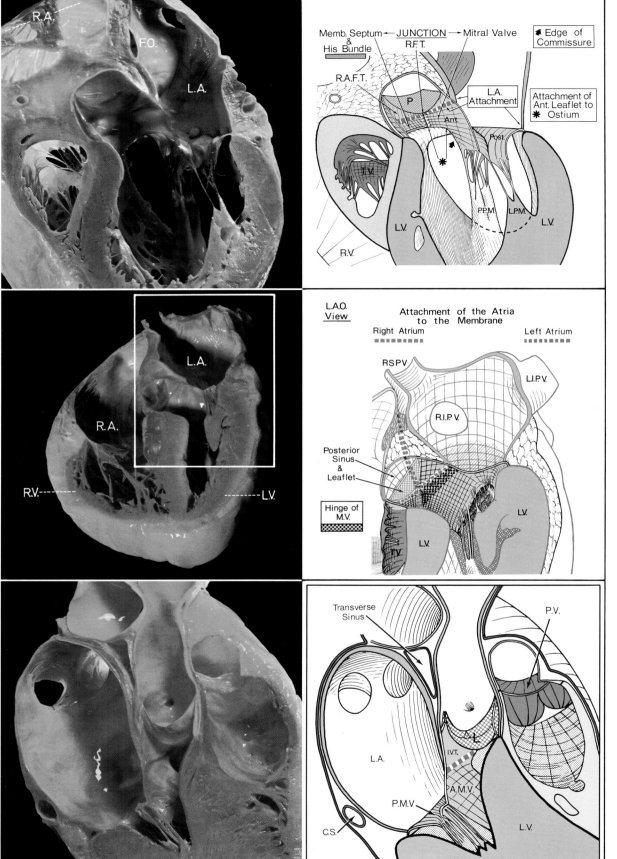

F. The Anterior Leaflet of the Mitral Valve and the Outflow Tract of the Left Ventricle

The four segments of the attached border are described on page 38. We will first examine their relationship to the outflow tract and then assess the anatomic implications in mitral valve replacement in general and the role of mitral valve replacement as the sole treatment of subaortic stenosis in particular.

Specimen A: 1 and **2**: This specimen has been transected in a near horizontal plane. Both segments are on page 105. Here the lower segment is seen in a nonattitudinal L.A.O. view. The mitral valve leaflets are in their systolic position. A window is present in the posterior wall of L.V. Observe: (a) **The right ostial attachment** is found at the attachment of the anterior leaflet of the mitral valve to the ostium of L.V. It normally extends 10 mm between the right fibrous trigone and the inferior commissure. Variations are seen in this length: A reduction will not bring the leaflet into greater proximity to the anterior wall of L.V. during systole. (b) The edge of the commissure is 10 mm in length; its sharpness may be an additional anatomic factor in the production of turbulence which results in fibrosis and calcification in the area of the right fibrous trigone (R.F.T.)—Lev's disease. (c) **The junctional attachment** at the right fibrous trigone is to the right and above the muscle wall of the outflow tract. The attachments of the right and left atria on the opposite side of the A.V. membrane are indicated by the interrupted blue and red lines. (d) Only the right half of **the intervalvular segment** of the attached border of the anterior leaflet is seen.

Specimen B: 3 and **4**: L.A.O. view: The rectangular area in **3** is shown in **4**. This specimen, which occupies the next page, has been transected in a plane which is elevated 45° above the horizontal as it is directed anteroposteriorly. The inferior segment is seen here, demonstrating the relationship of **the right half of the intervalvular part of the attached border** to the ostial slope of L.V. In passing, note: The membranous septum and the muscular septum of L.V. form an obtuse angle.

Specimen C: 5 and **6**: A transection has been carried out in the axis of the ascending aorta from 45° to 210°. A nonattitudinal view of the left segment is seen. (a) The left half of the anterosuperior attachment of the left atrium to the A.V. membrane is indicated by the interrupted red line in the drawing; it is behind the dark ridge, produced by the hinge of the valve, in the photograph; this is the **left half of the intervalvular part of the attached border of the anterior leaflet**. It is posterior to the ostial slope—the proximity of the two is minimized because the transection is to the left of the greatest prominence of the slope. The right half of the attachment may be seen in **63—4–6**.

Note: Atrial arrhythmias have been ascribed to lipomatous hypertrophy of the interatrial septum (Hutter and Page). The area where the fat develops—behind the posterior aortic sinus—is seen in the lower segment of Specimen B: it has been dissected away in the upper segment, **55—4**.

Specimen B: 1–6: The inferior segment is seen from a superior A.P. view in **1, 3, 5**, and **6**.* The superior segment has been rotated anteriorly on its transverse axis and is seen from a P.A. view in **2** and **4**. **The intervalvular part of the attachment: The right half** is seen in the inferior segment; following transillumination of the anterior leaflet of the mitral valve it appears as a darkened line X in **5** and **6; the left half** is in the plane of examination in the superior segment. Visually replace the upper segment on the lower segment of the specimen and note the relation of this part of the attached border of the anterior leaflet of the mitral valve to the ostial slope. **The left ostial attachment** of the anterior leaflet is seen in the superior segment; it is between the left fibrous trigone and the superior commissure: It is apparent that reduction in its length will not reduce the antero-posterior dimension of the outflow tract.

Comment: (1) During ventricular systole, the mobile segment—the portion removed in valve replacement—is in the plane of the ostium. Forming the posterior wall of the critical part of the outflow tract is the intervalvular segment of the attached border of the anterior leaflet—the prominence of which will be increased by the seat of a prosthesis placed in a subannular position. In conclusion, it cannot be postulated that variations in the normal attachment of the anterior leaflet will affect the degree of obstruction in subaortic stenosis. Other explanations are needed to account for the apparent correction of infundibular hypertrophic subaortic stenosis by valve replacement alone.** (2) The outflow tract may be only 10 mm in A.P. dimension in an adult. The intervalvular segment of the attached border of the anterior leaflet forms the posterior wall of the tract. When a mitral valve prosthesis is placed in a subannular position, significant obstruction may result from the seat of the prosthesis. The size of the outflow tract should be assessed prior to mitral valve replacement; this will determine whether the seat of the prosthesis should be placed below the valve remnant—the position preferred if periprosthetic leak is to be avoided—or above the remnant if outflow tract obstruction from the seat of the prosthesis is feared. Faced with a small outflow tract, I have placed a mitral prosthesis with the part in relation to the posterior leaflet in a "subannular" position and the part in relation to the anterior leaflet in the "supra-annular" position. When subannular placement is used, ventricular systole produces an impacting force in contrast to the distracting force exerted on a prosthesis placed in a supra-annular position.

_____

*   The drawings are made from the areas within the squares in **3** and **4**.

** In systole the reduction in size and the configurational change of the cavity of L.V. effect disalignment of the papillary-chordal complex—the resulting abnormal anterior motion of the anterior leaflet of the mitral valve effects both mitral regurgitation and outflow tract obstruction. This information has resulted from echocardiography, which promises to be as important in the comprehension and treatment of disease in the future as the invasive techniques have been during the past three decades.

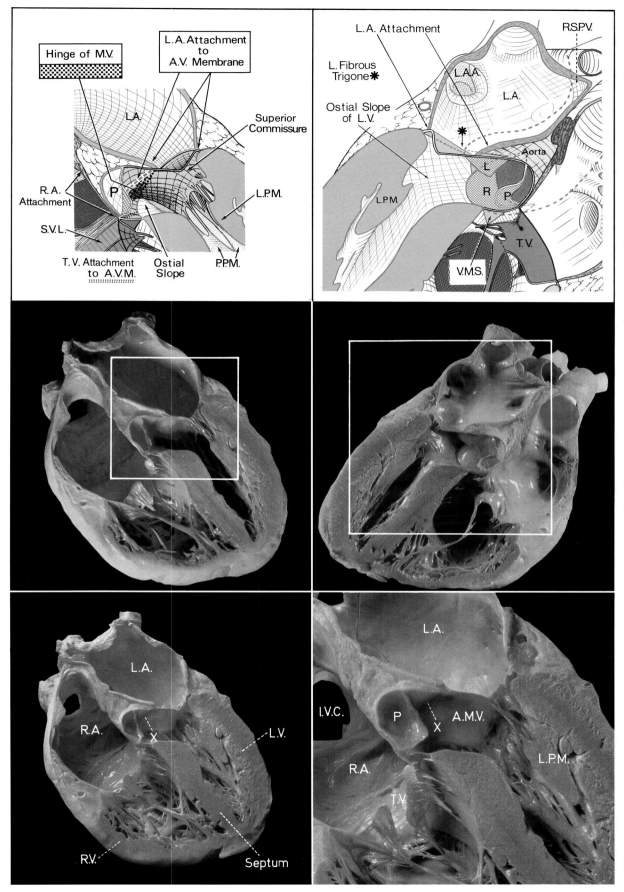

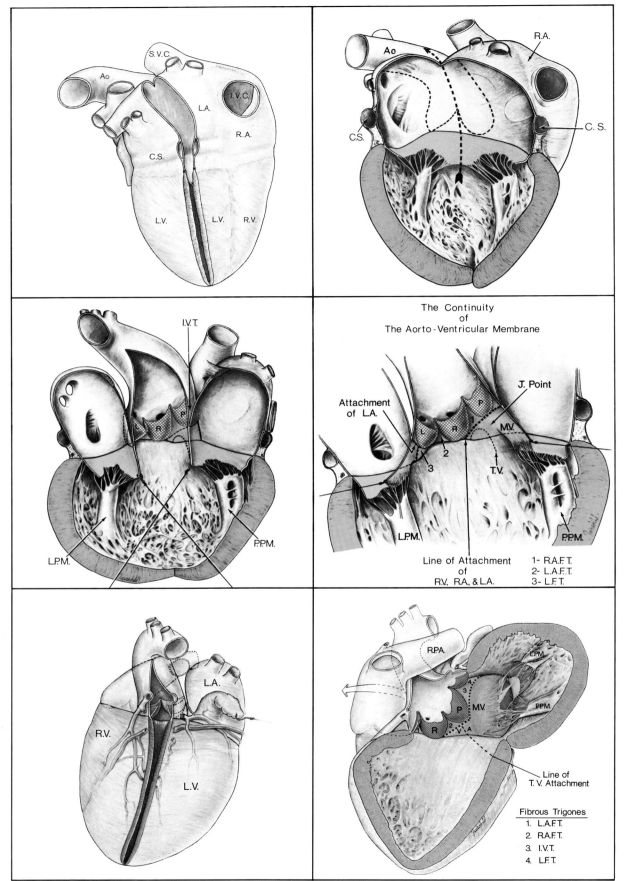

G. The Mitral Valve Leaflets—Components of the Aorto-Ventricular Membrane

Specimen A: **1–4:** An inferior view: In **1**, the incision passes through the middle of the posterior leaflet of the mitral valve and the posterior walls of the atrium and the ventricle. In **2**, the margins of the incision are distracted. The arrow indicates the next incision to be made which results in **3**. It passes through the anterior leaflet of the mitral valve, the adjoining anterior wall of L.A., the intervalvular trigone (between the left and posterior aortic sinuses), and the aorta. **4**: The halves of the anterior leaflet of the mitral valve are everted, demonstrating its relationship to the other components of the A.V. membrane. Note the sites where fistulae into the adjoining chambers may (very rarely) develop following aortic or mitral valve replacement. The tricuspid attachment (T.V.) to the membranous septum is often not linear but semicircular.

Specimen B: **5** and **6**: The incision, used at autopsy, passes through the middle of the left aortic sinus. In these specimens, note the relation of the mitral valve leaflets to the aorto-ventricular unit.

H. Periprosthetic Leak—Anatomic Considerations

(1) **The suitability of tissues for suture placement:** The attachment of the anterior leaflet at the left fibrous trigone and the upper part of the right fibrous trigone and the thickened A.V. membrane between the two provides stronger material than does the attachment of the posterior leaflet where, certainly, no tough annulus exists and the leaflet tissue itself may be thin and calcification (see page 51) may present an additional problem. When the preferred subannular placement has not been selected, for many years I have routinely used buttresses of teflon felt on the sutures.

(2) **Inappropriate removal of leaflet tissue: Excessive removal** of the posterior leaflet results in the insecure placement of sutures in the muscle of the ventricle or in the subvalvular membrane. **Inadequate removal** of the anterior leaflet, in particular, may result in placing the sutures in its thin nonappositional portion.

(3) **The inappropriate size of the prosthesis**: Two valves occupy the ostium of L.V. which, in mitral regurgitation, is often enlarged (which may be reversible following valve replacement) allowing insertion of an unduly large prosthesis; this may (1) distort the aorta and disalign the aortic leaflets producing regurgitation, (2) protrude into and obstruct the outflow tract, and (3) increase the tension on the sutures and increase the hazard of periprosthetic leak.

(4) The **systolic reduction in the size of the ostium of L.V.** may exert a shearing strain on the sutures related to it.

(5) **Suture fatigue fracture** may result in a false aneurysm due to separation of the abdominal aorta and a postrenal aortic vessel prosthesis. Similarly, a periprosthetic leak may result years after the insertion of a valve prosthesis. The biological incorporation of a prosthesis is imperfect. In both operations, the strength and durability of the suture should not be ignored.

Chapter 5: The Left Atrium

Introduction

The terminology of the atria has been confusing. The words, auricle, atrium, and appendix (or appendage) are often interchanged. **Auricle** (L. auricula = ear) has long been used—presumably because of the fancied resemblance of the protuberance of the right-sided chamber to the ear of a dog. In the Grays Anatomy of 1893, the word auricle denoted the entirety of each chamber (right or left) which was divided into two parts, sinus and appendix. Approximately 4 decades later in Cunninghams Textbook of Anatomy (1931), the word **atrium** denoted the entirety of each chamber—however, the protuberances were termed the auricles. Today, another 4 decades later, in some medical writings auricle denotes the entire chamber, which is divided into atrium and appendix. Most authors use only the terms atrium and atrial appendage (auricle is discarded)—this practice is followed in this work. Use of the Greek word **atrium**, which roughly denotes the room where one pauses before entering the main hall, seems appropriate although the end diastolic volume of the left atrium is less than the stroke volume—i.e., the chamber acts as more than an atrium but also as a conduit during ventricular filling. The word left atrium denotes, herein, either the entire chamber when used in a general sense— or the chamber minus the appendage when anatomic relationships are described.

The junction between **the left atrial appendage** and the left atrium (the attachment of the appendage) is not only well defined but its circumference is often less than that of the remainder of the appendage. In closed mitral commissurotomy this fact may frustrate a surgeon—the terminal two phalanges will enter the atrium—but not the proximal interphalangeal joint!

The appendage has also been used as the avenue for a left heart decompression catheter. In either case the appendage is excised at its junction with the atrium. The related posterior division of the left coronary artery (the circumflex branch) must be avoided in this step. The arterial-appendageal relationship is highly variable: The specimens on page 61 indicate that closure of the appendage from within the atrium during operations on the mitral valve is highly dangerous. During open operations on the mitral valve, the artery may be encircled by suture. In two valuable articles, 7 fatalities were reported (Danielson *et al.* [1967]—3; MacVaugh *et al.* [1972]—4). The danger is greatest in relation to the superior commissure where the artery may be contiguous with the ostium of L.V.; however, arterial injury may occur in relation to the entire mitral division of the ostium: Large branches of the left coronary artery, extending to its posterior aspect in 23% and to the crux in an additional 12%, usually lie 10 mm above the ostium, however, exceptions occur and large right coronary branches may run in contact with the ostium.

The shape of the left atrium may be compared to an inverted, obliquely disposed earthen pot, the mouth of which is attached to the A.V. membrane. This attachment will be referred to as **the left atrial attachment**— there is no other attachment as the left atrium is apposed to the right atrium. Although the design of this attachment is simpler than that of the right atrium (to both the tricuspid and A.V. membranes), it has great clinical interest. This attachment consists of both the origin and insertion of most muscle fibers of the chamber. (With the exception of the interatrial muscle bundle [often termed Bachmann's Bundle] and a few scattered fibers which cross the interatrial plane, the muscles of each atrium are confined to its wall.) This attachment is a dynamic one—reflecting (a) the motion of the mitral valve and (b) the systolic movement of the ostium of L.V. towards the apex: To this latter motion, which draws the walls of the atrium apex-ward, is ascribed an important role in active (rather than passive) left atrial filling. This attachment may also be important in the pathogenesis of mitral regurgitation. The appositional tolerance of the mitral leaflets (measured by the appositional fraction described on page 52) may be exceeded by traction on the leaflets from below resulting in regurgitation. This occurs in left ventricular dilatation—the dilated walls exert traction on the chordae tendinae. When the left atrium enlarges, traction is exerted from above, by the left atrial attachment, on the A.V. membrane interfering with leaflet apposition.

Consistent with its higher pressure, the left atrium has a thicker wall than the right atrium (approximately 3 and 2 mm). Myocardial infarction of the atria, in contrast to that of the ventricles, is more common in the thinner chamber, albeit its thickest portion—the right atrial appendix.

Following its spatial examination, the left atrium may be divided into five, poorly demarcated walls: anterior, posterior, superior, left lateral, and right lateral (largely septal). As seen on page 64, all but the anterior have been used in the approach to the mitral valve. On the next page it will be seen that the superior approach must utilize the narrow strip of the superior wall between the interatrial band and the summit of the left atrium (between the superior pulmonary veins). An incision in the right lateral wall is usually used; however, the posterior approach, examined on page 62, merits attention and should be in the repertoire of every surgeon.

The relations of the left atrium are important, not only in surgery, echocardiography and in invasive studies, but in radiology and bedside diagnosis—two examples will be noted: (1) The left atrium is the posterior chamber of the heart—examine page 103. (The right atrium is the right lateral, the right ventricle the anterior, and the left ventricle is the left lateral [and apical] chamber.) As a result, early left atrial enlargement is recognized as a double density in a P.A. chest x-ray—not by alteration in the outline of the heart. (2) The relationship of the mitral leaflets to the atrial walls (see **52**—**1–4** and **53**—**1** and **2**) is relevant to the location of the murmurs which result from rupture of the chordae tendinae: When anterior leaflet chordae are ruptured, the jet strikes the posterior wall of the left atrium—this wall is anterior to the vertebral bodies—and the murmur is heard to the left of the spine or transmitted to the skull. In rupture of the chordae to the posterior leaflet, the extent of involvement determines the size and orientation of the prolapsing leaflet tissue and thereby the direction of the jet—characteristically the jet strikes the anterior wall (which is in contact with the aorta) and is transmitted along the aorta to the aortic area of auscultation. The maximal intensity of murmur may be heard in other areas, however—below the pulmonary area of auscultation or at the apex. Our knowledge of the anatomy and the physics of the location of murmurs is incomplete.

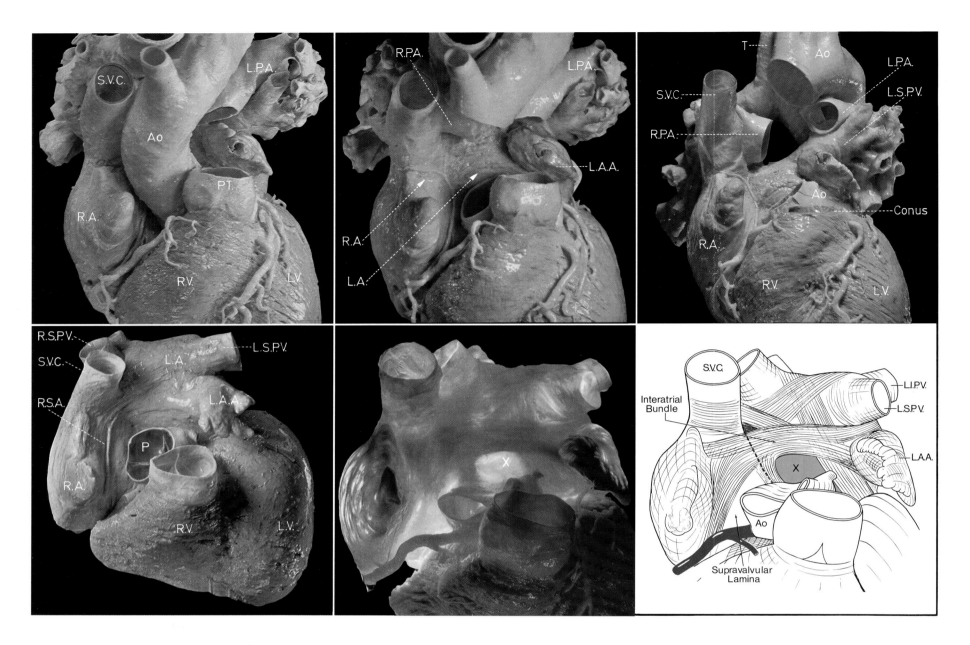

I. The Relations of the Anterior and Superior Walls of the Left Atrium

Specimen A: 1: Superior A.P. view: The pulmonary trunk, which has been excised, has a variable relationship to the left atrial appendage but is separated from the left atrium by the transverse sinus.

2: With the exception of its bulb, the ascending aorta has been excised. It is related to the anteromedial wall of the right atrium and the anterior wall of the left atrium (these walls are indicated by arrows); it is separated inferiorly by adipose tissue, superiorly by the transverse sinus of the pericardium.

3: A.P. view: The upper portion of the infundibulum (conus) of the right ventricle has been excised. An interior window in L.P.A. displays the related bronchus.
Observe: (a) The bifurcation of the trachea is high above the superior wall of the left atrium. (b) The left main bronchus is also above the atrium; its termination is posterior to the superiorly directed left superior pulmonary vein. (c) The left pulmonary artery winds above the left main bronchus; it is not in contact with the left atrium. (d) The right pulmonary artery lies on the superior wall of the left atrium. It is anterior and inferior to the right main bronchus. (e) The left atrial appendage is attached to the anterior wall of the left atrium—an unusual variation. (f) The highest portion of the left atrium is at the attachment of the left superior pulmonary vein.

Specimen B: 4: Superior A.P. view: The great vessels have been excised above the level of their sinuses.
Observe: (a) Behind the middle of the posterior aortic sinus (P), the anterior wall of the left atrium meets the anteromedial wall of the right at an obtuse angle.
(b) The right sinus node artery (R.S.A.) ascends on the anteromedial wall of the right atrium. (c) The anterior interatrial sulcus is indistinct, in contrast to the wedge-shaped, fat-filled posterior interatrial sulcus. (d) The adjoining halves of the posterior and left aortic sinuses are in relation to the lower portion of the anterior wall of the left atrium; the anterior half of the posterior protrudes into the right atrium. (e) The appendageal attachment to the atrium is just inferior to the attachment of the left superior pulmonary vein. These five features should be examined in Specimen A.

II. The Unprotected Area in the Anterior Wall of the Left Atrium

This area is a hazard in the superior approach to the mitral valve, located as it is below the interatrial bundle; the incision must not be below the latter; if placed inferiorly in the former, closure may be virtually impossible. This horseshoe-shaped, thin, poorly muscled unprotected area (marked by an X) is seen transilluminated in Specimen C, **5** and **6** (a superior A.P. view) in which the aortic bulb has been deflected anteriorly, and in Specimen D, **59—1**, which is an A.P. view of the atria which have been separated from their attachments to the tricuspid and A.V. membranes (see the anterior segment **176—5**).

Specimen E: 2: The interatrial is the largest muscle bundle of the left atrium. It extends into the anteromedial wall of the right atrium anterior to the superior vena cava where it overlies, and its fibers intermingle with those of the precaval bundle, the superior extension of the largest muscle bundle of that chamber—the terminal bundle. See this specimen following the initial frontal transection in **89—1** and **2**: On this page, a large part of the anteromedial wall has been removed. The interatrial bundle crosses the upper portion of the anterior wall of the left atrium; and from each of its ends, two rami partially encompass the orifices of the superior vena cava and the left atrial appendage.

III. Variation in the Conformation of the Left Atrium and in the Attachment of Its Appendage

Specimen F: 3: Superior view: The summit of the left atrium is seen between the superior pulmonary veins. Below this level, the interatrial muscle bundle (I.A.B.) marks the junction of the anterior and superior walls of the left atrium. The anterior wall is disposed in the frontal plane, meeting the anteromedial wall of the right atrium (which is marked by the arrow) at an obtuse angle. The orifice of the left atrial appendage is located largely on the lateral wall of the left atrium.

4: L.A.O. view: The left atrial appendage fails to cover the left coronary fossa.

Specimen G: 5: A superior view: The appendage is large and disposed in a sagittal plane providing a wall for the left coronary fossa. Its orifice is large, centered at the junction of the anterior and lateral walls of the left atrium; in the horizontal plane, it extends between the midpoint of both walls. Contrast the development of both the atrium and the appendage in specimens F and G. The interatrial muscle bundle presents a triangular upper surface to the left of the orifice of the superior vena cava.

6: L.A.O. view: The appendage has been retracted. In a frontal plane, its orifice extends from the left superior pulmonary vein to a point 6 mm above the ostium of the left ventricle. The posterior division of the left coronary artery runs in contact with its inferior attachment.

Comment: In the horizontal plane, the axis of the left main branch of the left coronary artery is directed anteriorly 20° in **3**, and 30° in **5**. In the frontal plane, this axis is directed inferiorly 15° in **4** an 45° in **6**. Wide variation is seen in (a) the axes of the left main branch and the proximal portions of its two divisions (see page 144) and in (b) the site of attachment of the left atrial appendage to the left atrium in both the horizontal and the sagittal planes. A variable relationship of the coronary arteries to the left atrial appendage results.

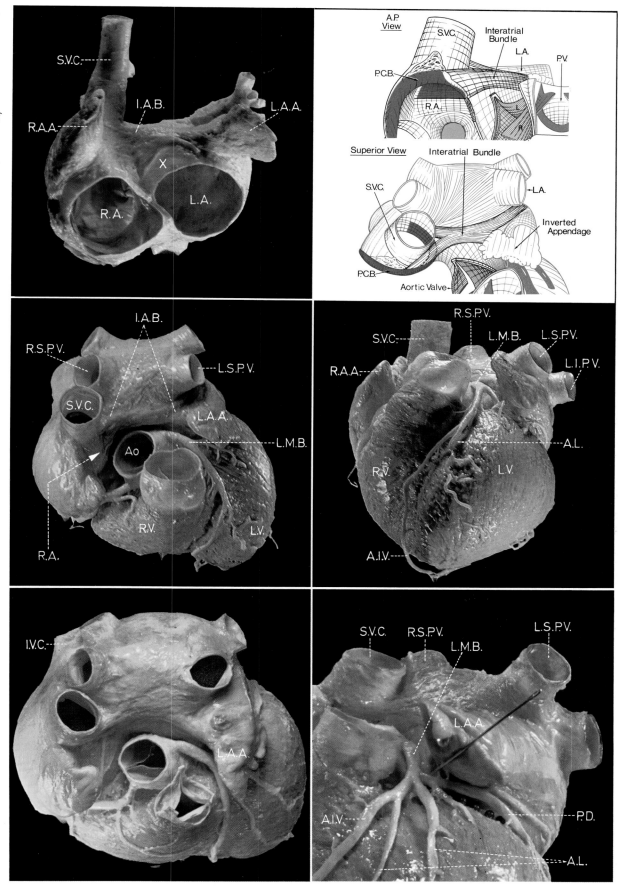

59

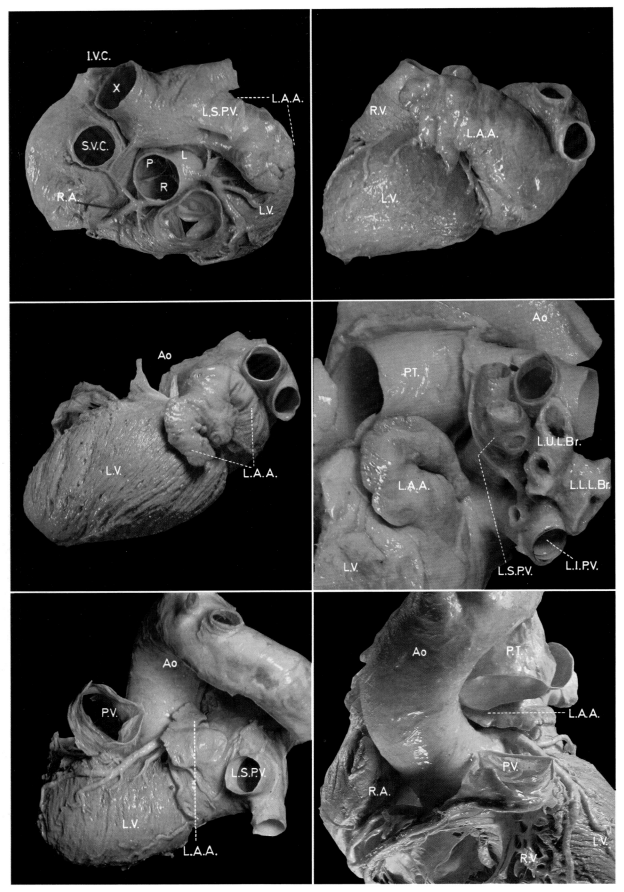

IV. Five Variations in the Configuration and the Axis of the Left Atrial Appendage

1: Superior view: The large atrial appendage has a large orifice, located entirely on the lateral wall of the left atrium underlying both left pulmonary veins. Its axis is **directed laterally.** A common right pulmonary vein (X) is present.

2: Left lateral view: The large orifice is located in the lateral wall. The axis of this large appendage is **directed anterosuperiorly.**

3: This strangely sculptured appendage has a posterior attachment, but its axis is **directed inferiorly.** (The right ventricle has been removed.)

4: Left lateral view: The C-shaped appendage is **directed superiorly** and to the right, underlying the pulmonary trunk. See the drawing on page 130.

5: A superior left lateral view shows an appendage with an attachment midway between the left superior pulmonary vein and the A.V. sulcus. However, **the appendage is inverted into the transverse sinus of the pericardium.**

6: A superior A.P. view of the same specimen, after removal of a segment of the pulmonary trunk, shows the inverted atrial appendage. It should be differentiated from the attachment of the appendage to the anterior wall (see **58—1–3**), a much less common variation. Inversion of the atrial appendage has been seen in approximately 30% of my specimens and frequently at operations. The tip of the inverted appendage may reach the right coronary fossa. No relationship is implied with the rare congenital malformation, juxtaposition of the atrial appendages, in which, in most cases, the right atrial appendage is inverted through the transverse sinus to lie, side by side, with the left atrial appendage. Less commonly (1:6—Charuzi *et al.*) right juxtaposition, wherein both appendages lie to the right side of the great vessels, occurs. The malformation portends the presence of grave associated abnormalities denoting faults in the early development of the heart, e.g. transposition of the great vessels, persistent truncus arteriosus, and common ventricle. Mathews *et al.* (1975) collected the 12 reported cases of right juxtaposition—3 were unassociated with severe defects—the simplest being a bicuspid valve. They state "contrary to previous views, this condition may not be accompanied by severe conotruncal abnormalities".

In a standard A.P. chest x-ray of a patient with mitral stenosis, the cardinal features of the disease are those of left atrial enlargement: (a) the presence of a double density; (b) a double contour, found protruding to the right of the cardiac silhouette. However, enlargement of the appendage may produce an added contour in the left heart border, inferior to that of the pulmonary trunk. This finding is helpful, giving the surgeon some indication of the size of the structure, should a closed mitral operation be contemplated. The site of its attachment, and particularly its axis, will, in addition to its initial size, determine whether or not appendageal enlargement will be identified in a given patient.

V. The Relation of the Posterior Division of the Left Coronary Artery to the Left Atrial Appendage

The Effect of the Course of the Posterior Division on the Relationships

This will be studied in two specimens with identical modes of origin (the left main branch, 2.0 mm in length, arises from an orifice midway between the annuli) and similar modes of termination (at the obtuse margin).

1: 210° view: The right atrium remains—black cloth fills the fossa (F.O.). The posterior division passes directly inferiorly to lie on the wall of L.V., situated only 2 mm from the ostium as it passes above the superior commissure of the mitral valve. The appendageal orifice is usually found in a line joining the left superior pulmonary vein and the superior commissure of the mitral valve; hence, it may be only a few millimeters above the latter. When **the artery courses on the surface of the ventricle**, its point of maximum proximity to the ostium is characteristically seen in relationship to the superior commissure. Hence, the artery and the appendage may be closely related to each other as seen in **59—6.**

2: A nonattitudinal left superior view: The posterior division passes from its origin to its termination, **applied to the atrial wall like a taut string.** It impinges on the attachment of the appendage.

Comment: These two variations in the course of the posterior division do not preclude its proximate relationship to the appendage.

The Effect of the Site of the Orifice of the Appendage on the Relationships

A high orifice is seen in two specimens, the one—**3, 4,** and **5,** and the other—**6.**

3, 4, and **5:** Following a frontal transection which passes through the branching portion of the pulmonary trunk, the anterior segment is seen in **3,** and the posterior in **4.** The atrial appendage is small and located at the junction of the anterior and lateral walls, high above the ostium of the ventricle, contiguous with the orifice of the left superior pulmonary vein (see **4**). However, as seen in **5,** which is an enlargement of **3,** the posterior division passes tightly around the orifice of the appendage.

6: In the specimen above (in **3, 4,** and **5**), the posterior division terminates as the posterior descending branch (a dominant left coronary artery), so its relation to a high-lying appendage might be deemed unremarkable. In this specimen, however, a high attachment of the appendage is associated with a posterior division that impinges on its inferior attachment, although the vessel is terminating as an obtuse marginal branch.

Comment: The posterior division and the atrial appendage at its orifice may be in contact regardless of the mode of termination of the former and the location of the orifice of the latter.

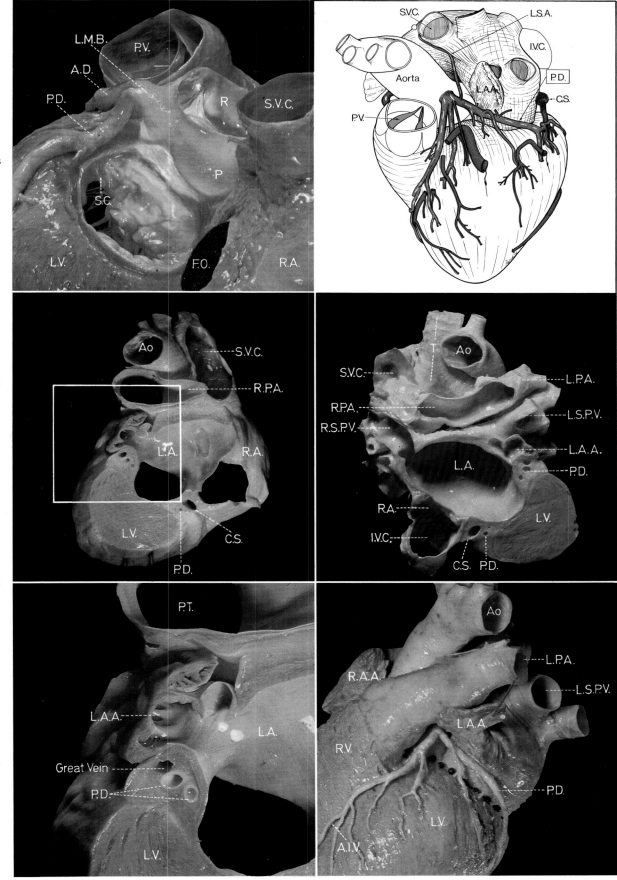

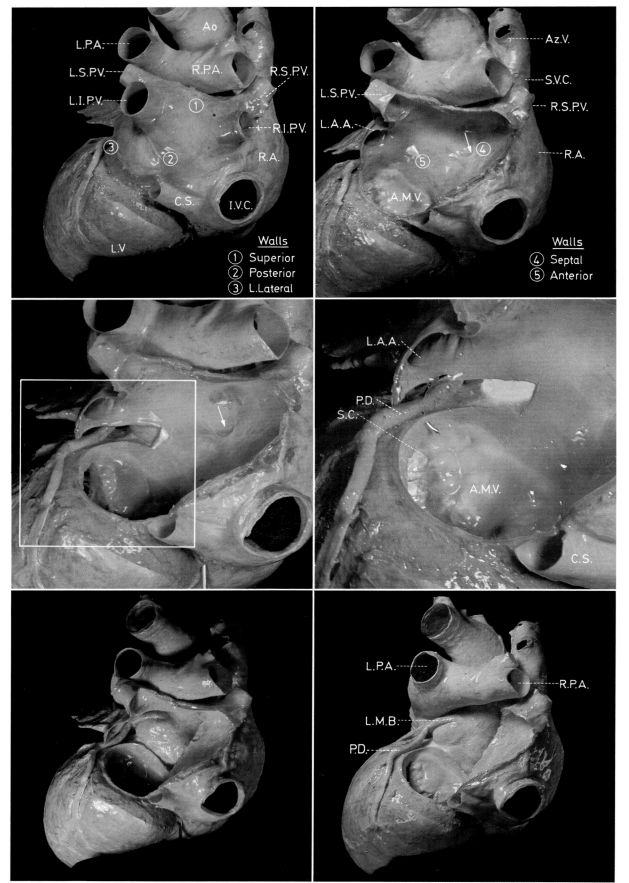

VI. The Five Walls of the Left Atrium

Specimen A: 1–6: In this progressive dissection, viewed from P.A., one can examine some of the anatomic features seen when the posterior approach is used for operations on the mitral valve.

1: The left pulmonary veins are higher than the right. The right pulmonary artery crosses the superior wall. The coronary sinus crosses the posterior wall.

2: The posterior wall and the posterior portions of the superior and lateral walls of the left atrium have been excised, affording a right-angle view of its anterior wall and an oblique view of its septal wall. The small atrial appendage has a small orifice in the anterior portion of the lateral wall.

3: Below the atrial appendage, a 1.0 cm wide rectangle of the adjoining anterior and lateral walls has been excised. The posterior division of the left coronary artery is related to the appendage above and the L.V. ostium below. The arrow marks the superiorly directed U-shaped upper border of the valvula foraminis ovalis: It is at the junction of the anterior and septal walls.

4: The area of the square outlined in **3** is shown with transillumination of the mitral valve and the left aortic sinus. A suture needle has been passed through the upper portion of the mitral valve and the artery, simulating the violation of the latter during mitral valve replacement. The fatal myocardial infarction resulting may be attributed to metabolic problems arising from the disease or the perfusion.

5: The anterior wall of the left atrium has been largely removed, showing the **proximity of the main branch of the left coronary artery to the left superior pulmonary vein and to the left atrial appendage.** This relationship is important: (a) In the performance of radical pneumonectomy for the treatment of carcinoma, in order to be well proximal to the tumor, I have, not infrequently, removed the portion of the left atrium to which the pulmonary veins are attached: The atrial wall is separated only by fat and connective tissue from the left main branch which could be injured. (b) When the superior approach to the mitral valve is used, the incision may be angled inferiorly along the course of the interatrial muscle bundle towards the atrial appendage, again placing the left main branch in jeopardy.

6: The anterior and left lateral walls have been removed. Note the relation of the former to the aorta and to the left coronary artery. In this specimen a common variation is seen; the orifice of the artery is located in the posterior half of the left aortic sinus (which is more correctly termed—left posterolateral). Just anterior to the superior commissure of the mitral valve, the posterior division, which terminates as an obtuse marginal branch, effects contact with the ostium of L.V. Compare this specimen with **61—1**. In both, the course of the posterior division is similar despite the disparity in the lengths of the left main branch.

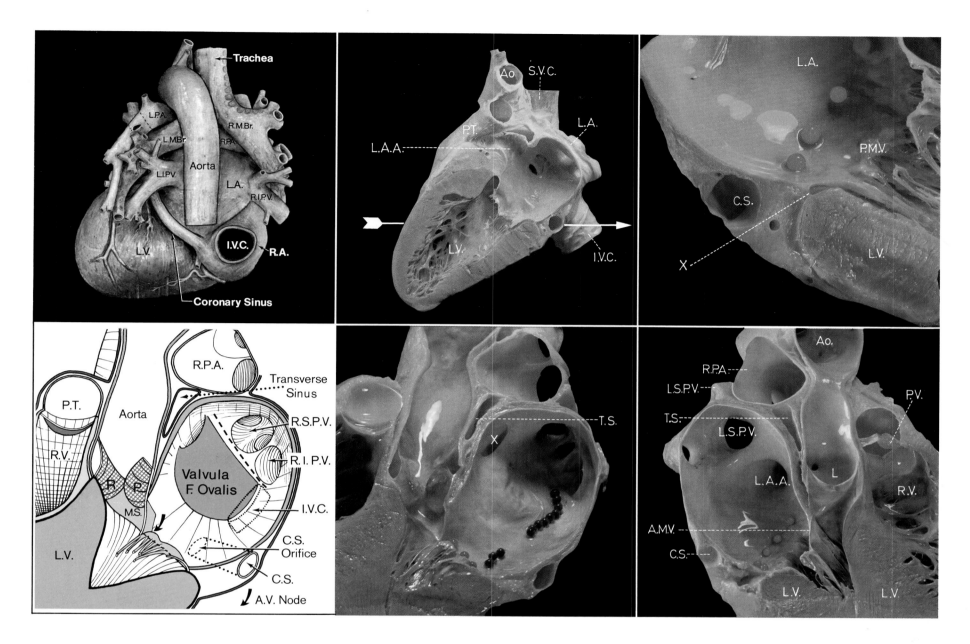

VII. The Relations of the Coronary Sinus to the Left Atrium

Specimen B: 1: P.A. attitudinal view: (a) **The axis of the coronary sinus in the frontal plane**: The coronary sinus enters the junction of the inferior and medial walls of the right atrium after coursing behind the ostium of the left ventricle at an angle of 45° above the horizontal. (b) The left atrium continues the direction of the left ventricle—posteriorly, to the right, and superiorly—as a result, the left pulmonary veins are higher than the right.

Specimen C: 2 and 3

2. A left lateral attitudinal view of the right segment of a heart following an oblique transection. As a consequence of the axis of the left atrium, the posterior wall also faces inferiorly. The coronary sinus is on the posterior wall 10 mm from its attachment; however, because of the posterosuperior inclination of the wall, the coronary sinus is seen directly posterior to the ostium of the ventricle when examined in the A.P. (see arrow) and lateral planes.

3: This is a 1.5:1 magnification of the left segment. **In the average male, the coronary sinus is 10 mm in diameter and is 10 mm from the ostium of the ventricle.** The subvalvular segment of the A.V. membrane (X) is 2 mm in width. When the right coronary artery or a branch thereof, runs in the left posterior A.V. sulcus, it will be found between the coronary sinus and the ventricle; in contrast, a major element of the left coronary artery is frequently between the sinus and the left atrial wall (see page 190).

VIII. The Relation of the A.V. Node to the Left Atrium

Specimen D: 4, 5, and 6: An oblique transection in the axis of the ascending aorta: The right segment is seen in **4** and **5** and the left in **6**. Lateral views are used. See 129—**3–6**.

(a) The A.V. node is in jeopardy during mitral valve replacement and injury to it, rather than metabolic derangements, may be the cause of some arrhythmias seen postoperatively. The beads in **5** mark the structures on the opposite side of the septum: the three lower blue = orifice of coronary sinus; red = ostium of L.V.; the upper red = the A.V. node. (b) in **5**, the upper blue beads = the orifice of the inferior vena cava: Extending anterosuperiorly from its orifice is the membranous valvula foraminis ovalis (orange in **4**) which may be lacerated by retraction during mitral valve operations—a septal defect may be acquired. A probe patent foramen ovale is present (X in **5**). (c) The transverse sinus (T.S.) is at the junction of the anterior and superior walls— the right pulmonary artery courses over the superior wall.

6: Observe: (a) The orifice of the atrial appendage is found, as is usual, in a line between the superior pulmonary vein and the superior commissure of the mitral valve (which is seen below the most superior red bead); in this specimen the orifice is close to the vein. (b) The characteristic prominent ridge between the orifice and the vein is well seen. (c) The summit of the atrium is between the superior pulmonary veins. A similiar view with a drawing of this segment can be seen—**54**—**5** and **6**.

IX. Comments on the Five Approaches to the Mitral Valve

With the exception of the anterior wall, each of the five walls of the left atrium has been used for an incision to enter the chamber.

(1) **In the most popular incision,** the right lateral wall (see page 98) between the right pulmonary veins and the septum is divided. In **63—4**, the interrupted line between the valvula foraminis ovalis and the right pulmonary veins indicates the initial part of the incision. If the atrium is small, the interatrial sulcus is developed; however, as described on page 154, this exposes to injury a sinus node artery with a counterclockwise course. To expose the valve, the right atrium and septum are retracted to the left; the caval attachments tether the right atrium and atrial septum and limit this retraction and, particularly when the left atrium is small, poor exposure of the valve and trauma to the septum result. As the septum may be largely membranous, it may be perforated and if the perforation is unrecognized, an atrial septal defect will be acquired. It has been the custom to attempt circumvention of this problem by extending the incision into the inferior part of the posterior atrial wall, above (and avoiding) the coronary sinus. Unfortunately, the intrapericardial segment of the inferior vena cava is short, wide, and relatively fixed—the exposure remains poor. At Toledo Hospital we untether the superior vena cava. This modification was devised by Dr. H.M. Foster Jr.

The anatomy of this maneuver can be seen on pages 131 and 132. Between the superior vena cava and the anterior and antero-inferior surface of the right pulmonary artery, a rectangular extrapericardial zone is present; it lies between the right lateral pericardial reflection in the retrocaval recess and the superior pericardial reflection in the transverse sinus. These pericardial reflections are divided and the superior vena cava is freed up to a level above the azygos vein. The incision in the lateral wall of the left atrium is extended into the superior wall below the pulmonary artery; this superior extension divides the right half of the superior wall. Now, gentle retraction displaces the untethered upper right atrium, the upper atrial septal wall, and the adjoining anterior wall of the left atrium to the left. The mitral valve faces to the right and posterosuperiorly; the axis of view is nearly perpendicular to its plane—better exposure results. In contrast, when the incision is carried into the posterior wall, the valve is distant, its plane is oblique to the view of the surgeon and vigorous retraction is needed, particularly when the left atrium is small. A sinus node artery with a clockwise course will not be divided by this modified, or superolateral approach. During the past 18 months at Toledo Hospital, mitral valve replacements have been performed in 63 patients with one death. One cannot minimize the importance of the careful monitoring of the many physiologic parameters used during and following these operations, nor the strict attention paid to detail in the management of the airway; however, attention to these anatomic principles with the attendant simplification of the operative procedure (which not only reduces the pump time, but allows precise removal of the diseased valve and meticulous insertion of the prosthetic valve) are important if the best results are to be obtained in the seriously ill group of patients selected for operation.

If a left superior vena cava is present in the adult heart—a not uncommon anomaly—it is of interest that a rectangular extrapericardial zone is present on the anterior wall of the left pulmonary artery; it corresponds to the area on the right pulmonary artery (the site where the superior vena cava has been mobilized). The vestigial fold of the pericardium can be thought of as the anterior wall of an aborted left retrocaval recess (page 132).

(2) **The posterior incision** is made vertically in the posterior and superior walls midway between the left and right pulmonary veins. Extension of the incision superiorly may injure the right pulmonary artery as it lies on the superior wall anterior and at an inferior level to the "right bronchus". Similarly, injury may befall the coronary sinus inferiorly. (a) This incision provides good exposure of not only the mitral valve, but also of the anterior and septal wall of the left ventricle. Therefore, the incision should be considered in the correction of infundibular hypertrophic subaortic stenosis. (b) Atrial myxoma are easily removed (1) with precise excision of the origin of the pedicle, which is usually in the septal wall—this may be important in the prevention of recurrence and (2) with less risk of fragmentation of the tumor and the attendant embolization and possibly of implantation. Awareness of the entity and its clinical features plus the inclusion of echocardiography in the study of "mitral valve disease" should make preoperative diagnosis routine—the surgeon may therefore choose the best approach. The danger of intraoperative asystole due to tumor occlusion of the mitral orifice must be gauged in each case—this may contraindicate the posterior approach however. (c) As the aorta is not clamped, the coronary circulation is maintained; for this reason, and also because of the superior location of the atriotomy when the patient is rotated ventrally, the danger of air embolism is reduced. (d) The sinus node arteries are only very rarely transected by the incision. (e) The incision is easy to close. In the presence of atriomegaly, substantial reduction in the size of the atrium may be accomplished by the removal of demilunar margins of the atrial wall on both sides of the incision prior to closure of the latter.* Reduction in atrial size will reduce the transit time of blood in the chamber, and warrants attention as a measure to reduce the incidence of thrombo-embolism following valve replacement. However, (f) the morbidity following the posterolateral thoracotomy incision exceeds that of median sternotomy. (g) The latter incision also can be effected more quickly in a gravely ill patient in whom asystole is a threat. (h) When concomitant aortic valve replacement is needed, the median sternotomy incision is used.

(3) **The transseptal approach:** Transverse incisions are made first in the right atrium, then in the atrial septal wall. This has been advised when a sternotomy incision is used and the left atrium is small. However, the following anatomic considerations apply: (a) The atrial septum is an area for the development of collateral circulation, a matter of relevance when valve replacement is necessary in a patient with occlusive arterial disease. (b) Internodal bundles connecting the S.A. and A.V. nodes may be divided which may increase the likelihood of postoperative arrhythmia**. (c) The incision in the septum must be made and closed with care, especially when the membranous component of the septum is large, or an atrial septal defect will result. (d) The axis of exposure is oblique to the surface of the valve, in contrast to the relatively perpendicular axis that results when the superior vena cava is untethered as described in the first approach. (e) A cramped view results particularly in a small female patient.

(4) **The superior approach** passes above the junction of the anterior and superior walls. The location of the right pulmonary artery on the superior wall and the aorta in relation to the anterior wall (pages 58, 59, 124, and 125) demonstrates how these structures will require dissection and displacement to expose the area for the incision. When the sinus node artery arises from the left coronary artery, it usually runs intramurally through the interatrial muscle bundle. If, to facilitate its closure, the incision is made through the interatrial muscle bundle, loss of the artery will usually result. Incisions made more inferiorly will pass through the unprotected area in the anterior wall; warnings have been issued that these are virtually impossible to close, which is not surprising in view of the anatomic appearance of the area. See the three articles of Myer, Saksena, and Robinson and their respective colleagues.

(5) The **left lateral approach** will be discussed on page 159.

---

* Le Roux and Gotsman, in a valuable paper, show the result of atrial reduction carried out using not a posterior but the more usual incision described on this page in (1).
** Three pathways are present; the posterior running in relation to the sulcus terminalis will certainly be divided—the middle (passing obliquely across the upper septum) will frequently be divided, while the anterior is free of danger as it crosses the anteromedial wall of the right atrium—see references—(1) James. (2) Meredith and Titus.

Chapter 6:
The Right Ventricle

Introduction

A. If, for descriptive purposes, the septal wall is considered a part of the aorto-ventricular unit, the right ventricle has anterior, posterolateral, and inferior walls, and tricuspid and pulmonary ostia. **We then can describe five attachments:** (1) anterior, (2) posterolateral, (3) inferior, (4) tricuspid or posterior, and (5) pulmonary or superior.

B. In setting in place **the inferior attachment** on page 68, a word is encountered, the **crux**, which qualifies as a vestigial term. The latter should be "defined" as the persistence in the description of adult anatomy of a designation only appropriate during a fleeting period of fetal development. The word, crux, is assigned three meanings by Webster: "(1) a cross, (2) anything very puzzling or difficult to explain, and (3) a crucial point". Examination of the inferior aspect of the heart reveals relationships of crucial importance. However, it is hoped that these will not be deemed very puzzling after examination of the following four pages. Although a variety of crosses was used in heraldry, the essential structure consisted of an upright supporting a horizontal beam, that is, the two members cross at right angles. This would imply that the interatrial and interventricular grooves form a line, and the posterior right and left atrioventricular sulci also form a line, and the two lines are coordinates of a point. Of one, however, uses the unit concept, either to progressively remove portions of the heart ending with the unit (which is represented in the inferior view by the left ventricle), or if one begins with the unit and adds the chambers, it is apparent that the term, **crux**, is not descriptive of the relationships in this area. In reality, as seen in the inferior view in **68—2**, the interatrial sulcus extending inferiorly meets the posterior left A.V. sulcus at a right angle, and the posterior I.V. sulcus extending superiorly meets the posterior right A.V. sulcus at a right angle. The A.V. sulci are parallel, but the right is inferior to the left. Also, the interatrial and interventricular sulci are parallel, but the latter is to the right of the former. A diagonal line joins the right-angled junctions. This line is the posterior margin of what will be described herein as the posterosuperior process of the left ventricle. When the unit concept is utilized, and the true anatomy of the crux realized, the relationships of the septal leaflet of the tricuspid valve are easily perceived and the wide separation of the latter from the mitral valve is recognized.

C. **The posterior attachment,** formed by the septal leaflet of the tricuspid valve, is divisible into membranous and muscular components. The former, the attachment to the membranous septum, has been discussed in Chapter 2. At this time, we will examine the latter, the attachment of the leaflet to the left ventricular (or septal) muscle wall. The importance of the relations of this component to the neighboring arteries and to the A.V. node in tricuspid valve replacement will be seen.

D. **The posterolateral wall** of the right ventricle most commonly extends between the left anterior and the right anterior fibrous trigones, placing it anterior to only the right aortic sinus. Three common and two uncommon variations affect the aortic sinus-ventricular wall relationship.

Common variations: (1) On the right—**the posterior limit of the attachment** of the posterolateral wall to the A.V. membrane may be located, not inferior to the right and posterior aortic annular commissure, its usual site, but shifted posteriorly, at times, to almost reach the nadir of the posterior annulus. (2) On the left—**the size of the infundibulum** is independent of the general size of the right ventricle. (a) Its size is mainly determined by the axis of the plane of the pulmonary ostium. When this plane is almost horizontal, a small infundibulum results. When it extends anterosuperiorly (e.g. at a 45° angle), a large infundibulum occurs. (b) In a minority of specimens, the posterior wall of the infundibulum extends above (the left ventricular component of) the A.V. unit—a larger infundibulum is the consequence. (3) **The normal right ventricle varies in size and shape;** it may be large and balloon around the aorta, or it may be meager and, in large part, relatively distant to the latter. The right ventricle wraps around the A.V. unit, therefore, the positive occurrence of any of these three variations will increase both the area of contact and the degree of proximity of the ventricular wall to the aorta.

Uncommon variations: (1) Variations occur in **the relative size of aortic sinuses;** involvement of the right and posterior sinuses will exert an obvious effect on the relationship. An example will be shown. (2) **Annular rotation on the ostium,** though rare, has a pronounced effect on the aortic sinus-ventricular wall relationship as seen on page 25.

E. The two valves of the left ventricle are found in a single ostium. The valves of the right ventricle, on the contrary, are afforded two well-separated ostia. The term, tricuspid ostium, is used to denote the **margins** of the inflow valve orifice, which is composed of the posterolateral, anterior, and inferior walls of the ventricle and the site of attachment of the septal leaflet of the tricuspid valve to the A.V. unit. The superior margins of the posterolateral, anterior and the ventricular septal walls form a circular outlet, the pulmonary ostium. To this the pulmonary trunk is attached. The delicate pulmonary annuli are attached to the internal surface of both the right ventricle and the trunk.

F. The muscles of the right ventricle may be divided into three groups: (1) **the trabeculae,** (2) **the papillary muscles of the tricuspid valve,** and (3) **the infundibular muscles.** The sinus of the ventricle is highly trabeculated, particularly at the apex. The infundibulum is relatively glabrous, varying with the degree of segmentation of the septal band. The papillary muscles of the tricuspid valve will be termed superior, anterior, and inferior. The superior, is usually located immediately inferior to the nadir of the right aortic annulus, receiving chordae from the anterosuperior leaflet. The anterior and inferior papillary muscles, attached to the anterior and inferior walls, respectively, provide insertion for the chordae from the remainder of the nonseptal leaflets of the tricuspid valve. Almost all of the chordae from the septal

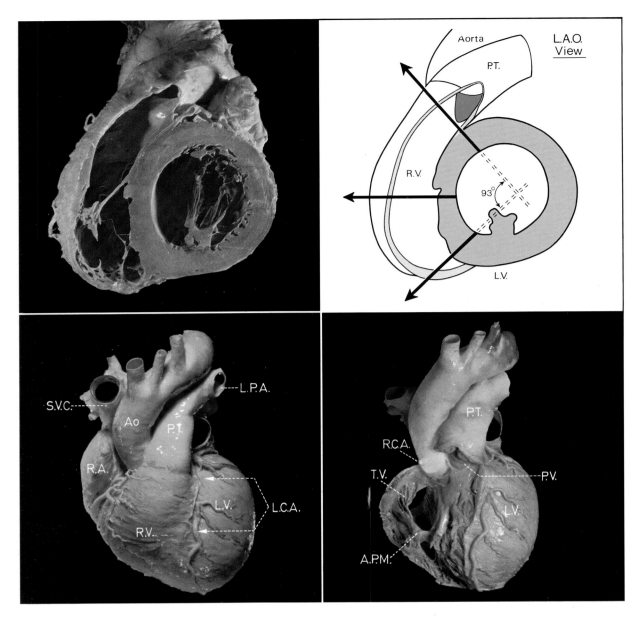

A. Preview

I. The Contour of the Ventricular Septum

The right ventricle wraps around the A.V. unit, extending between the right anterior and left anterior fibrous trigones, that is, 120° in the horizontal plane. In birds, the envelopment may be 180° (see page 16). In animals, the left ventricle has a conical shape; in man, the shape of the left ventricle is more variable and complex; however, the septal wall of the left ventricle, is usually strongly curved. The upper portion of the latter wall is directed superiorly and anteriorly, while the lower portion is directed anteriorly, inferiorly, and to the right. Knowledge of this contour is essential in the clinical examination of the septal wall and its arterial branches.

Specimen A: 1 and **2**: L.A.O. view: This specimen is transected at right angles to the plane of examination. Arrows are directed at right angles to the surface of the septal wall—superiorly at the pulmonary attachment and inferiorly at the attachment of the inferior wall of the right ventricle to the unit. These arrows form an angle of 93°, and provide an expression of the slope of the septum. A third arrow is extended at right angles to the ventricular portion of the membranous septum (which is not shown in the photograph). Knowledge of the contour of the ventricular septum is important in appreciating the variable location of murmurs found in the different anatomic types of ventricular septal defects. Each of the three arrows can be used to simulate the direction of **the jet of blood which passes through a defect** located at the three sites. (a) Approximately 5% of isolated ventricular septal defects are found inferior to the fibrous trigone between the posterior and right anterolateral pulmonary leaflets. These defects have been termed supracristal; however, due to the ambiguity of the term crista (supraventricularis), just referred to, the term subpulmonic, which is favored by Baron (1968), seems preferable. The maximal intensity of the murmur is heard at the pulmonary area; radiation superiorly to the clavicle and suprasternal notch occurs. (b) The maximum intensity of the murmur due to a defect in the membranous septum is heard over the fourth sternocostal junction. (c) In the presence of the least common type, the low defect, the maximum intensity of the murmur is heard as low as the xiphoid process.

Specimen B: 66—3 and **4** and **67—1–6**

3: Superior left anterior nonattitudinal view. The left atrial appendage has been removed—its orifice appears black. The specimen is otherwise intact.

4: The following have been removed: (1) the right atrium; (2) the anterior and posterolateral walls of the right ventricle with the exception of rims in relation to the pulmonary and tricuspid valves. Observe: (a) The inferior wall is attached to the receding antero-inferior surface of the left ventricle. The posterior or septal wall of the infundibulum faces upwards and anteriorly and continues the contour of the left ventricle—the right ventricle wraps around the left ventricle.

leaflet are attached with or without the intermediation of small papillae to the septal wall; a few pass to the inferior papillary muscle.

The **muscles of the infundibulum** are divisible into the **septal band** and the **parietal band**; only these terms are used herein. The junction of these two bands is often indicated by a raphe or a ridge extending from the superior papillary muscle to the nadir of the posterior pulmonary leaflet. This junction has been termed the **crista supraventricularis**. The word, crista, denotes a crest, and this characteristic is only seen if a sagittal section passes through this junction point. The term, crista supraventricularis, also has been used by Tandler to designate what is here described as the parietal band. Also, other workers have used the term to comprise the entire infundibular musculature. An extension of the septal band, the moderator band, is usually seen extending inferiorly to the site of attachment of the anterior papillary muscle to the anterior wall. The parietal band extends across the tricuspid orifice onto the anterior wall, fading out above the area of the attachment of the anterior papil-

lary muscle. The terms, parietal and septal bands, are in reality quite specious. They could, with reason but without facility, be replaced by the terms, infundibular portion of the posterolateral wall of the right ventricle and the posterior wall of the infundibulum, if one condition could be applied—namely, that portions of both pass onto the anterior wall. This applies particularly to the latter band or wall—a moderator band is usually present and segmentation above its level frequently results in large trabeculae. Certainly in normal hearts, stout, easily definable ridges may intrude into the ventricular cavity at the junction of the sinus and infundibulum. If the terms, septal and parietal bands, are reserved for these ridges, the observer is faced with a descriptive dilemma when the ridges are, as often occurs, not present.

II. The Five Attachments of the Right Ventricle to the Aorto-Ventricular Unit

1: The pulmonary trunk and valve have been removed. The specimen is rotated, and we view it from above in the axis of the ascending aorta. The black beads (P.V.) mark the site of the pulmonary valve attachment. **The posterior wall of the infundibulum** extends from the latter attachment inferiorly to the moderator band (M.B.), which projects anteriorly to the remnant of the anterior wall of the right ventricle (X). **The anterior papillary muscle** (A.P.M.) arises from the anterior wall and the anterior extremity of the moderator band. Its origin is closer to the tricuspid valve than it is to the attachment of the anterior wall of the right ventricle to the septum. This is the usual pattern in humans. It is often erroneously stated that it is attached to the anterior wall near the latter's attachment to the septum or to both the anterior and septal walls at their junction.

2: The specimen is rotated more posteriorly. **The septal wall continues the contour of the left ventricle.**

3 and **4**: Further posterior rotation enables us to see that the pulmonary and tricuspid attachments underlie the left anterior and right anterior fibrous trigones, respectively. The color-coding identifies the three aortic annuli.

4: Commencing at the pulmonary or superior attachment, proceed in a clockwise manner and note **the five lines of attachment of the right ventricle** to the unit and then note **the two margins of apposition of the right atrium** to the left atrium. The right atrium is apposed, not attached to the left atrium, and it has been removed therefrom by dividing the interatrial muscle bundle and dissecting through the appositional plane. The upper portions of the ventricular and atrial septa (shown in white) face superiorly. Not only does the right ventricle wrap around the left ventricle but the right atrium wraps around the left atrium.

5 and **6**: The specimen is further rotated and is viewed with the apex below. Three of the attachments are marked by beads and in **6**, all are indicated by the numbers which correspond to those seen in **4**. The inferior papillary muscle (I.P.M.) is separated from the inferior wall and held in its normal position by a needle. A segment of the tricuspid leaflet is excised, revealing the large ventricular portion of the membranous septum. The right and left coronary arteries identify the right and left aortic sinuses and annuli; note the left anterior fibrous trigone between the two. The superior papillary muscle (S.P.M.), indicated by the yellow bead, is below the nadir of the right aortic annulus. The right half of the right aortic sinus is related to the sinus or inflow tract of the right ventricle and the left half to the infundibulum. The septal wall is strongly curved as it recedes towards the inferior attachment of the right ventricle. Note the elliptical shape of the tricuspid ostium.

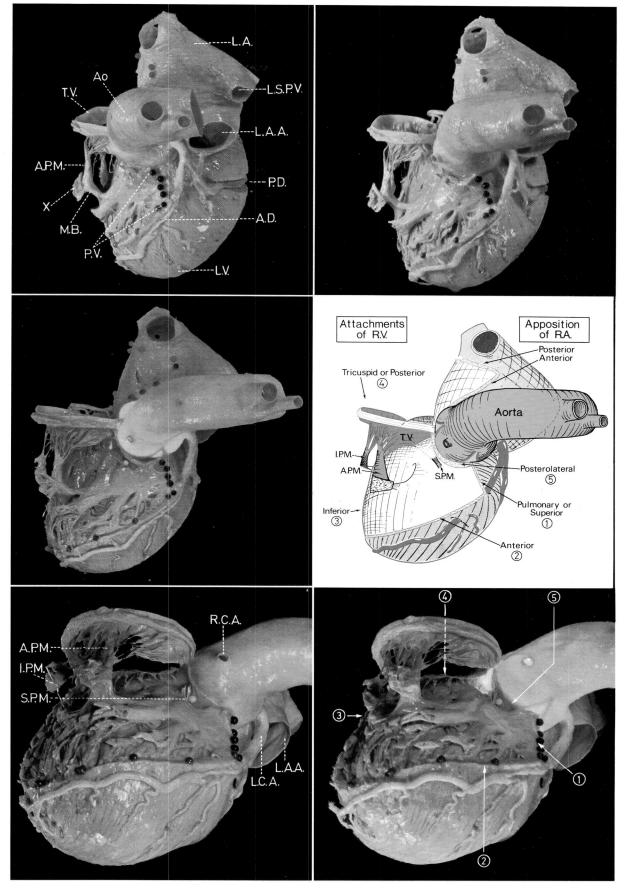

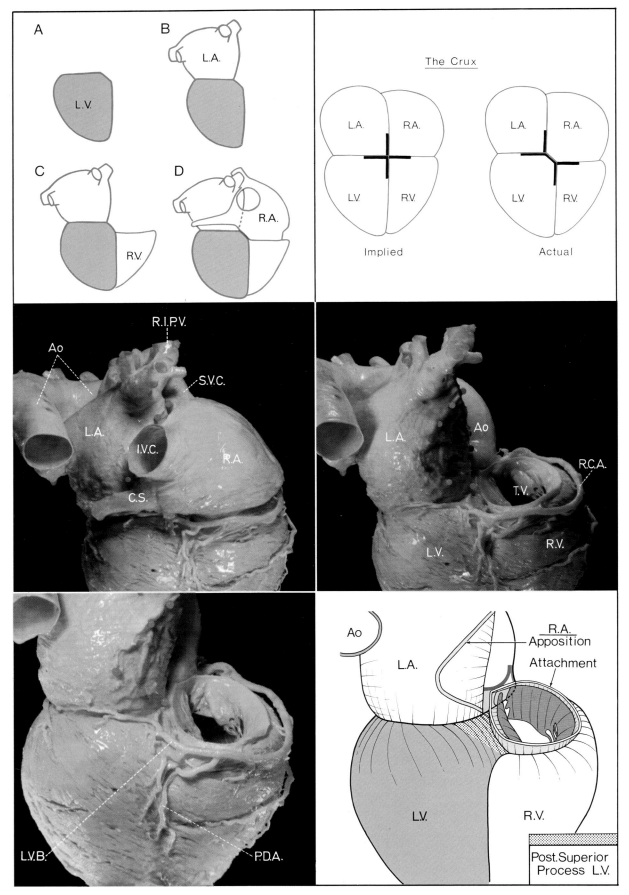

B. The Attachment of the Inferior Wall of the Right Ventricle to the Aorto-Ventricular Unit

I. The Crux of the Heart—Its Definition

1: (A) The left ventricle is viewed in the plane of its ostium. (B) The left atrium is attached in relation to the inner aspect of the ostium. (C) The right ventricle is applied and viewed in the plane of the tricuspid ostium, which is inferior to the ostium of the left ventricle. The interventricular sulcus, so formed, is to the right of the left atrium in this view. (D) The right atrium is applied to the other chambers. It wraps around the left atrium, placing the posterior interatrial sulcus even further to the left of the posterior interventricular sulcus.

2: First we see the implied relationship and then the actual relationship of the four chambers at the crux.

Specimen A: 3–6: Now examine the inferior view of the specimen featured on the last two pages and observe the features diagrammed above.

3 and **4**: The right atrium is removed from the left. The area of apposition on the latter is shown by the shadow, and its margin is delineated by the red beads. On page 67, we saw that the upper portion of the atrial septum was directed superiorly, and now we see that its lower portion is directed inferiorly. **The right atrium wraps around the left atrium**.

5 and **6**: A more superior view: The posterior descending artery (P.D.A.) identifies the posterior interventricular groove. Observe: (a) The left atrium is attached to the aorto-ventricular membrane in relation to the inner aspect of the ostium of the left ventricle. (b) The ostium of the left ventricle is above and distant to the attachment of the inferior wall of the right ventricle to the A.V. unit, represented here by the left ventricle. The promontory between (1) the attachment of the septal leaflet of the tricuspid valve to the A.V. unit, (2) the ostium of the left ventricle, and (3) a line drawn from the latter to the upper end of the posterior interventricular groove will, in this work, be called the **posterior superior process of the left ventricle.** The A.V. node artery and the posterior septal artery almost invariably course over this area. The continuing left ventricular segment of the right coronary artery may traverse it, as it does in this specimen, or pass at a lower level to reach the posterior wall of the left ventricle. On the next page, the hearts are shown with their arteries in place, because the anatomy of the crux has great relevance in the study of their course and mode of branching. The word crux has one virtue, brevity; however, if it is to be used, it should designate, **not a point, but a region or area where the chambers effect their maximum proximity posteriorly,** although each does not effect contact with the other three as the term suggests. This area, the space between the chambers, is filled with fat and can be seen in frontal transections on pages 102 and 104.

II. Variations in the Attachment of the Inferior Wall

69—**1**: Four basic types are seen. In **Type A**, the posterior right A.V. sulcus is staggered a short distance below the posterior left A.V. sulcus. The apices are approximately at the same level. **Type B**: The apex of the right ventricle is elevated. **Type C**: The (tricuspid) ostium of right ventricle is markedly depressed below that of the left. In **Type D**, both the apex is elevated and the tricuspid ostium is depressed.

2: Tracings of the four photographs **3–6** are shown in the same sequence. The type of variation they represent is indicated. The measurements of **the ostial-apex length of the ventricles** were made. The relations of the right to the left expressed as a percentage are: **3**—88%, **4**—83%, **5**—60%, and **6**—66%. The relation of the apices of the ventricles to each other, as described on page 28, is not without clinical significance; however, more relevant to the anatomy of the crux is the relation of ostial heights as these determine the size of the posterior superior process separating the left ventricular ostium from the posterior I.V. sulcus.

5: In this small (180 gram) heart, the distance between the most medial red bead in the posterior left A.V. sulcus and the blue bead (A), at the right-angled junction of the posterior right A.V. sulcus and the upper end of the posterior I.V. sulcus is 23 mm. The distance between the blue beads A and B, marking the upper and lower end of the sulcus, is 52 mm. These measurements indicate the dimension of the specimen and the matter under discussion.

6: The posterior left A.V. sulcus is 25.2 mm from the I.V. sulcus.

The arteries and the crux: Observe: (a) A statement that an artery "crosses the crux" must be viewed with caution. For example, in **3** and **5**, the dominant right coronary artery reaches the junction of the posterior right A.V. sulcus and the I.V. sulcus, then continues as a left ventricular artery (L.V.B.) passing directly onto the posterior wall of the left ventricle, below the left A.V. sulcus and the posterior superior process.
(b) When the crux is thought of as a cross, it would seem a natural consequence for the A.V. node artery to always arise from the artery that supplies the posterior descending branch and many statements to this effect are found in medical writings; however, cognizance of the actual disposition of the crux anticipates the disposition seen in **4** and **6**. The right coronary artery supplies the posterior descending branch (P.D.A.) and the left, the A.V. node branch (A.V.N.A.). The "balanced" pattern thus depicted was observed in 17 of 100 dissections*.
(c) The posterior interventricular groove is often not recognizable, (see **4**) hence identification of the posterior descending branch may be difficult. The variations in this branch are discussed on page 167; on this page, **3**, **5**, and **6** represent three different examples of the retro-ventricular type. Each is common.

---

* See page 166 for the definition of "balanced" and dominant.

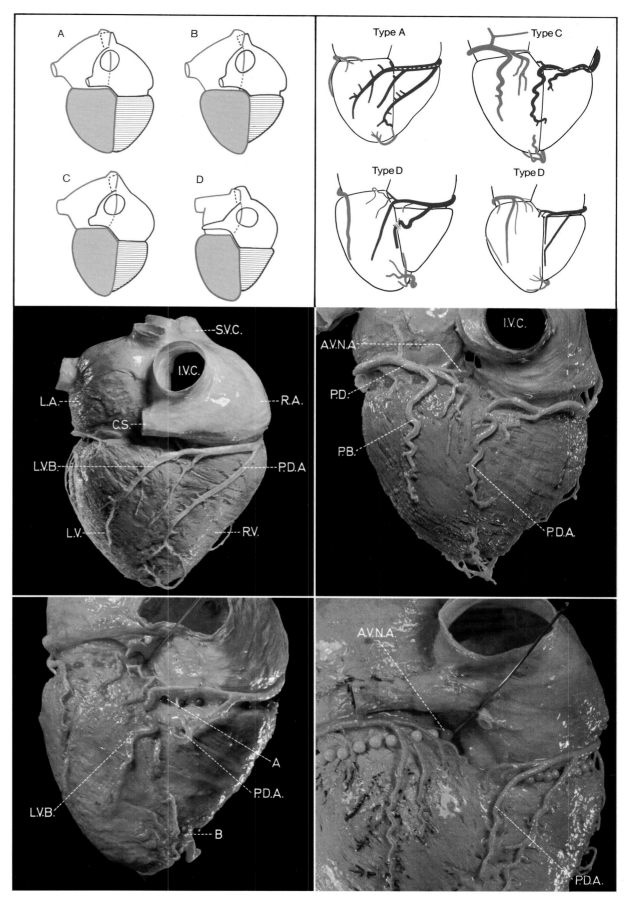

69

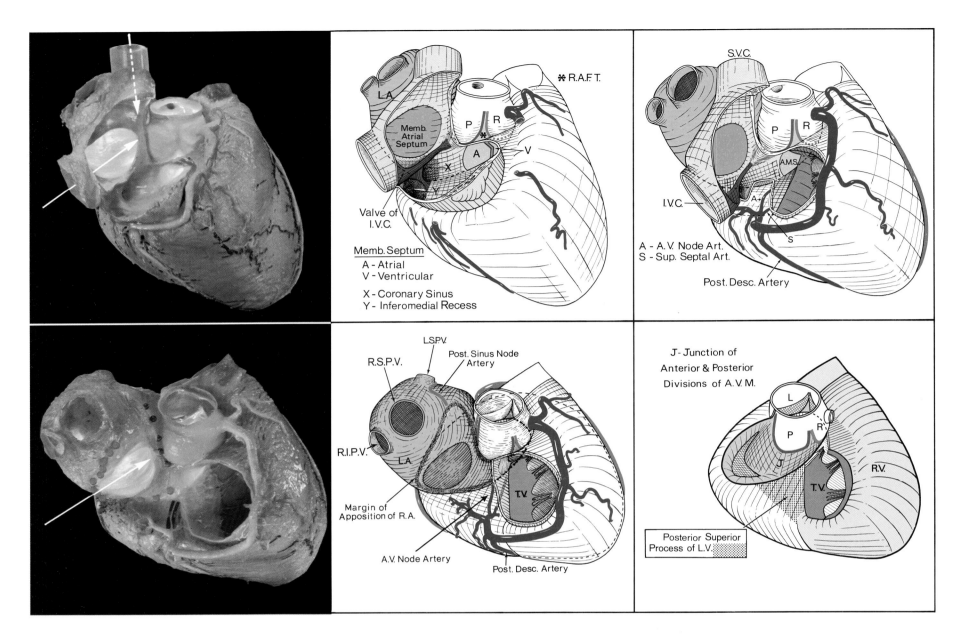

Valve of
I.V.C.

Memb. Septum
A - Atrial
V - Ventricular

X - Coronary Sinus
Y - Inferomedial Recess

A - A.V. Node Art.
S - Sup. Septal Art.

Post. Desc. Artery

R.S.P.V.

LS.P.V.

Post. Sinus Node
Artery

R.I.P.V.

L.A.

Margin of
Apposition of R.A.

A.V. Node Artery

Post. Desc. Artery

T.V.

J - Junction of
Anterior & Posterior
Divisions of A.V.M.

Posterior Superior
Process of L.V.

C. The Posterior or Tricuspid Attachment of the Right Ventricle to the Aorto-Ventricular Unit

As described on page 65, the attachment of the septal leaflet of the tricuspid valve to the A.V. unit is divisible into membranous and muscle components; the latter will be examined now.

Specimen A: 1–6

1 and **2**: Nonattitudinal right lateral view: The lateral, much of the posterior, and the anteromedial walls of the right atrium have been removed. The inferior wall of the right atrium lies above and lateral to the posterosuperior process of L.V. The coronary sinus orifice, at the junction of the inferior and posteromedial (or septal) walls, is medial to the inferomedial recess or fossa (see page 93). The major component of the atrial septal wall is membranous; it is transilluminated in **1** and **4** and shown in orange in **2**, **3**, and **5**.

3: Following further removal of the right atrium, including the inferomedial recess but not the coronary sinus orifice, we expose the posterosuperior process of the left ventricle across which the superior septal and the A.V. node arteries run.*

4 and **5**: The large, upper portion of the right atrium has been removed: Small portions remain: (1) a segment covering the apex of the triangular posterosuperior process—the superior septal artery runs between the two structures; (2) a rim attached to the tricuspid and A.V. membranes. In **4**, the blue and red beads indicate the anterior and posterior margins of apposition of the atria. The most anterior red bead is at the lower attachment of the right fibrous trigone and indicates the location of the A.V. node—its artery is seen running to it. In **5**, the margin of the apposition of the right to the left atrium (pink) is indicated by a blue strip. The membranous portion of the atrial septum (orange) is disposed in the axis of the inferior vena cava, as shown by the arrows in **1** and **4**. The axes of the venae cavae (**1**) form an obtuse angle.

6: After removal of the atria and the attachment of the posterolateral wall of the right ventricle to the A.V. membrane, note the latter in its entirety and the posterosuperior muscle process of the L.V.

Conclusion: (a) The tricuspid and mitral valves are widely separated by the posterosuperior process of L.V. (b) The muscle component of the septal leaflet attachment is 2.0 cm from the coronary sinus and 0.7 cm from the A.V. node and its artery. The attachment crosses the superior septal artery which is en route to supply the first division of the right bundle branch of the conduction system. (c) The course of the main trunk of the right coronary artery is variable; in this heart, it is distant to the muscular attachment of the leaflet. However, on the next page the contiguity of the two evinces the potential hazard to the artery during replacement of the tricuspid valve. (d) The axis of the sinus venarum of the right atrium crosses the left atrium at an angle of 60°.

* To avoid confusion, the traditional term, superior septal, is used—the spatially correct term is posterior septal—see page 86.

The Relation of the Right Coronary Artery to the Posterior Superior Process of the Left Ventricle

Specimen B: 1: Right lateral view: With the exception of rims at its attachments, the right atrium has been removed. The right coronary artery passes posteriorly, superiorly, and to the left over the posterior portion of the posterior superior process of L.V. (P.S.P.). Not a U, but obtuse-angled bend is seen in the artery at the site of origin of the A.V. node branch. In arteriography, the right lateral view is useful in studying the right coronary artery in this area.

Specimen C: 2: The inferior view: In the middle of the posterior right A.V. sulcus, the right coronary artery bifurcates into the posterior descending artery (P.D.A.) and the left ventricular branch (L.V.B.); the latter and all its elements exhibit no deflection as they cross the crux: This vessel has been reputed to always present a U-shaped bend, which is directed anterosuperiorly into the crux; from the apogee of this bend, the A.V. node artery arises. (It has also been postulated that the bend is caused by the inward pressure of the posterior interventricular vein during fetal development.) This conformation may well occur; however, in the majority of the specimens I have studied the vessel passes either below the posterior superior process or across its periphery to reach the left ventricle. (In arteriograms, a bend is often not seen.) However, it is important to note that striking incursions of the artery (L.V.B.) into the crux may occasionally be encountered.

Specimen D: 3 and 4: Nonattitudinal R.P.O. view: A green oxygen catheter has been inserted into the posterior interventricular vein, which is 3.5 cm posterior to the apex of the right coronary artery, which is in contact with the right fibrous trigone. The vein lies directly under the pericardium, which forms the floor of the crux. The artery hugs the margins of the triangular posterior superior process; its contact with the tricuspid and left ventricular ostia places it in jeopardy from injudiciously placed sutures during the replacement of either valve.

Specimen E: 5 and 6: Nonattitudinal right lateral view: The right atrium has been incised, leaving a small segment in relation to the apex of the posterior superior process. Again, the right coronary artery passes arteriorly over the process. A 5 mm-long A.V. node branch is present.

Conclusion: When the right coronary artery reaches the crux, it exhibits a variable relation to the tricuspid ostium and the ostium of L.V. It may (a) run in contact with both, resulting in a sharp angulation directed towards the right fibrous trigone, or (b) present a straight course from the posterior right A.V. sulcus to the posterior wall of the left ventricle, or (c) pursue a variety of courses between the two just described. The cause of death following cardiac operations often remains obscure—careful examination of the coronary arteries is important.

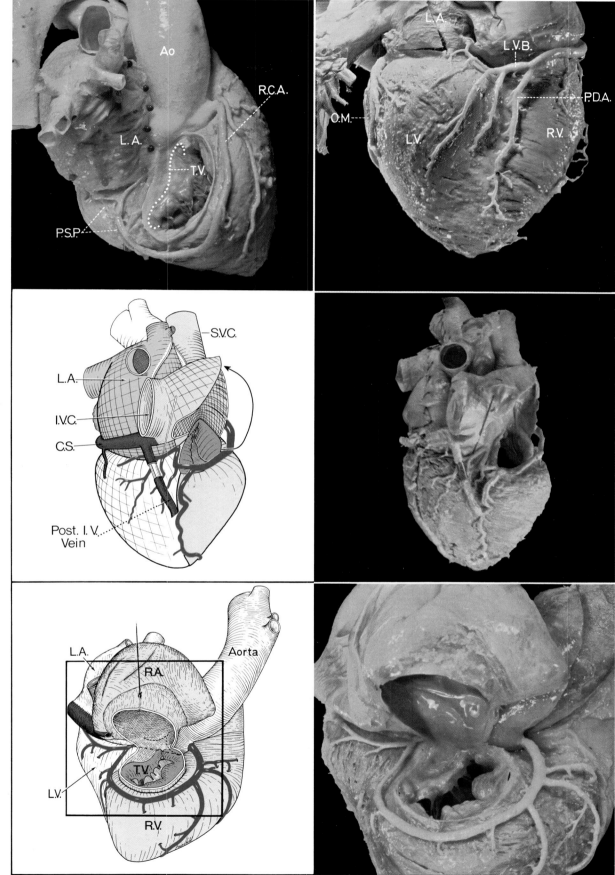

71

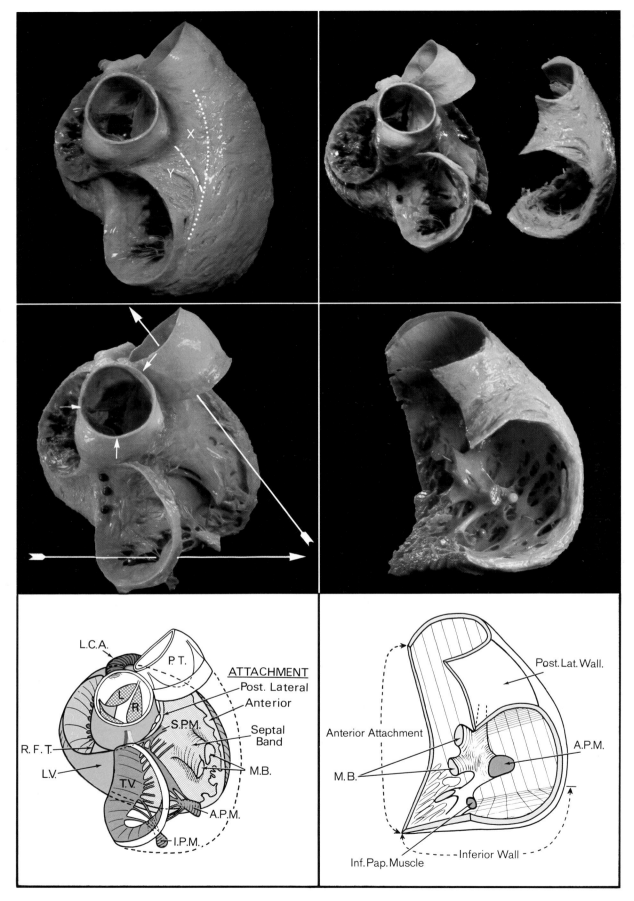

D. The Posterolateral Wall of the Right Ventricle and Its Attachment to the Aorto-Ventricular Unit

Specimen A: After removal of the atria and the great vessels above their sinuses, a superior right lateral view is seen in **1**, **2**, **3** and in **5**, the drawing of **3**.

1: The posterolateral wall, extending between the pulmonary and tricuspid ostia, is demarcated from the anterior wall by the dotted line. It is divided into infundibular (X) and sinus (Y) portions. Though both face posterolaterally, the infundibular portion faces more posteriorly than does the sinus portion. The sinus portion projects over the anterosuperior leaflet of the tricuspid valve and also faces superiorly. It is demarcated from the anterior wall by a furrow which is best seen in **73—3**.

2: Leaving rims at the tricuspid and pulmonary ostia, the three walls of the right ventricle have been divided at the site of their attachment to the A.V. unit. The walls are separated as a unit.

3 and **5**: Study **two determinants of the aortic sinus-ventricular wall relationship:** (a) **The relative size of the aortic sinuses** can be gauged by the distance between the aortic annular commissures, which are indicated by the short arrows in 3.* The measurements are right 26 mm, posterior 20.1 mm, and left 23.2 mm. (b) **Posterior shift of the attachment of the posterolateral wall to the A.V. membrane:** The posterior limit of this attachment usually underlies the right and posterior annular commissure. Here it is 12.0 mm past this point and only 7.0 mm from the nadir of the posterior annulus. The area of contact between the right aortic sinus and the wall parallels the increased size of the sinus: The decreased size of the posterior sinus diminishes the effect of the posterior shift of the wall attachment to the A.V. membrane on the relation of the posterior sinus to the right ventricle.

4 and **6**: P.A. view: The posterolateral wall roughly forms a trapezoid. The moderator band (red bead) is attached to the anterior wall, forming an angle of approximately 60° with the anterior papillary muscle (yellow bead). A large trabeculum passes inferiorly to the inferior papillary muscle (blue bead). The third portion of the right bundle branch terminates at the apex of the above angle. The excitory impulse first reaches these two papillary muscles. Note the parallel in the left ventricle, where the two bundle branches first reach the two papillary muscles.

The posterolateral wall of the right ventricle and the adjoining pulmonary ostium and sinuses are in contact with the left half of the right aortic sinus and left anterior fibrous trigone. Between these structures, dense connective tissue is present; sharp dissection may be needed for its division. Since no cord-like structure can be found, I suggest replacement of the term "conus tendon", which has been used to designate this connection, with the term infundibular or conus fascia.

* The arrows in **3** showing axes of the orifices are for future reference.

Specimen A—1–4

1 and **2**: After removal of the free wall, the specimen is viewed nonattitudinally with the apex below. The line of attachment of the posterolateral wall is seen. The bifid moderator band is a continuation of the septal band, the lower margin of which is in the sinus of the ventricle! This is also shown in **72—3**.

3: Superior right lateral view: The sinus portion of the posterolateral wall forms a hood over the tricuspid valve. A furrow marks its junction with the anterior wall of the right ventricle. The large size of the infundibulum is suggested in this nonattitudinal view.

4: Right lateral view: In this attitudinal photograph, observe three determinants of the aortic sinus-ventricular wall relationship. (1) The **infundibulum is large**; the plane of the pulmonary ostium meets the horizontal at a 45° angle. (2) The **large size and bulging conformation** of the right ventricle is evidenced here by the elevation of the tricuspid ostium in relation to the aorta and by the examination of **3**. (3) The **posterolateral attachment is shifted posteriorly**; it is only 7.0 mm from the right fibrous trigone; this, coincidentally, reduces the size of the atrial division of the membranous septum—the septum as a whole is small because the posterior aortic annulus is only 5 mm above the ostium of L.V.

Specimen B: 5 and 6

5: A nonattitudinal, superior L.A.O. view: A membranous segment of the posterolateral wall is present. I have observed this relatively often in humans and also in horses and bears. This is a possible cause of an aneurysm of the right ventricle when pressure in the chamber is high. The characteristic location is indicated by the orange triangle. The pulmonary ostium is well shown from this vantage point. From the three segments of the pulmonary trunk which remain, the pulmonary annuli extend inferiorly onto the internal surface of the right ventricle.

6: Nonattitudinal R.P.O. view of the same specimen after removal of the tricuspid valve: Note the attachment of the tricuspid leaflets, the septal to the muscular and membranous septa, and the anterosuperior to the membranous segment of the posterolateral wall of the right ventricle.

A very rare congenital malformation, the partial or complete absence of muscle of the right ventricle, was described and termed the **parchment heart** by Osler in 1905; however, Uhl described a case in 1952 and in some writings the term Uhl's anomaly is used. In most of the few cases reported, major segments of the wall have been involved; however, in 1964, Reeve and MacDonald predicted that instances of lesser involvement would be found. And Gould *et al.* then reported such a case in a 57-year-old man where two small areas of membrane were found; one in relation to the tricuspid valve measured 4.0 by 2.5 cm. The dimension seen in my material is approximately 2 cm². Aneurysmal-like dilatation of the right atrium (Tenckhoff *et al.*) and the atrial appendage also occur (Goodwin).

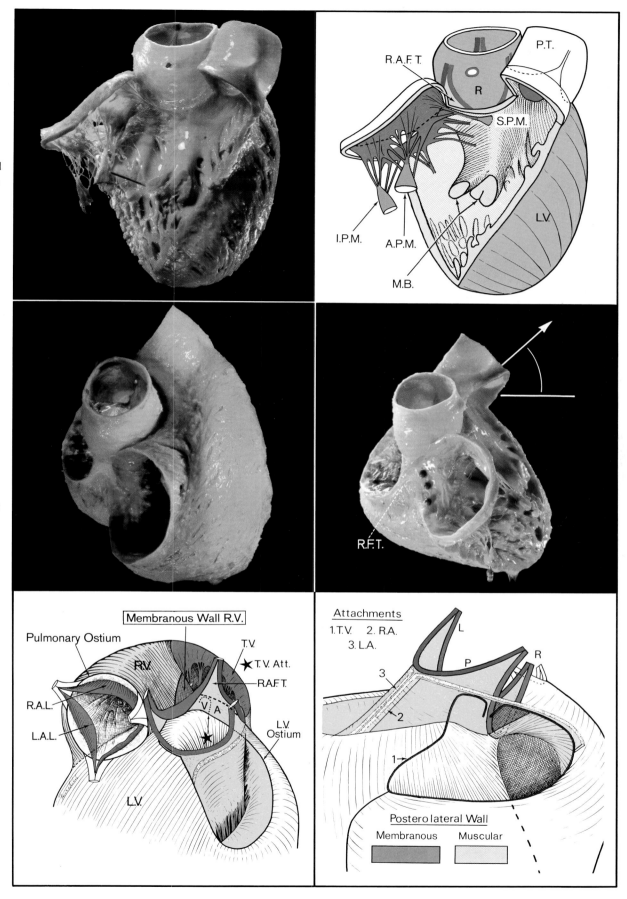

73

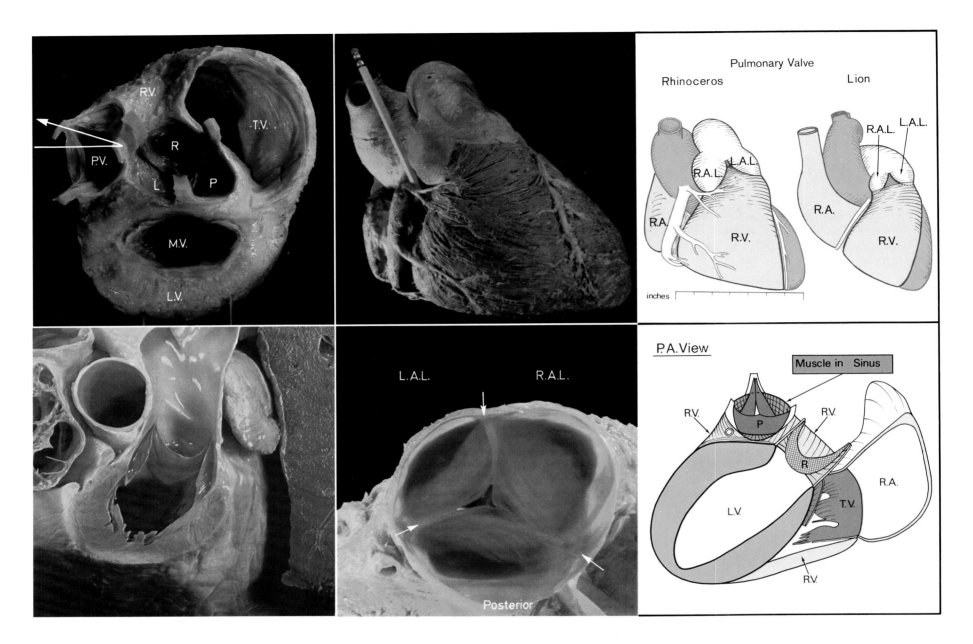

Pulmonary Valve

Rhinoceros   Lion

P.A. View

Muscle in Sinus

E. The Pulmonary Attachment of the Right Ventricle to the Aorto-Ventricular Unit

I. The Pulmonary Ostium and the Pulmonary Valve

1: The **ostrich heart** is examined from above and posteriorly. The great vessels, down to their annuli, and the atria have been removed. First review the anatomy of the pulmonary valve of the rhea, horse, and rhinoceros on page 16. In the rhea, the right ventricle wraps around the left to a degree which places the pulmonary valve leaflets and sinuses in the same disposition as those of the aortic. This phenomenon is less marked in the ostrich; the line between the ends of the right anterolateral pulmonary annulus is angled 20° anterior to the transverse. This can be compared with the angle seen in the human heart in **5**. The muscle in the aortic sinuses appear dark from blood staining.

2: **Rhinoceros:** Examine this specimen at a later stage of dissection in **16—6**. The pulmonary ostium is not round,

but tricornuate. The major portion of the pulmonary annuli is attached to muscle: The interannular fibrous trigones of the pulmonary valve are greatly reduced in size. The anterior trigone is shown in the drawing **3**, where this specimen is shown in contrast to the heart of a **lion,** wherein the arrangement of the pulmonary valve is identical with that seen in human hearts, to which we now return.

4: Anterosuperior View: This specimen appears in **125—3.** The line of transection crosses the infundibulum (of R.V.), the pulmonary ostium and trunk—the trunk is attached to the ostium—the leaflet attachment crosses the ostium. The atrial appendages are shown: The right transected, the left below the trunk. The posterior- right anterolateral pulmonary commissure adjoins the aorta.

5: The pulmonary valve of the specimen, which will be seen in **6** and **75—1–6**, is seen at a right angle to our plane of examination. The commissures between the annuli are marked by arrows. Muscle is present in each

of the sinuses between the leaflets and the pulmonary ostium.

6: The P.A. view demonstrates the incision made preparatory to the dissection seen on the next page. Three truncated triangles of the pulmonary trunk remain; attached to these are the leaflets on either side of the small interannular trigones.

Comment: (1) The pulmonary valve, with its extensive attachment to muscle, seems ill-suited from an immunologic basis for an allograft and poorly constructed for removal and replacement as an autograft. (2) In congenital pulmonary stenosis (see photographs: [a] Hudson, page 1891 [b] Parker) the leaflet tissue forms a truncated cone or dome with a distal orifice—the surgical re-creation of the normal anatomy is not possible. In isolated pulmonary stenosis, the effects of pulmonary regurgitation are rarely significant; hence, the functional result is satisfactory. In the tetralogy of Fallot, this insufficiency may be a factor in cardiac performance.

1 and **2**: The specimen is now examined from the same perspective as **74—6**. The muscle between the pulmonary annuli and the pulmonary ostium is shown in orange in **2**.

3 and **4**: The valve is tipped posteriorly to display the muscle in the posterior sinus to better advantage. The translucent leaflets are transilluminated from below in **3**. In **4**, the two anterior leaflets are deflected from the lumen, displaying their attachments in the interior of the ventricle and to the pulmonary trunk above; the anterior interannular trigone between the pulmonary annuli can be seen.

5 and **6**: The leaflets, except for a rim at their attachment to the inner surface of the ventricle, have been excised. The term "pulmonary annulus" denotes the fibrous attachment of each of the pulmonary leaflets. However, they are much less sturdy than the aortic annuli. The term pulmonary ring or annulus, used in reference to the entire valve, is quite inappropriate. There is a circular pulmonary ostium of the right ventricular muscle and three fibrous annuli from which the leaflets are suspended. On page 9 comments are found on the use, in this work, of the word annulus.

II. The Division of the Right Ventricular Chamber—the Sinus and the Infundibulum

Both the right and left ventricles have been divided into inflow and outflow segments. In order to evaluate the validity of this concept, we should first re-examine the left ventricle. In the horizontal transection in **53—6**, the shape of its cavity in systole roughly resembles a right-angle triangle—the base, hypotenuse, and perpendicular, are formed by the lateral and septal walls and the mitral valve, respectively. The chamber is not divisible into two discrete anatomic parts. A narrowed outlet, however, is present; it has been called either the vestibule (a chamber between the door and the interior of a room), or the infundibulum (L.=funnel), or less often the conus (Gr.=konus=cone). As seen in **116—4–6**, the walls of this outlet is formed anteriorly by the often intruding, ostial slope of the ventricle; however, in contrast to the right ventricle, the posterior wall is formed by the anterior leaflet of the inlet valve. The ingress and egress valves are in a single ostium.

In the right ventricle, an anatomically recognizable outflow tract, the infundibulum or conus, is present; it separates the inflow and outflow valves; its walls are muscle; below it is the inflow tract or sinus. The axes of the orifices of the two divisions roughly form an angle of 60°—see **72—3** and **73—1**. On the next page (76) we will examine the walls of the infundibulum and on page 77 we will study the degree of demarcation between the infundibulum and the sinus. On page 78 elevation of the pulmonary ostium and coincident elevation of the posterior wall is seen. On page 79 the attachment of the ostium is seen separated from the A.V. unit.

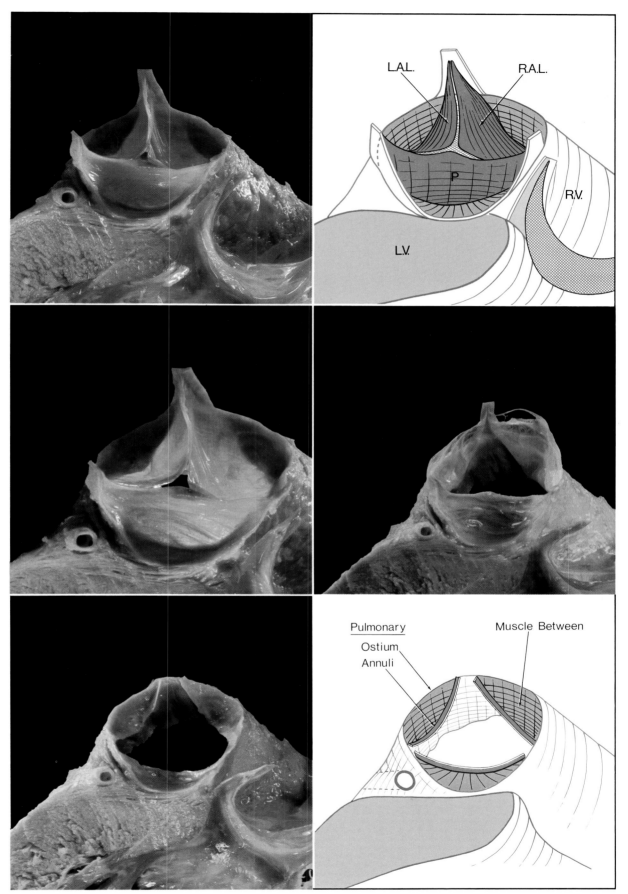

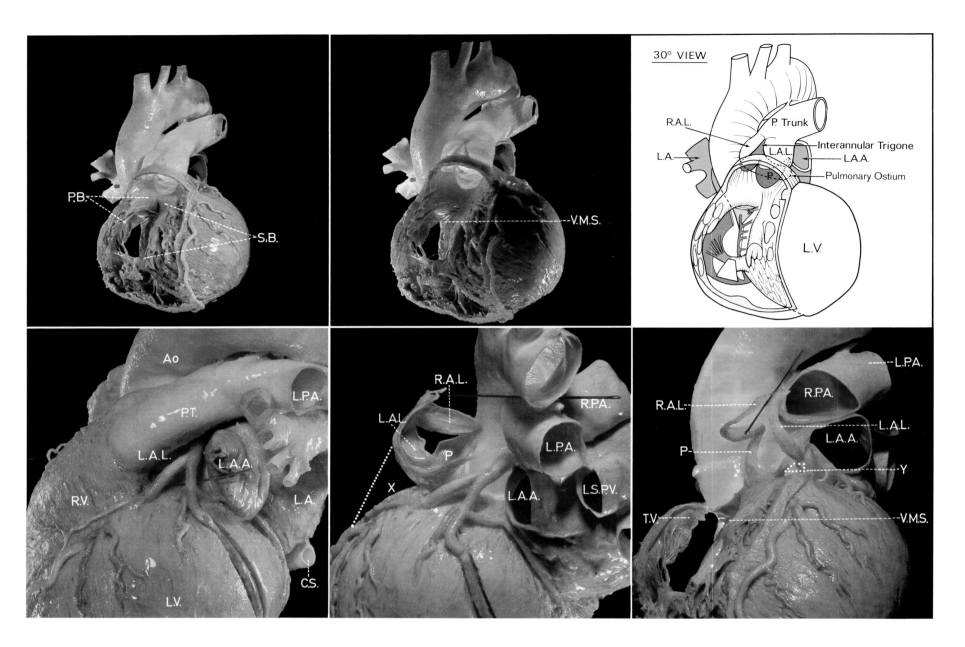

III. The Walls of the Infundibulum

In this work, the free wall of the right ventricle has been divided into anterior, posterolateral, and inferior walls: The upper portion of the infundibulum is a relatively tubular structure, hence this simplistic division requires elaboration. This will be carried out in **Specimen A—1–6**.

The Posterolateral Wall of the Infundibulum

1, **2**, and **3**: A 30° view: The anterior wall of the right ventricle has been removed. Observe: (a) The location of the septal (S.B.) and parietal (P.B.) muscle bands in this view. The latter runs in the posterolateral wall whose outer surface essentially faces in the directions indicated by its name. (b) **The pulmonary ostium—the round opening in the muscular wall of the right ventricle—** is indicated in **3**, and its anterior half is seen in **2**. (c) The posterior and right anterolateral pulmonary leaflets are seen below the posterior part of the ostium. (d) In **2** with interior lighting, the pulmonary annuli and the anterior interannular trigone are seen.

The Left Lateral Wall of the Infundibulum

4: An elevated left lateral view of the intact specimen: Inferior to the left anterior pulmonary sinus (L.A.L.), the wall of the infundibulum faces laterally. This is a part of what I have termed the anterior wall of the right ventricle. It may also be designated as the left lateral wall of the infundibulum.

5: An elevated L.P.O. view: The left atrial appendage (L.A.A.) and the pulmonary trunk, excluding the site of the pulmonary annular attachments, have been removed, as has the triangular portion of the anterior wall of the right ventricle just examined in **4** and labeled here as X.

The Supraseptal Portion of the Posterior Wall of the Infundibulum

The upper portion of the ventricular septum forms almost the entire portion of what may be termed the posterior wall of the infundibulum. The latter also pos-

sesses, in this specimen as in most, a small supraseptal portion—see area Y in **6**.

6: L.A.O. view: Observe: (a) The pulmonary annuli are located in the following order from above downward: the right anterolateral (R.A.L.), the left anterolateral (L.A.L.), and the posterior (P.). (b) The supraseptal portion (Y) underlies the adjacent parts of the posterior and left anterolateral annuli.

Comments: Consistent with its functional role, the muscle wall of the normal right ventricle is neither thick nor sturdily structured. This relative friability probably explains the infrequent use of left lateral atriotomy for open operations on the mitral valve entailing, as this approach does, cannulation of the right ventricle through the anterior wall of the infundibulum. In the same context, a cardiac catheter passed from the right femoral vein tends to become engaged by the left lateral or the supraseptal walls of the infundibulum—perforation may result.

IV. The Demarcation of Sinus and Infundibulum

Specimen B: 1, 2, 3, and **4:** Attidudinal lateral views: Transection: Nearly sagittal through (1) the lateral 1/3 of the right anterolateral pulmonary leaflet, (2) the middle of the right and the right portion of the left aortic leaflets, (3) the posterior superior process of L.V. (P.S.P.) and (4) the anterior leaflet of the mitral valve anterior to the commissures (A.M.V.).

The Infundibulum: Observe: (a) The pulmonary ostium extending anterosuperiorly at an angle of 45° forms **its upper border.** (b) "The infundibular muscles form **the lower border**"—How precise is this statement? The free. 12 mm wide moderator band (M.B.), seen in **2** and **4**, is an extension of the septal band; however its lower margin is at a low level, well below the superior papillary muscle (of Lancisi or of Luschka) which also has been used as a point of demarcation between the infundibulum and the sinus. (c) The parietal band (see **1** and **3**) projects anteriorly as a curved promontory above the tricupid valve; it fades out above the anterior papillary muscle. **It forms the posterolateral wall.** The curved oblique dotted line in **3** runs between it and the anterior wall. (d) The left lateral wall has been just defined. It is above the dotted line seen in **2**. (e) The **anterior wall** as indicated in **4** is much larger than the posterior. (f) The short **posterior wall** is in contact with the left half of the right aortic sinus. (Conus and infundibulum are synonyms.)

The Sinus: It is subdivided into a proximal part seen in **3** and the highly trabeculated **apical recess** seen on page 80. Observe: (a) The right (therefore the inferior) half of the right aortic sinus is above the sinus, which may roll over it as seen on **73—3**. (b) The superior, anterior, and inferior papillary muscles provide insertion for the chordae from the portion of the tricuspid valve which is in relation to the free walls of the ventricle. Most of the chordae from the septal leaflet are attached with or without intermediation of small papillae to the septal wall. Some pass to the inferior papillary muscle.

Do the Infundibular Muscles Demarcate the Divisions? In many normal hearts, they are often poorly developed and their margins, in lack of harmony with their definition, are often found in the sinus—the answer is often negative. **Other features:** (a) The proximal right pulmonary artery (R.P.A.) lies in the 60–240° plane; it is seen at an angle of 150° in this lateral (90–270°) plane. (b) Below the right pulmonary artery, the transverse sinus of the pericardium (green) covers the left sinus node artery which, in this instance, is superficial to the interatrial muscle bundle. (c) The membranous septum slopes to the right, superiorly and slightly posteriorly. (d) In the left atrium, the dots in **1** indicate the junction between the septal and posterior walls. The membranous portion of the former is seen transilluminated in the photograph. (e) The coronary sinus is sectioned just to the left of its termination.

Specimen C: 5 and **6**: The superior cavo-atrial angle (see page 7) and the pulmonary ostium are found in a low horizontal line; both the right atrium and the infundibulum are short, in contrast to the specimen on the next page. The axes (arrows) will be discussed on page 79.

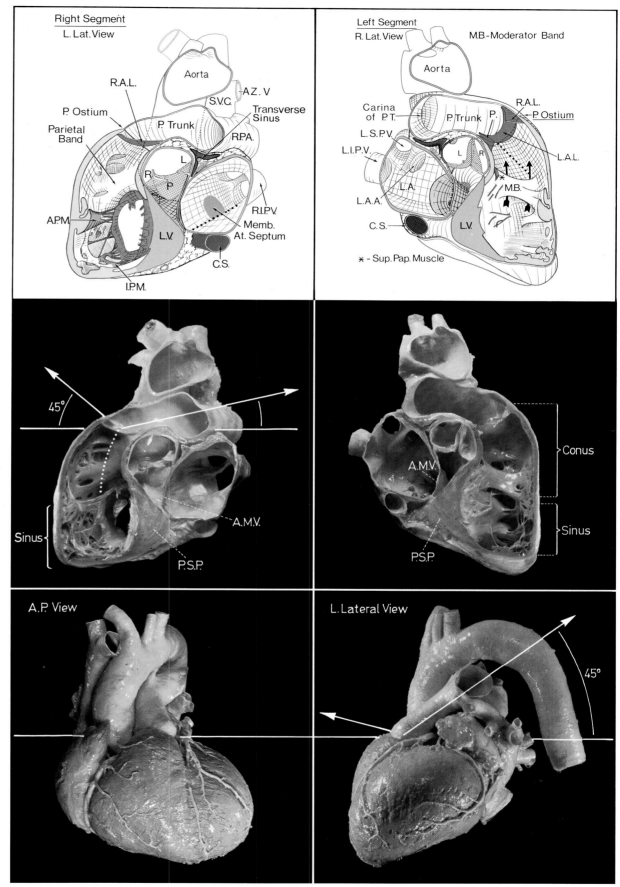

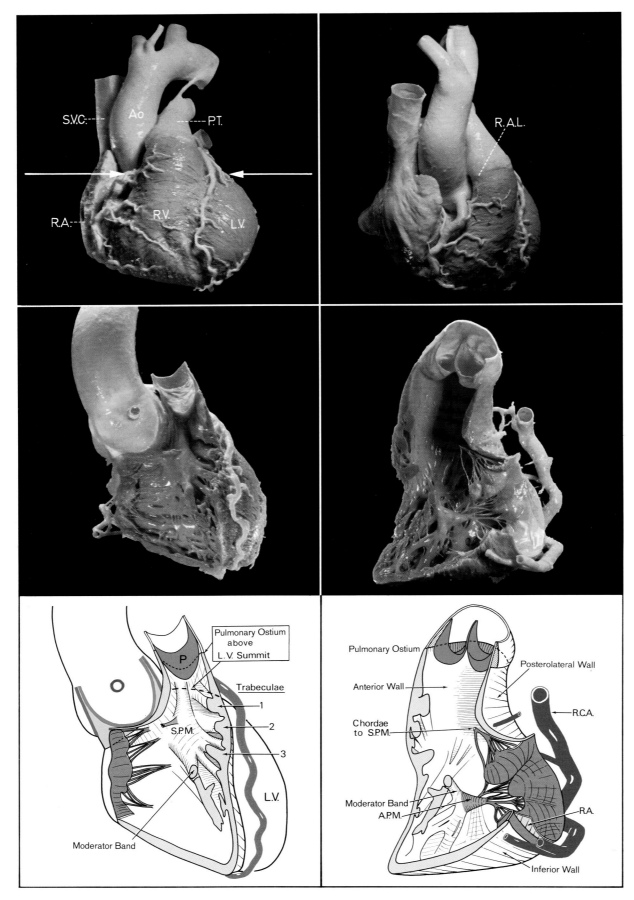

V. Variations in the Infundibulum

The Elevated Pulmonary Ostium

Specimen A 78—1–6 and **79—1** and **2**

1: A.P. view: The infundibulum rises high above the upper surface of the left ventricle and the level of the right coronary artery orifice, which are indicated by arrows.

2: Superior R.A.O. view: The infundibulum rises above the level of the right aortic sinus. The gently curved anterior wall meets the posterolateral wall beneath the nadir of the right anterolateral leaflet of the pulmonary valve (R.A.L.).

After transection of the pulmonary trunk above its sinuses and removal of the atria, the anterior, posterolateral, and inferior walls are separated from the A.V. unit, leaving the posterior leaflet of the pulmonary valve and the septal leaflet of the tricuspid valve on the posterior segment. The posterior segment is seen in **3** and **5** and the anterior in **4** and **6**.

In **3** and **5** observe: (a) The pulmonary ostium is elevated above the left ventricle. Below the entire posterior annulus, a large supraseptal portion of the posterior infundibular wall is present.* (b) Three large trabeculae are present in the septal band, which terminates as the moderator band.

In **4** and **6**: (a) The pulmonary leaflet attachments cross the pulmonary ostium. (b) The anterior papillary muscle is low in the ventricle. (c) In the anterior wall, the trabeculae run vertically and are usually not prominent. (d) The infundibular portion of the posterolateral wall faces posterolaterally—the sinus portion, which forms a mantle over the tricuspid valve, as seen on page 72, faces almost superiorly. (e) On page 65, we noted the factors affecting the aortic sinus-ventricular wall relationship. The large infundibulum is related to the aortic wall above the right aortic sinus. (f) In this 310-gram heart, the right coronary artery measures 8 mm in diameter. The left main coronary branch measures 6 mm at its origin. Both vessels appeared entirely normal at subsequent detailed examination, and there was no evidence of any abnormality, such as aortic insufficiency, to account for their large size. This is cited as an example of the considerable variation in size of coronary arteries. Precise information is lacking regarding the normal range of caliber of coronary arteries: In this atlas, considerable variation is seen—see pages 174–175. Lars Bjork (1965) reported the occurrence of "ectasia of the coronary arteries" in the tetralogy of Fallot. In a 24-year-old patient—the hematocrit was 79%—"tortuous and 10- to 12-mm-wide arteries" were observed in an aortogram and at operation; they were otherwise normal. He also found ectasia of a lesser degree in two children. (g) In **6**, the muscle in the left anterolateral and the right anterolateral sinuses is colored orange.

---

*   The supraseptal portion of the posterior wall, seen on page 76, lies on the left side of a normally attached posterior pulmonary annulus.

1 and **2**: A posterior nonattitudinal view of the segment of the heart just examined displays the **elevation of the pulmonary ostium** and a segment of the posterior infundibular wall **above the level of the left ventricle**. The lighting in **1** was used to demonstrate a feature not related to this discussion; namely, the presence of elevation of the subvalvular segment of the aorto-ventricular membrane; additional views of this specimen and a discussion of this subject are on page 48.

Depression of Infundibular Attachment

Specimen B: **3**, **4**, **5**, and **6**: Turn to **51—1** and **2** and note the details and description of the initial transection. Return to this page and note in **79—3** and **4**, after removal of the fat, that the infundibulum, not the pulmonary ostium, is attached to the left ventricular component of the A.V. unit. (In **3**, the tissue between the left atrium and the pulmonary artery (R.P.A.) and the fat in the posterior A.V. sulcus have been removed; an artifactitious depression of the left atrium results; its orientation in **4** is correct).

Comment: The posterior wall of the infundibulum may extend above the left ventricle (Specimen A) or the two structures may be separated by fat (Specimen B). Hence in the operative correction of the tetralogy of Fallot, removal of muscle of the posterior wall of the infundibulum may result in perforation of the right ventricle; on page 172 it will be seen that division of the large left superior septal artery may occur at the same time.

VI. The Axes of the Pulmonary Ostium and the Pulmonary Trunk

It has been indicated previously that one determinant of the size of the infundibulum is the axis of the pulmonary ostium (see pages 72 and 73). The axes of the ostium and the trunk are important in diagnosis. Examine each of these two axes and their interrelationship in four specimens: the first is seen here—**79—3**, the second and third on page **77—3** and **6**, and the fourth on pages 176 and 177. The following may be inferred: (a) The elevation of the axis of the trunk is greater when the infundibulum is poorly developed. (b) The infundibulum is less well developed in the presence of a horizontal heart, which is exemplified by the third (**77—6**) and fourth (pages 176–177) specimens. Note the angle formed by the ostial and trunk axes in the four specimens—112°, 122°, 107°, and 105°, respectively.

Clinical Implication: (a) (1) In the presence of a more horizontal axis of **the pulmonary trunk**, a cardiac catheter, seen in A.P. fluoroscopy, remains at a near horizontal level as it passes from the right ventricle through the pulmonary valve into the pulmonary trunk; its location cannot be determined from its height. (2) The axis of the trunk becomes more horizontal as the diaphragm moves cephalad; this occurs in the supine and often sedated patient during cardiac catheterization. (b) A decrease in the angle of elevation of the pulmonary trunk exaggerates the degree of its superimposition on the left pulmonary artery in A.P. angiocardiography. (c) In optimal radiographic studies, an elevated view is used—see page 123.

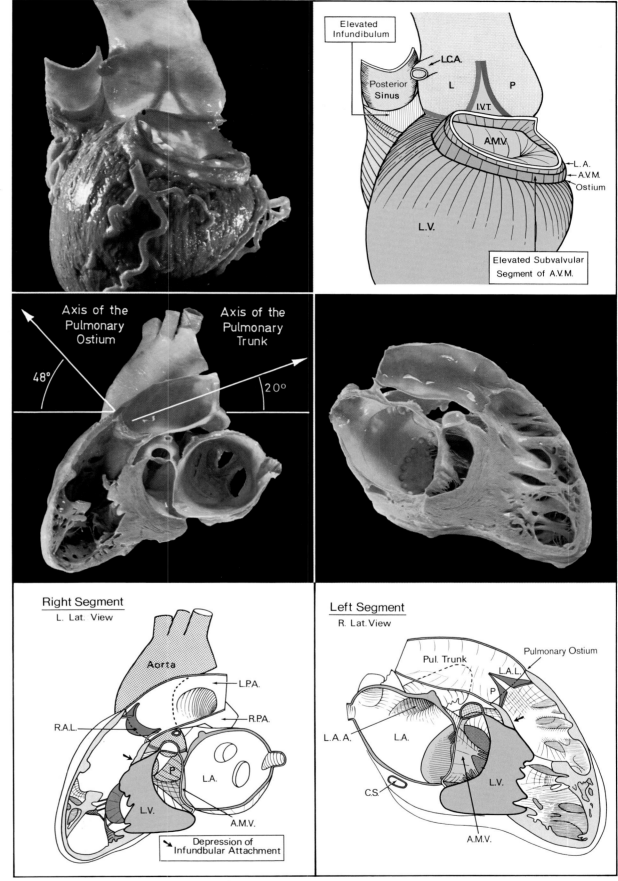

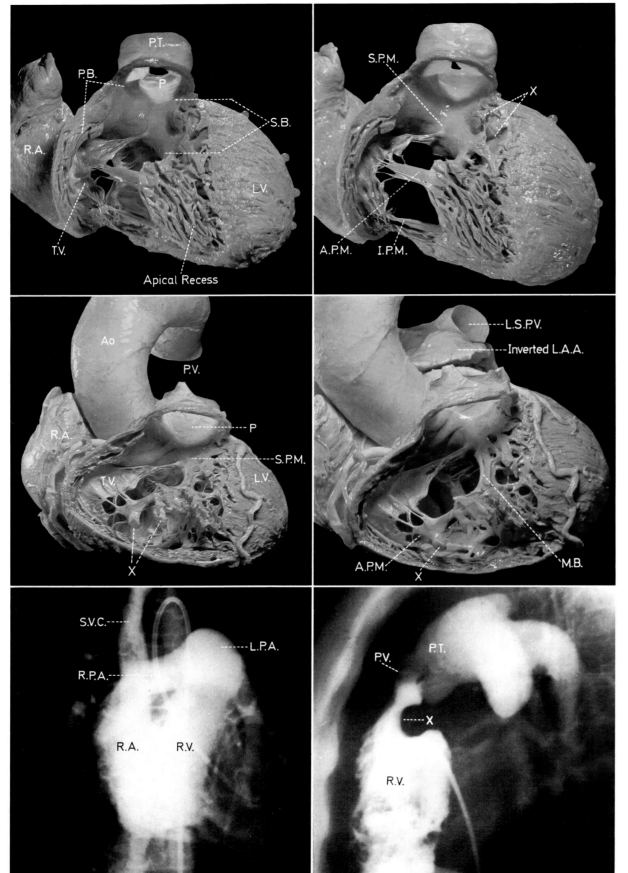

F. The Muscles of the Right Ventricle

Specimen A: 1 and **2**: The anterior and inferior walls have been removed. Observe: (a) The trabeculae at the apex have been sectioned to reveal their profusion. (b) The posterior, right anterolateral, and left anterolateral pulmonary leaflets are transilluminated and their locations are well seen in **2**. (c) A line drawn between the superior papillary muscle (S.P.M.) and the nadir of the posterior pulmonary leaflet demarcates the parietal and the septal bands. (d) This line is 23.0 cm in length, in contrast to specimen B, where shortening of the posterior wall of the infundibulum is present. (e) The septal band (S.B.) extends inferiorly to the anterior papillary muscle (A.P.M.). (f) Large trabeculae (X) are present below the pulmonary valve on the left. (g) The large parietal band (P.B.) projects over the anterosuperior leaflet of the tricuspid valve. (h) The base of the anterior papillary muscle is 43 mm from the tricuspid orifice and 37 mm from the anterior interventricular groove.

Specimen B: 3 and **4**: A.P. and superior A.P. views: Observe: (a) The superior papillary muscle is only 13.2 mm below the posterior pulmonary leaflet, an example, in a normal heart, of **shortening of the infundibulum**; this is seen in the tetralogy of Fallot. (b) The septal band is fragmented into multiple small trabeculae, which extend forward between the lower border of the moderator band and the pulmonary valve. (c) A free **moderator band** (M.B.) reaches the anterior wall to the left of the anterior papillary muscle, which is attached to the anterior wall by two trabeculae (X). (d) The parietal band is poorly developed. (e) The **anterior papillary muscle** (A.P.M.) is located 33 mm from the tricuspid orifice and 52 mm from the anterior interventricular groove.

5: An A.P. view following simultaneous caval injections: Seen from this view, the right ventricle presents a truncated triangular shape, with the base inferiorly. However, when viewing a ventriculogram, this triangularity may not be noted. Since the septal and anterior walls meet at an acute angle anteriorly, the A.P. dimension is small at their junction and the apical area is frequently occupied by trabeculae. Hence, in contrast studies, the right ventricle may present a rectangular shape extending from below, upward, and to the left.

6: A left lateral view is seen of a selective right ventriculogram in a patient with pure pulmonic stenosis. The hypertrophied infundibular muscle (X) bulges into the ventricular cavity just below the stenotic pulmonary valve. This bulge is frequently termed the crista supraventricularis, as indicated on page 65.
Note the comments on the relation of the septal arteries to the operative correction of the tetralogy of Fallot which appear on page 172.

Specimen C: 1–6: The following have been removed: (1) the left atrium, (2) the free walls of L.V. in all but **5**, (3) the pulmonary trunk and sinuses in all but **6**, and (4) the anterior and inferior walls of the right ventricle.

1: Nonattitudinal R.A.O. view: The **septal band** consists of multiple large fasciculi. These require division in operations for the correction of the tetralogy of Fallot. A fasciculus extends vertically, through the junction of the parietal and septal bands; it descends from the nadir of the posterior pulmonary leaflet to the superior papillary muscle and then on to the anterior wall just above the attachment of the duplicated **anterior papillary muscle**, the base of which is 43 mm from both the tricuspid orifice and the anterior interventricular groove. The **parietal band** has a well-defined, large lower fasciculus which courses just above the tricuspid valve leaflets and a secondary higher fasciculus.

2: A.P. view: The level of attachment of the anterior papillary muscle in this specimen is below that seen in the first specimen on the preceding page. The septal and parietal bands together extend like a horseshoe downward and forward to reach the anterior wall; hence, **the dimension of the anterior wall of the infundibulum is greater than the posterior.** The transilluminated pulmonary leaflets are seen at 12 o'clock.

3: The line of attachment of the inferior wall of the right ventricle to the unit is inferior and horizontal in the photograph. The tricuspid orifice is vertical. The **inferior papillary muscle** is between the inferior attachment and the anterior papillary muscle.

4: The two bands of the infundibular muscle pass to the anterior wall, forming with it the boundary of **the infundibular ostium.** The infundibular muscles may hypertrophy; e. g., in right ventricular diastolic overloading, this orifice may be reduced to a few millimeters in diameter—this process is seen in instances of ventricular septal defects which progress into a pink tetralogy. Infundibular muscle obstruction occurs as an isolated congenital malformation but is much more commonly seen in association with (a) ventricular septal defects, (b) pulmonary valve obstruction, and (c) the combination of (a) and (b).

5: An infero-anterior view: Note the marked development of the trabeculae at the apex and separation of the anterior papillary muscle from the latter. Permanent pacemaker electrodes are "engaged" by these trabeculae in this, **the apical recess of the right ventricle.**

6: Superior A.P. view: In the examination of contrast studies, one should recall that **the right ventricle, like the left, has a zone of maximum dimension.** It extends, as indicated by the arrow, from the attachment of the septal leaflet (X), in the plane of the tricuspid ostium. In angiocardiography, the contrast will be maximum in this zone.

The tricuspid leaflets throughout present multiple small cusps—there is no suggestion of a division into three leaflets.

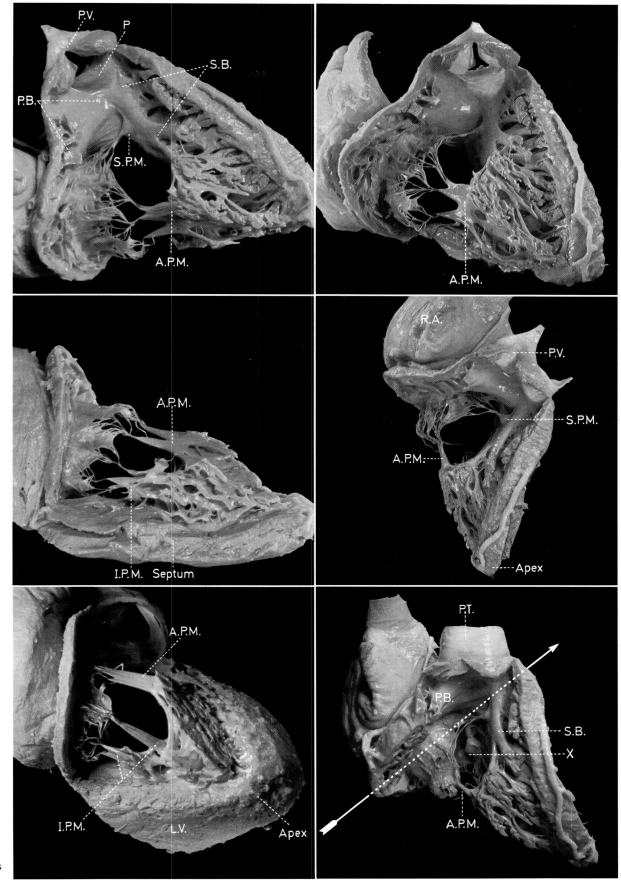

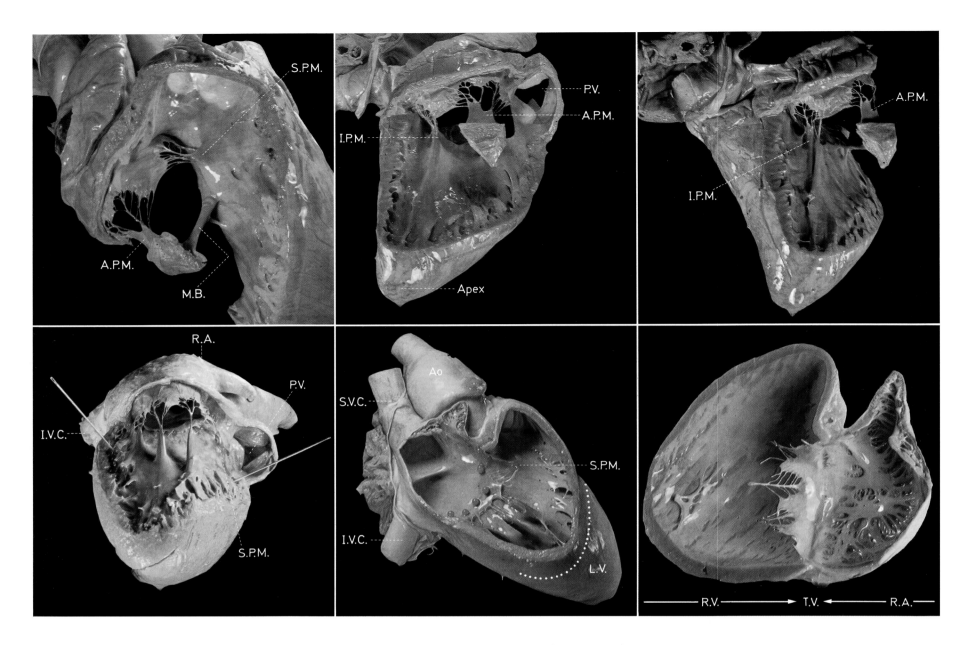

G. The Tricuspid Valve

I. The Tricuspid Valves
of Four Animal and Four Human Hearts

On page 16, the tricuspid valve in a bird (rhea) can be seen and its muscular anterolateral unicusp noted.

1, 2, and 3: Himalayan Mountain Goat. The right ventricle is seen after removal of the inferior wall and the anterior wall with the exception of an island at the site of attachment of the anterior papillary muscle. **1**: Anterosuperior view: The pulmonary valve is at 12 o clock. **2**: An apex view. **3**: Posterior view. Observe: (a) The superior papillary muscle is located at the junction of the infundibulum and sinus. (b) A free moderator band passes to the smooth, triangular anterior papillary muscle, which is close to the tricuspid orifice. (c) The inferior papillary muscle is attached to the septum. (d) The walls are atrabecular. (e) A small anterior, and large superior and inferior leaflets are present.

4, 5, and 6: Black Bear *(Ursus americanus)*—two specimens.
4: The apex view following removal of the anterior and inferior walls: The chordae from the nonseptal leaflets are attached to a single, small superior papillary muscle and to four conical papillary muscles which are attached to the septum. This arrangement is a characteristic of this species. The needles are placed at right angles to the septal surface, one below the pulmonary valve, and one just above the inferior attachment. The angle formed by the axes of the needles (110°) is indicative of the degree to which the right ventricle wraps around the left. This may be compared to a human specimen on page **66** where the same measurement was 93°.

5 and 6: An oblique transection passes through the right atrium and ventricle of this specimen. The lowest papillary muscle is not visible. The red beads indicate the attachment of the septal leaflet. In **6**, the right anterolateral segment is shown, demonstrating the highly characteristic arrangement of the leaflets in this species. Forty

specimens have been examined, and the appearance shown here is one of the few constants observed in the anatomy of the tricuspid valve. In **5**, observe the sharp ridge in the right atrium passing from the medial to the posterior wall; it should be recalled when the tuber of Lower of human hearts is studied.

The hearts of avia, and mammalia below the primate level exhibit atrabecular internal surfaces in all chambers except the right atrium, and in this chamber, seen in **6**, the pattern is less exuberant than that seen in humans. There is little to remind one of the muscles of the human infundibulum which are so often strongly marginated and multiple, and the contrast in the sinus is even greater. In the goat heart, the superior and inferior leaflets are both prominent and the anterior leaflet is small; this pattern is only one of the many which may be seen in human hearts.

1: Zebra: The inferior view: An island (X) of the anterior wall remains. To this island the anterior papillary muscle and the moderator band are attached. The former is close to the tricuspid orifice and the latter is long and free but of small caliber. The leaflets are five in number. The superior (1), anterior (2), and an antero-inferior (3), are equal in size. A smaller inferior leaflet (4) is present. The septal cannot be seen. The inferior papillary muscle is attached to the septal wall.

2: The Porcine Heart: L.A.O. view: The anterior and inferior walls of the right ventricle and large portions of the left ventricle have been removed. The anterior papillary muscle is again close to the tricuspid ostium. The large size of the moderator band, characteristic of this species, is seen.
In conclusion: (a) In the hearts of these four animals the ventricles exhibit a conical shape, which is unlike that seen in humans. The apex is formed strictly by the left ventricle and is widely separated from the right ventricle. (b) In all specimens, the inferior papillary muscle is attached to the septum. (c) With the exception of the bear, the anterior papillary muscle is attached to the anterior wall, closer to the tricuspid valve than is usual in human hearts. (d) In the bear, the counterpart of the anterior papillary muscle is formed by four separately based muscles which are attached not to the anterior wall but to the septum. The dispositions (b) and (c) are seen in the human hearts **3** and **4**, respectively, and multiple anterior papillary muscles are seen in **4**, **5**, and **6**, although they remain attached to the anterior wall.

The Tricuspid Valve of Four Human Hearts

3: R.A.O. view: A strip of the anterior wall of the right ventricle (Y) remains; the anterior papillary muscle is attached to it. The remainder of the free wall of the ventricle and the pulmonary valve has been removed. The aortic valve leaflets are at 11 o'clock. **The base of the inferior papillary muscle is attached to the septal wall.**

4: The upper component (A.P.M.[1]) of the duplicated anterior papillary muscle is only 15 mm from the tricuspid ostium; it is attached to the triangular island (X) of the anterior wall of the right ventricle which remains. The lower component (A.P.M.[2]) is confluent with and meets the moderator band (M.B.) behind the strip of unremoved anterior wall (Y). A drawing and a different view of this specimen should be seen in **153—1** and **2**.

5: Nonattitudinal A.P. view: A large triangle of the anterior wall and the inferior and posterolateral walls remain. The red beads mark the anterior interventricular groove. Observe: (a) There are 6 small anterior and 2 small superior papillary muscles. (b) A large anterosuperior leaflet is present—a common finding in human hearts.

6: R.A.O. view: Duplication of the anterior papillary muscle is seen. The upper muscle bifurcates, and its lower limb passes below the level of the lower anterior papillary muscle.

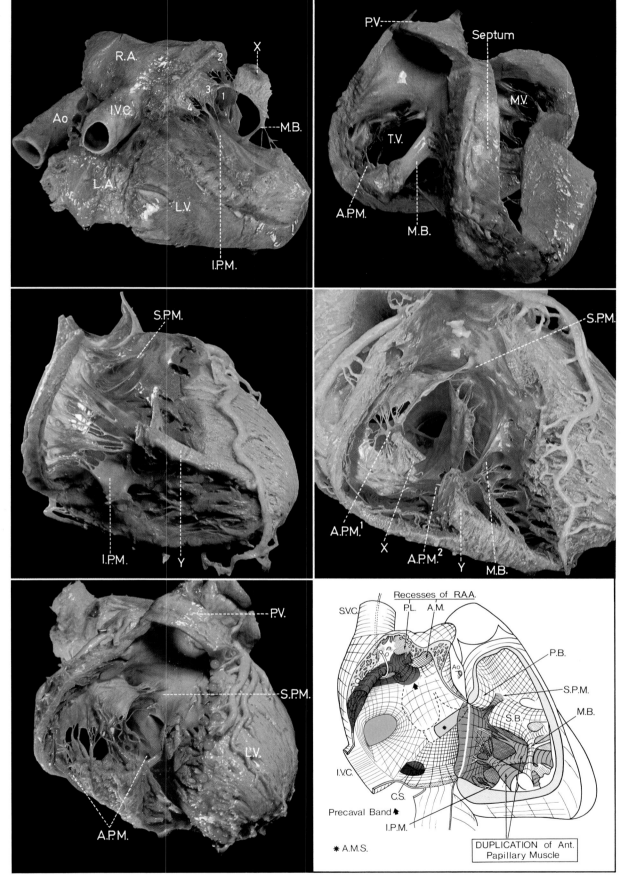

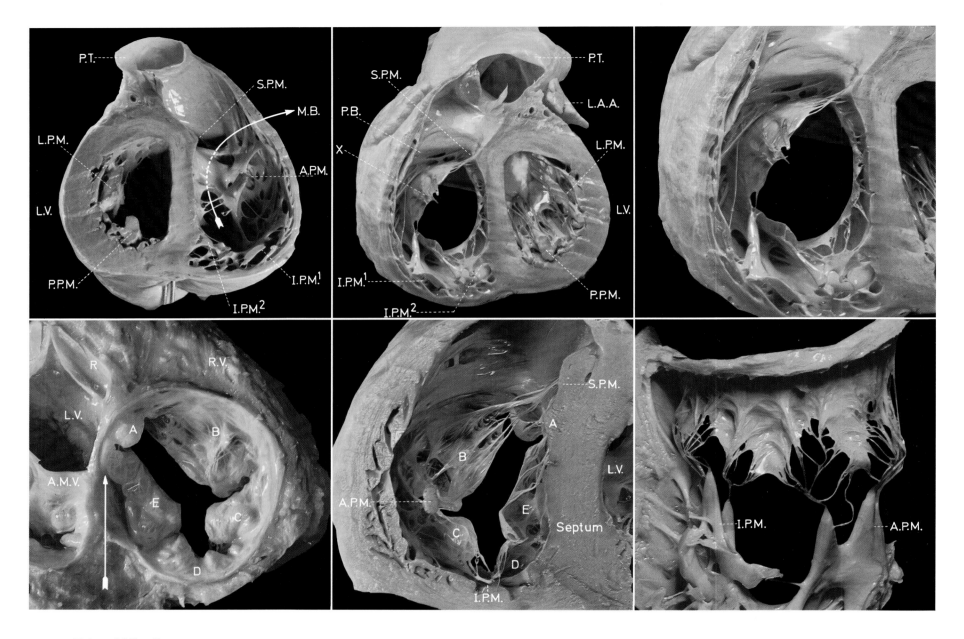

II. The Tricuspid Leaflets

Specimen A: 1, **2**, and **3**: Transection has been carried out in the R.A.O.-L.P.O. plane. In **1**, the left anterior segment is viewed from R.P.O.; in **2** and **3**, the right posterior segment is seen, not strictly from L.A.O. (45°), but from 30° to afford visualization of the septal leaflet, the attachment of which is to the left of the septal margin and, hence, not well seen at 45°. The plane of the tricuspid ostium meets the plane of an L.A.O.-R.P.O. examination at a right angle. In **2** and **3**, first note that **the tricuspid ostium or orifice is elliptical.** It can be divided into medial (or septal), inferior, anterior, and superior portions. The line of transection has passed through the base of the superior papillary muscle (S.P.M.), the chordae from which extend to **the antero-superior leaflet** which is in relation to the entire superior and the upper 90% of the anterior portion of the orifice. From the apex of this leaflet (X), chordae pass to the anterior papillary muscle (A.P.M.). Two **inferior papillary muscles** are present. The first (I.P.M.[1]) receives chordae from the anterosuperior and the inferior leaf-

lets. The second (I.P.M.[2]) is attached to the septal wall and receives chordae from the septal and inferior leaflet. In current terminology, the first leaflet described here would probably be designated as the anterior, although a large portion of it is related to the superior portion of the tricuspid ostium. In the L.A.O. view, the parietal band seen passing above the tricuspid ostium (in **2**) is at a right angle to the plane of examination. The septal band is parallel to this plane; hence, with the exception of the moderator band (M.B.), it is not seen. The latter crosses to the anterior wall at a right angle to the plane of examination. The details of the left ventricle of this specimen are on page 121.

Specimen B: 4: R.P.O., **5**: L.A.O. The leaflets are in a position approaching systolic; they are at a right angle to this L.A.O.-R.P.O. plane and are seen from both its aspects. Three papillary muscles are present. The point indicated by the arrow in **4** is the junction of the muscular and membranous components of the septal leaflet. It is, of course, located on the ostium of the left ventricle.

The membranous attachment is frequently interrupted, but usually the upper component is continuous with the anterosuperior leaflet. In a minority of specimens, a separate superior accessory leaflet is present, as we see here designated by the letter A. An anterosuperior (B) and a smaller antero-inferior (C) leaflets are present. An inferior leaflet (D) and a septal leaflet (E) also appear. This specimen demonstrates the difficulty in attempting to identify the three leaflets usually described.

Specimen C: 6: The inferior view of the specimen seen on page 81 shows the presence of multiple small leaflets which are seen throughout the entire valve. The appearance is similar to that seen in the bear heart on page 82, although in the latter the pattern is more geometric. The inferior papillary muscle is attached to the inferor wall of the ventricle (**81—3**).

Specimen D: In this heart, seen in a nonattitudinal manner, the anterior and inferior walls of the right ventricle have been removed with the exception of a strut in each wall at the site of attachment of the anterior and inferior papillary muscles. At this stage of dissection, the specimen is seen in **1** from a left superior view, **3** an apex view, and **5** an inferior view. The views in **2**, **4**, and **6** approximate those in **1**, **3**, and **5**; however, the posterolateral wall has been removed, and the plane of examination parallels the plane of the valve orifice. The **anterosuperior leaflet** is the largest; it is best seen in **1** and **2**. It is attached by chordae to the superior and anterior papillary muscles. **The superior papillary muscle receives no chordae from the septal leaflet.** The **anterior leaflet** (X) seen best in **3** and **4**, is considerably smaller. Chordae from it are attached to the anterior and the inferior papillary muscles. From the inferior view (**5** and **6**), note that only a band of leaflet tissue passes from the anterior to the septal leaflet—no "cusp" is present.

Apart from the present topic, note the large main septal artery arising from the upper part of the anterior interventricular groove in **1** and **2**. Two other views, one in a drawing, are found in 172—**3** and **4**.

Conclusion

1. The arrangement of the tricuspid leaflets is simple in one respect only: In systole, their nonappositional portions are disposed in a single plane.

2. The largest leaflet is usually anterosuperior, not anterior.

3. The inferior may be absent.

4. The number of leaflets is highly variable: Three leaflets are not seen with adequate frequency to justify the term tricuspid.

5. The pattern seen in this specimen, demonstrating a large anterosuperior, a smaller anterior, a septal, and no inferior, is commonly seen.

6. The septal leaflet has been discussed on pages 12-14. Its attachment is highly variable. In many specimens, an important gap is present between it and the anterosuperior leaflet.

7. *Cuspis*, in Latin, indicates a point or a pointed end or apex. *Tricuspid* suggests three triangular leaflets. The leaflets are often not triangular—in this regard, tricuspid is often not descriptive.

8. Three leaflets have been termed anterior, posterior, and medial. These terms result from examining the heart in a nonattitudinal manner with the apex inferiorly and the septa in a sagittal plane. The (spatially) correct terms are anterosuperior, inferior, and septal (or medial).

9. The leaflets are thin and delicate as indicated by (a) transillumination in **3** and (b) their transparency in **2**—with surface lighting, the black background is visible in the leaflet directly below 12 o'clock. *Clinical Inference:* A normal leaflet—divided to facilitate transatrial exposure of the right ventricle—is difficult to repair.

10. In contrast to the mitral valve, (a) the tricuspid chordae are attached to the margins and the entire ventricular aspect of the leaflets and (b) the papillary muscles protrude freely into the ventricular cavity.

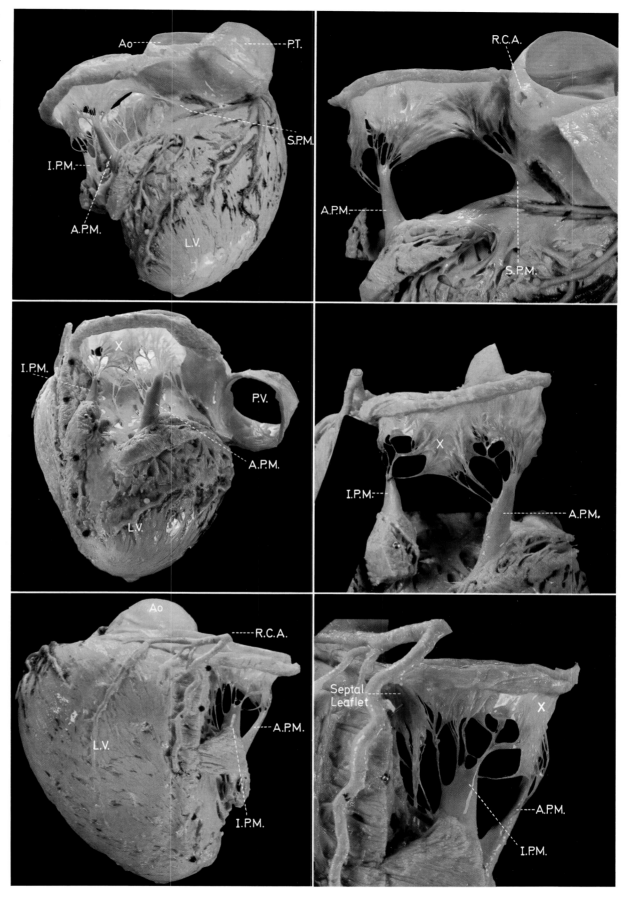

H. The Surface Connections of the Cardiac Chambers

If **the atrioventricular sulcus** is defined as the fat-filled space, roofed by the pericardium, between the atria and the ventricles, it is immediately evident that it provides an imperfect reference point. Its shape and size vary in different locations and its upper and lower margins, the lines of pericardial reflection, vary with the amount of fat present—in the hearts of wild animals and humans of similar good health, the fat is meager and a prominent sulcal depression is present between the atria and the ventricles—this condition is usually only seen in children—its absence in adults is, in part, a reflection of the present plague-producing Western nutritional habits. The cause of description would be served if we could speak of **the atrioventricular junctions** in reference to both the left and right heart. On the left, (pages 46–49) the subvalvular segment of the A.V. membrane intervenes between the left atrium and the left ventricle; therefore, the two chambers do not, in fact, meet. On the right (pages 94–95), the atrium and ventricle are separated by the supra-ostial segment of the tricuspid membrane. The term A.V. junction cannot, therefore, be proposed as an alternative; accordingly, when the term A.V. sulcus is used, its shortcomings must be recognized; certainly, in connection with the coronary arteries, its use is often associated with considerable imprecision, both conceptual and descriptive—the statement that an artery runs in the A.V. sulcus cannot be considered definitive.

The A.V. sulcus is interrupted anteriorly by the aorta, and description would be facilitated if the crux (seen in cross section on pages 102 and 104) were considered an interruption in the sulcus posteriorly. We may then recognize a right and a left A.V. sulcus. The **left A.V. sulcus** is divided into three parts; in each, the subvalvular segment of the A.V. membrane intervenes between the atrium and the ventricle. (1) The **posterior left A.V. sulcus** is related to the posterior walls of the left atrium and the left ventricle (see page 63). (2) The **lateral left A.V. sulcus** is related to the lateral walls of the left atrium and left ventricle. (It is seen in **94—4** and **42—3**.) (3) The **left coronary fossa** has been defined on page 6 and is seen on pages 188, 202 and 209. Frontal transections appear on page 19, **102—1, 2** and **104 – 3, 4.** Its junction with the lateral left A.V. sulcus appears in a transection on page 50. The **right A.V. sulcus** is also divided into three parts, and in each, the supra-ostial segment of the tricuspid membrane intervenes between the atrium and ventricle. (1) The **posterior right A.V. sulcus** is related to the inferior walls of the right atrium and ventricle. (2) The **anterior right A.V. sulcus** is related to the lateral wall of the right atrium and the anterior wall of the right ventricle. (3) The walls of the inverted wedge-shaped upper portion, which I call the **right coronary fossa,** are: the anteromedial wall of the right atrium, the posterolateral wall of the right ventricle, and the aorta. The right A.V. sulcus is examined on page 96. Following this examination we may assay the definition and note the right and left extremities of the A.V. sulcus.

Turn to **98—2–4** and note (a) that the right atrial attachment in relation to the right ventricle extends to the vertical level of the right/posterior aortic commissure; (b) Posterior to this point, the right atrium, forming the wall of the right coronary fossa, is related only to the aorta. As noted in the index, the left coronary fossa is seen on many pages. It is found before and after removal of the left atrium in **206—1–4** and **20—1–2,** respectively. Observe: (a) The left anterior extremity of the left atrium/left ventricle attachment is found at the nadir of the left aortic annulus. (b) In reality, the left coronary fossa incorporates a part of the left A.V. sulcus rather than constituting a part thereof—its floor, roof, and medial walls are formed by the left ventricle pulmonary trunk and aorta.

The crux was defined on page 68 as a region or an area—not a point, as its name might imply. On that page the posterior superior process of L.V. is seen connecting the posterior right, and posterior left A.V. sulci: This process, therefore, and the inferior wall of the right atrium (and the pericardial floor) form the major walls of the crux—the non-septal part of the right lateral wall of the left atrium forms a small part of the walls of crux as seen in 102 and 104.

The Interatrial Sulci

It has been seen (page 58) that the **anterior interatrial sulcus,** is, in reality, not a groove or a sulcus (L., a furrow) but an obtuse-angled junction. The posterior interatrial sulcus, as we shall see in the next chapter (page 98), is a fat-filled, shallow, wedge-shaped area resulting from chamber apposition. It may be seen before dissection in **131—1** and on page 154 following dissection. Note that the extent of the posterior sulcus may be exaggerated by a dissection which separates the apposed atria. This principle is utilized by the surgeon, when necessary, in the exposure of the mitral valve. Passage of sinus node arteries through the upper part of the posterior sulcus adds to its importance.

The Interventricular Sulci

We can now examine the validity of the terms, anterior and posterior interventricular sulci. On page 30, we may observe that the sulci are, in fact, not grooves but both result from the junction of surface contours of the ventricles. Indeed, the terms, **anterior and posterior interventricular junctions,** are appropriate: Substitution of (the English word) groove for junction results in inaccuracy: Substitution of (the Latin word) sulcus only obfuscates this inaccuracy; nevertheless, these traditional terms are used herein. **The anterior interventricular sulcus** extends from the left coronary fossa, whose anterior border is formed by the pulmonary attachment of the right ventricle, to the apical incisura. This sulcus may be divided into a distinct upper and a less distinct lower half: Both result from the fact that the right ventricle wraps around the left ventricle. Examine the sulcus and incisura (their presence and their absence) on pages 28 and 29, 30, 31, 36, 53 (**5** and **6**), 54 (**3**), 55 (**3**). The sulcus, along with its related artery, may be seen on pages 59 (**3** and **4**). In the dissection on pages 66 and 67, the upper end of the

sulcus may be precisely noted, coincident to noting the relationship of the anterior interventricular artery to the sulcus—the latter relationship is also clearly shown in the dissection on page 78. The term, anterior interventricular artery is appropriate: The artery courses between the ends of the sulcus. The course of the related artery may be (1) intramural, (2) epicardial, and (3) aerial. The degree of proximity of the artery to the sulcus, therefore, varies accordingly. The term, **posterior interventricular sulcus,** is used to denote the line of attachment of the inferior wall of the right ventricle to the A.V. unit—the posterior interventricular junction—see pages 68 and 69. A sulcus, demarcating the essentially uniplanar adjoining walls of the ventricles, is rarely recognizable. Its ends, in particular the apical incisura, may also be unrecognizable (see page 28). When visible, these ends may be used to plot the sulcus and identify a related artery.

Addendum

Branches enter the septum at the five sites of attachment of the right ventricle to the aorto-ventricular unit. These may be examined in a clockwise fashion, from above. (1) the **left superior septal branch** arises at a right angle from the retropulmonary portion of the anterior division of the left coronary artery, penetrating the septum behind the pulmonary or superior attachment. (2) The **anterior septal branches:** Six or more vessels arise from the deep surface of the anterior interventricular branch, to enter the septum in relation to the anterior attachment. (3) The **inferior septal:** Four to six short branches are seen in relation to the inferior attachment. (4) The **posterior septal:** Two branches are commonly seen here, (a) the A.V. node branch and (b) a 30 to 40 mm artery, which, traditionally is termed the ramus septi superiorus. This branch, if viewed in an attitudinal mode, is better termed a posterior septal branch (5) A **right superior septal branch** may arise from the proximal right coronary artery, extend inferiorly, entering the septum at the attachment of the posterolateral wall.

Chapter 7: The Right Atrium

Introduction

The divisions of the atrium: (A) **From a spatial viewpoint,** the right atrium may be divided into lateral, inferior, medial, and posterior walls. The medial wall is subdivided into posteromedial (or septal) and anteromedial portions. (B) **From an embryologic viewpoint,** the right atrium may be divided into two parts. (1) The **sinus venarum** is derived from the right horn of the sinus venosus; its wall is smooth. (2) **The body:** (a) The area of its wall roughened by the musculi pectinati and the appendage are derived from the right half of the primitive atrium. (b) The smooth-walled band bordered anteromedially by the attachments of the chamber is derived from the right half of the atrio-ventricular canal. This classic division is not an attempt to effect concordance between embryologic concepts and gross anatomic observations—its practical value will be discussed. The lateral, inferior, and anteromedial walls form the body; the posterior and septal walls form the sinus venarum which is dominated by the orifices of the superior and inferior venae cavae. The venae cavae form a pivotal part of the anatomy of the right atrium—review the dissection on page **7**. During a period in development of the human fetus, in adult reptilia and birds, the right and left venous valves guard the junction between the sinus venarum and the body of the atrium. In the human heart, the left venous valve regresses; occasionally, remnants persist on the septal wall. Three derivatives of the right venous valve provide the semblance of a partition between the two divisions. (1) The interior projection of the **terminal muscle bundle** (the crista terminalis) is most prominent superiorly and continues in front of the orifice of the superior vena cava as (2) a prominent ridge, which I term the **precaval muscle bundle.** The crista terminalis becomes less prominent inferiorly and in only 15% of specimens is it continuous with (3) **the valve of the inferior vena cava** (the Eustachian valve). This crescentic valve attached to the inferior wall, projects superiorly from the anterior margin of the orifice of the vena cava.

The Body of the Atrium: The tricuspid ostium may be divided into superior, anterior, inferior and septal parts (see **84**—**2** and **3**). To the tricuspid membrane in relation to its first three parts, the anteromedial, lateral, and inferior walls of the body of the right atrium are sequentially attached. From its attachment, **the inferior wall** extends posteriorly to the orifice of the inferior vena cava and medially to the ostium of L.V. Laterally, it merges imperceptibly with the lateral wall along a line which projects posteriorly to the sinus venarum. **The coronary sinus** is derived from the left horn of the sinus venosus, and it would appear more consistent with this derivation if it emptied into the sinus venarum—it doesn't—it empties into the body of the atrium at the medial attachment of the inferior wall. The valve of the coronary sinus (the valve of Thebesius) is derived from the right venous valve and is often confluent with the valve of the inferior vena cava. **The lateral and anteromedial walls** extend superiorly and meet at an acute angle which is inflated to form the (superior) atrial appendage. The anteromedial wall sweeps superiorly without interruption into the atrial appendage; however, beyond the attachments of the lateral and inferior walls, a ridge projects which contains (what I term) the **anterior vertical muscle bundle.** The ridge and its contained muscle fade as they extend to the crux. The atrioventricular sulcus is between the ridge and the right ventricle. Its floor is formed by a thin band of the wall which I term **the supravalvular lamina.**

The Posteromedial or Septal Wall of the Right Atrium: The septum primum is represented in the adult heart by the membranous portion of the septal wall.
On the right side of the septum primum, the septum secundum develops and is represented by the septal muscles of the right atrium. In this work, the term **membranous portion of the atrial septum** denotes that the membrane is adherent to the left side of the septum. When the term **valve of the foramen ovale** is used, it is implicit that a probe patent foramen ovale is present in the specimen being examined. Wide variation occurs in the relative development of the two primitive septa: (a) The area of the wall covered by muscle may be large or small—a small or a large membranous portion of the septal wall results. (b) Membrane forms the floor of the "fossa ovalis". However, if a fossa, i.e., a depression, is to exist, margination of the floor is necessary. Regardless of the size of the persisting membranous component, if the muscle is thin, virtual absence of the fossa results. The terms **fossa ovalis** and **membranous portion of the atrial septum** are therefore not synonymous. When a fossa ovalis exists, wide variation in the degree of muscle development results in corresponding degrees of prominence of its margins.

The word "fossa" in medical writing denotes a depression, pit, or cavity; this is a Latin word (for ditch), so it seems not unreasonable to use a Latin word, "limbus" (=border or margin), for the margin of the fossa. Limbus, however, may be confused with the Anglo-Saxon word "lim" = limb, because the margin and the contained muscle has been divided into superior and inferior parts; these two parts have been incorrectly deemed the two limbs of the fossa, with the crotch above. In connection with the divisions of the limbus and its bands into superior and inferior, we see another example of assigning terms to the heart when it is viewed with the apex below and the septa in vertical planes. The long axis of the fossa is not transverse; although it is usually not oriented vertically but antero-superiorly, it is preferable to replace the terms "inferior" and "superior" with anterior and posterior. I retain the term, limbic muscles, although they could be termed the marginal muscles. The fossa ovalis is usually elliptical in shape. It may be circular or be long and narrow. The word "oval" is imprecise if reference to the outline of an egg is implied; usually its ends are symmetrical; if not symmetrical, it is more horseshoe-shaped than oval. The floor of the fossa, most often, merges with the medial wall of the inferior vena cava, although limbic muscles may intervene; when these muscles are prominent, a ridge is present and the margins of the fossa become circular—the annulus of Vieussens.
A promontory is present between the orifices of the venae cavae—it is largely on the septal wall, although it may extend onto the posterior wall. The degree of its prominence parallels the degree of development of the muscles in the septal wall. It is best termed the promontory of the right atrium. It has great clinical significance, and I have long used the term "Tuber of Lower" for its designation—this term appears in this work, although I have virtually avoided eponyms. The Latin word tuber denotes a promontory, swelling or protuberance—on page 98 we see a structure in human hearts which meets this semantic qualification; however, a successful defense for the use of eponyms in anatomic description is impossible; a testimony to the problems which follows their use is found in the scholarly monograph of Franklin (1947); 42 pages are devoted in tracing the history of the term, Tuber of Lower, in the years subsequent to its description by Lower in 1669.

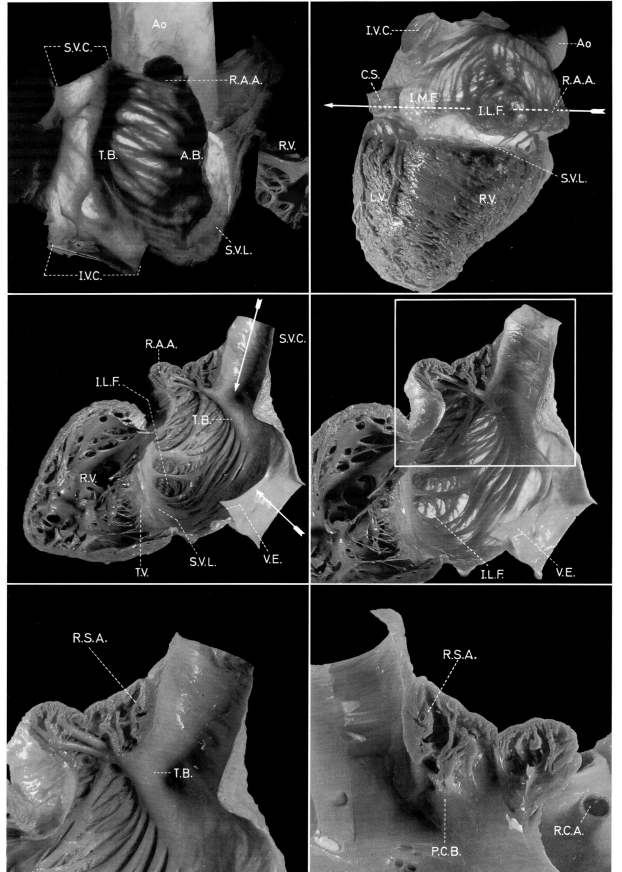

A. The Lateral Wall of the Right Atrium

I. Its Muscles

Specimen A: 1: Right lateral view of a transilluminated right atrium: The **terminal muscle bundle** (T.B.) descends between the superior and the inferior cavo-atrial angles, demarcating the sinus venarum posteriorly and the lateral wall: The pectinate muscles pass obliquely anteriorly, joining it to a second muscle bundle which we will term the **anterior vertical muscle bundle** (A.B.). In the (superior) right atrial appendage, muscle trabeculae extend forward, joining the two "vertical" muscle bundles. Anterior to the anterior vertical bundle, a thin muscle wall extends around the tricuspid valve ostium. This we shall call the **supravalvular lamina** (S.V.L.): It is normally covered by fat in the A.V. sulcus.

Specimen B: 2: The acute margin is examined with combined lighting. The thin supravalvular lamina and the anterior vertical muscle bundle extend inferiorly, and in a few specimens, both reach the crux. (The arrow is for future reference.)

Specimen C: 3: The right segment is seen following an oblique vertical transection passing through the venae cavae posteriorly and the right ventricle anteriorly. The left segment is seen on page 99. Observe: (a) The axes of the venae cavae (shown by arrows) form an obtuse angle (review page 7). (b) In this heart, the valve of the inferior vena cava (V.E.) is membranous—it may contain muscle. (c) On the external surface of the atrium, the terminal bundle is poorly marked by the sulcus terminalis. In contrast, a prominent ridge (see page 96) marks the junction of the anterior vertical bundle and the supravalvular lamina. On the internal surface, seen here, the converse is true, the terminal bundle presents a prominent ridge—the crista terminalis—the anterior vertical bundle merges imperceptibly with the confluent supravalvular lamina and the tricuspid valve leaflets (T.V.). (d) Near the midpoint of the tricuspid valve, the deep **inferolateral atrial appendage or fossa** (I.L.F.) appears. (e) The junction between the right atrium and the right atrial appendage is ill-defined—in this work, appendage denotes the anterosuperior protrusion of the atrium, an anatomic feature rather than an anatomic subdivision.

4: The sectioned valve of the inferior vena cava (V.E.) is seen here, but to better advantage in **3**; we can see, however, that the terminal muscle bundle is not continuous with the valve inferiorly; it ends in the midportion of the atrium. As seen here and in **3**, the inferolateral fossa or appendage (I.L.F.) is highly trabeculated.

5 and **6**: The right and left halves of the superior cavo-atrial junction are now shown. The area in the square in **4** is seen in a 1:1 scale in **5**; observe that the crista terminalis (T.B.) reaches its maximal development anterior to the orifice, at its junction with the precaval band. In **6**, a line drawn between 9 and 3 o'clock passes through the right sinus node artery (R.S.A.) and possibly the medial end of the sinus node itself—the artery runs through it.

II. The Precaval Muscle Bundle

Specimen D: 1 and **2**: A nonattitudinal antero-inferior view of the posterior segment resulting from a frontal transection: Observe: (a) Anterior to the orifice of the superior vena cava, the strongly ridged terminal bundle (T.B.) becomes **the precaval bundle,** which then continues for a short distance in the anteromedial wall before terminating in the posteromedial (or septal) wall of the right atrium. (b) The tuber of Lower (T.L.), the protruberance between the two vena cavae, is not prominent in this specimen. (c) The 18 × 14-mm valvula foraminis ovalis (orange) is also relatively small in relation to the distance between the two venae cavae and is disposed more transversely than normal. (d) The vertical dimension of the valve of the inferior vena cava (V.E.) is 4 mm. Variations in these features should be noted in all specimens. Examine other views of this dissection in **59—2**.

Specimen E: 3 and **4**: The right atrium is viewed from below after a flap has been made and turned inferiorly. The line of inspection is nearly in the axis of the inferior vena cava as we look directly into the 20-mm, circular, transilluminated, membranous portion of the atrial septum in the floor of the fossa ovalis. The view is somewhat obscured by remnants of the fenestrated valve of the I.V.C. (V.E.), which are seen in the photograph but not in the drawing. The line of section passes obliquely through the terminal bundle. The precaval band passes anterior to the superior vena cava orifice, gaining attachment to the medial wall of the right atrium. From the precaval band, the (poorly named) "sagittal" bundle extends anterolaterally, dividing the right atrial appendage into two compartments, posterolateral and anteromedial. Either compartment may serve as a good site for the engagement of an atrial pacemaker catheter.

Specimen F: 5: Nonattitudinal R.A.O. view. Two horizontal incisions, one through the superior vena cava (S.V.C.) just below the anterior pericardial attachment (X), and the other through the right atrium below the right atrial appendage, have been joined posteriorly. The resulting segment is everted and in it note the prominent precaval and sagittal (Y) bundles and the two compartments of the appendage. The membranous portion of the atrial septum has been transilluminated. It extends almost to the superior vena cava orifice—the atrial septum is largely membranous: The fossa ovalis and the inferior vena cava orifice are usually coterminous.

6: Right lateral x-rays are seen in atrial diastole and systole, following simultaneous injection of contrast into the venae cavae. The caliber of the superior cavo-atrial junction (transverse arrows) is reduced in systole due to contraction of the terminal and precaval bundles. The incisura at the inferior cavo-atrial junction (vertical arrow) is produced by the valve of the inferior vena cava, which is oriented in a frontal plane. These two phenomena represent the persistence in the adult heart of the valvular function of the right venous valve.

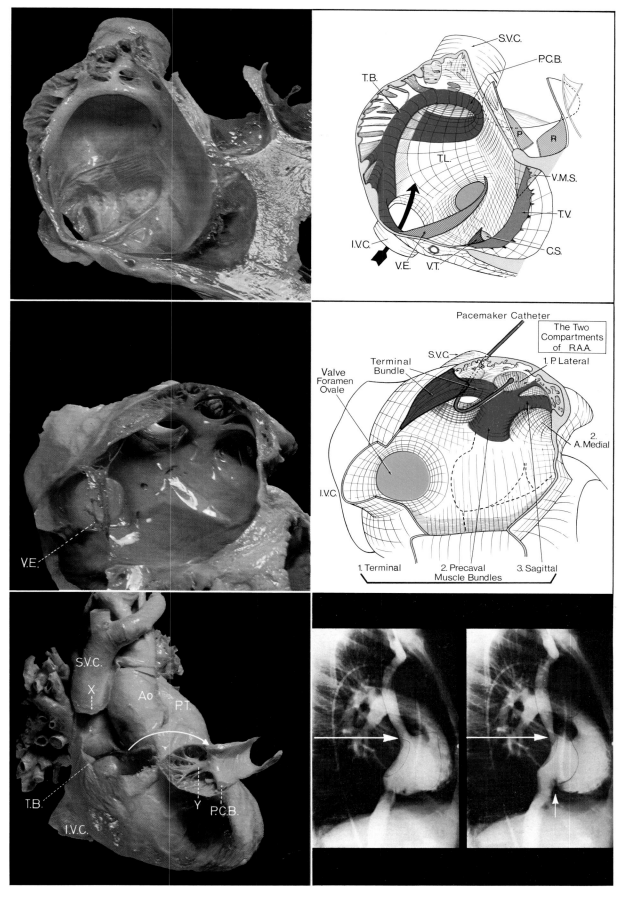

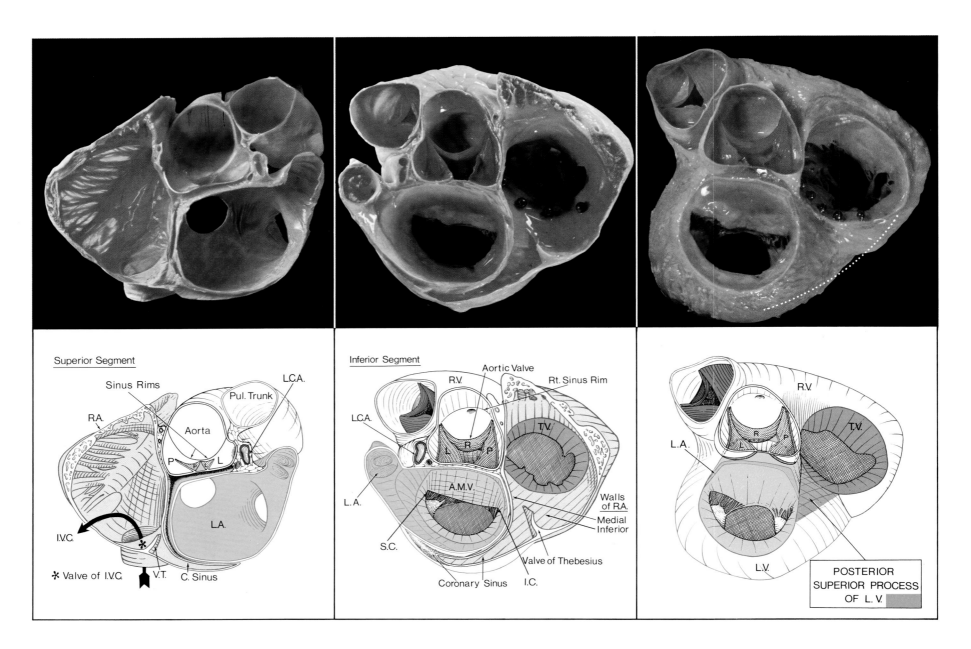

Superior Segment

Sinus Rims — L.C.A.

Pul. Trunk

R.A.

Aorta

P L

L.A.

I.V.C.

✷ V.T. C. Sinus

✷ Valve of I.V.C.

Inferior Segment

Aortic Valve

R.V. Rt. Sinus Rim

L.C.A.

L R P

T.V.

L.A.

A.M.V.

Walls of R.A.

S.C.

Medial Inferior

Valve of Thebesius

Coronary Sinus I.C.

R.V.

L R P

T.V.

L.A.

L.V.

POSTERIOR SUPERIOR PROCESS OF L. V.

B. The Inferior Wall of the Right Atrium

Specimen A: 1–6

I. The Coronary Sinus and Its Orifice

We will now carry out a transection through the coronary sinus which, as noted on page 63, is located on the left atrial wall 10 mm beyond its inferior attachment and directed to the left and superiorly at a 45° angle. These facts indicate the location in the atrium and direction of this transection in the frontal plane.

2 and **5**: The transection passes through the left and posterior aortic sinuses posteriorly and through the aorta, high above the right aortic sinus anteriorly. Recall that the aortic sinuses are all in an A.P. plane, the obliquity of which (in relation to the horizontal) is determined by the annular axis (see page 22). Hence, we can deduce that the line of transection passes obliquely, superiorly, and anteriorly. These descriptions are not mere dry tedium; in addition to providing spatial

orientation here, they serve as a reference: The view and dissection seen in **3** is similar to those found, not only in this but in other works—these have often been used for the portrayal of the fibrous skeleton. Observe: (a) The right atrium and the coronary sinus form a unit that wraps around the left atrium. (b) The **coronary sinus orifice** is located: (1) At the junction of the medial and inferior wall of the right atrium (note that these walls continue into the coronary sinus); (2) Opposite the inferior commissure of the mitral valve which is 10 mm postero-inferior to the attachment of the junction of the divisions of the A.V. membrane to the ostium of the left ventricle, which in turn is the location of the A.V. node. It is sometimes simply stated that the commissure is 10 mm posterior to the latter, just as it is sometimes stated that the His bundle runs anteriorly and inferiorly. Both statements ignore the spatial disposition of the right half of the ostium of the left ventricle—it is directed anterosuperiorly. (c) **The valve of the coronary sinus (V.T.)** is oriented anterosuperiorly—hence, it is divided in this transection.

II. The Borders and the Relations of the Inferior Wall

(a) The **anterior border**: Its attachment to the tricuspid membrane extends from the ostium of the left ventricle to the acute margin. (b) The transection in **1** and **2** has divided **the lateral border** where the inferior wall merges imperceptibly with the lateral wall of the atrium. (c) Its **posterior border** skirts the inferior vena cava orifice and its valve—seen better in **91—5** and **6**. (d) As shown in **90—2–3** and their underlying drawings, the inferior wall is related to the crux and the posterosuperior process of the left ventricle. The tricuspid and the left ventricular ostia are not in a single plane; the former is both anterior and inferior to the latter. Hence, the inferior wall of the right atrium is not a simple flat plane; it is convex inferiorly and to the left—again see **91—5** and **6**. The posterior limit of the inferior wall and coronary sinus is indicated by the dotted line in **3**.
Note: The four valves are often seen from the perspective of **3** which fails to demonstrate the wide separation of the tricupid and mitral valves.

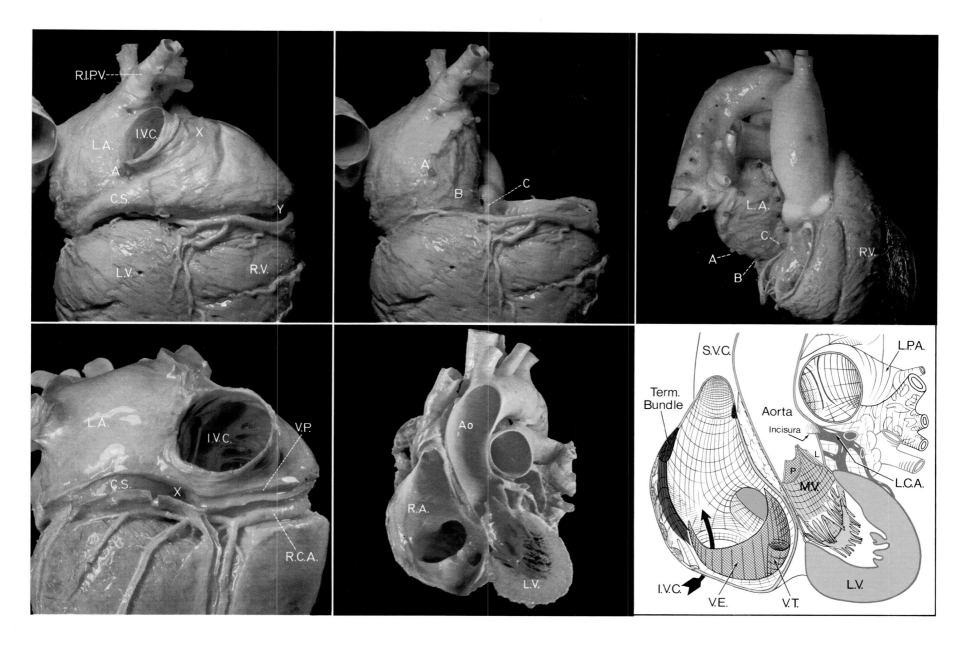

Specimen B: 1–3

In **1** and **2**, the inferior aspect of the heart is seen after the heart has been rotated to the left. The right atrium has been removed in **2** and in **3** which is the 300° view. In **3**, the blue and red beads mark the anterior and posterior margins of atrial apposition. The adjacent blue and red bead C = the right fibrous trigone. In **1**, **2**, and **3**, bead A = the angle between the coronary sinus (C.S.) and the inferior vena cava (I.V.C.); bead B = the coronary sinus orifice; bead C = the A.V. node. Observe: (a) In **1**, the semicircular posterior border of **the inferior wall** extends between bead A and point X, at the anterolateral margin of the inferior vena cava orifice. The lateral border extends between points X and Y. The anterior border is obscured by the right coronary artery. (b) As a consequence of the wrapping of the right atrium around the left atrium, the orifice of I.V.C. is close to the right inferior pulmonary vein (R.I.P.V.). (c) As seen in **3**, the right portion of the ostium of L.V. is directed superiorly and anteriorly, and the coronary sinus orifice

is postero-inferior to the A.V. node and anteromedial to the orifice of I.V.C.

Specimen C: 4: The inferior view: The roofs of the coronary sinus and the small cardiac vein (V.P.) have been removed. Observe: (a) The center of the coronary sinus orifice (X) is 10 mm above the left ventricle. This is a variable relationship. The orifice may straddle the junction of the left ventricle and atrium. (b) The small cardiac vein (V.P.) and the right coronary (R.C.A.) lie on the supravalvular lamina—a component of the inferior wall. The vein is almost always, as shown, postero-inferior to the artery.

Specimen D: 5 and 6: An A.P. view of the posterior segment following a frontal transection. Observe: (a) The transection passes through the inferior wall of the right atrium just anterior to the large valve of the inferior vena cava (V.E.), whose attachment forms the posterior border of the inferior wall. (b) The valve, attached to the crista terminalis and the anterior margin of the deep

fossa ovalis, forms an incomplete partition between the sinus venarum and the body of the atrium. The cornua of the crescentic valve may be at the same level—when the medial cornu is the higher, as seen here, the valve is tilted superomedially—the opposite may occur (**92—1**). (c) The coronary sinus orifice is 10 mm postero-inferior to the attachment of the right fibrous trigone to the ostium. The posterior aortic sinus is often 10 mm above this point. These two measurements are useful in catheterization of the coronary sinus—although, apart from the size of the patient, the height of the posterior annulus is quite variable—see **11—6**. The nadir of the posterior aortic sinus is most often 1 cm to the left of the median plane (see page 100). (d) The coronary sinus valve is large. It is continuous with the valve of the I.V.C.—both are derived from the right venous valve. (e) The fossa ovalis is deep—the marginal or limbic muscles are massive in this small (210 gram) heart of an adult female. (f) The carina of the pulmonary trunk is prominent—see page 125.

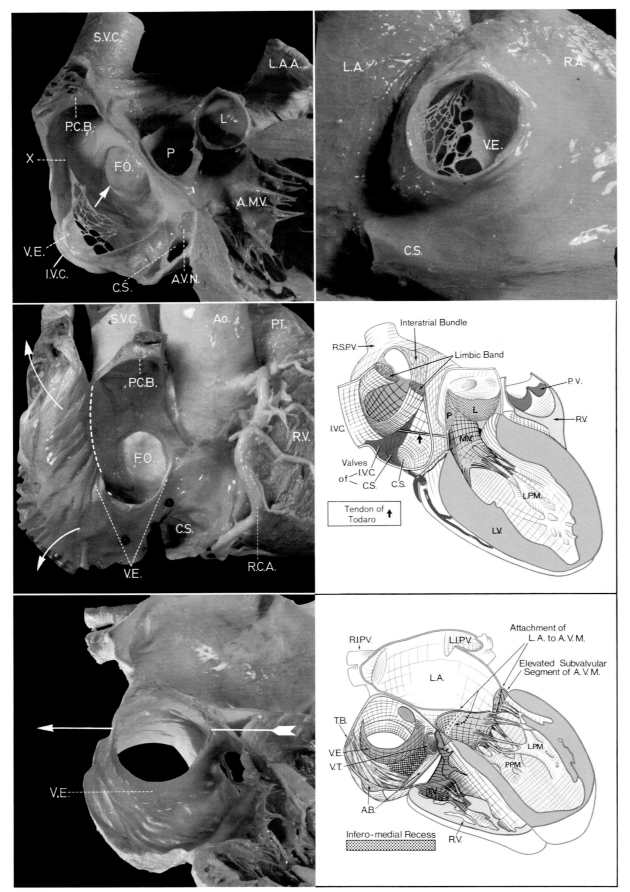

III. The Valve of the Inferior Vena Cava

Specimen A: 1–2: First examine **35—3–6**, where this specimen is seen following a frontal transection.

1: A.P. view: (a) The fenestrated valve (V.E.) extends superiorly onto the posterior wall of the atrium (X). It should not be confused with the network of Chiari which was believed by Chiari to develop from the septum spurium and right venous valve, and as may be inferred, in his 11 cases (described in 1897), the network extended between the inferior vena cava orifice and the precaval bundle and the upper atrial septum. (b) The diameter of the circular membranous floor of the fossa ovalis (F.O.) is 22.0 mm.
See the article of Powell and Mullaney.

2: Inferior view: The valve has been displaced across the orifice of the inferior vena cava which is seen in a 1:1 scale; its greatest vertical dimension (38.0 mm) exceeds the diameter of the orifice (30.0 mm)—this valve can hinder caval cannulation and ensnare venous emboli.

Specimen B: 3: R.A.O. view: The anteromedial wall of the right atrium has been removed. The lateral wall has been retracted following an incision through its anterior attachment and the zone anterior to the precaval bundle. In this wall, pectinate muscles are seen extending to the terminal bundle, which is indicated by the interrupted line. The typical concave upper margin of the valve is 15 mm above its convex attachment (which is marked by three beads) to the junction of the posterior border of the inferior wall and anterior half of the orifice (of I.V.C.). The valve is connected on the right to the terminal bundle, and on the left to the anterior margin of the fossa ovalis (the membranous atrial septum [F.O.] has been transilluminated). This photograph is intended to show that the valve may be sutured to the rim of an atrial septal defect, diverting two-thirds of the venous return into the left atrium. This unfortunate surgical misadventure is an example of the lack of attention to a simple facet of anatomy which was recorded by Eustachius in 1563.

Specimen C: 4: A nonattitudinal R.A.O. view: The **tendon of Todaro** passes from the right fibrous trigone to the valve (of I.V.C.) and may be encountered in dissections to display the A.V. node. Above, the stout interatrial and anterior and posterior limbic muscle bundles (or bands) have been divided obliquely. See the article on the tendon of Todaro by Vorboril.

Specimen D: 5 and **6:** Following a horizontal transection, the inferior segment has been rotated 45° on its transverse axis. Observe: (a) In **5**, the 18-mm-high, muscle-containing valve (V.E.) is seen lying with its cornua in a frontal plane—which is indicated by the arrow—its typical disposition. (b) In **6**, the anterior vertical muscle bundle (A.B.) extends to the medial wall of the atrium. (c) The inferomedial fossa (recess) is between this bundle and the valves of the coronary sinus and inferior vena cava. (d) In **6**, the subvalvular segment of the A.V. membrane extends superiorly in the axis of the left ventricle.

IV. The Two Fossae or Appendages of the Inferior Wall of the Right Atrium

Catheters are passed daily into the heart, either for diagnostic purposes or caval cannulation at operation. The presence of fossae or recesses, in which they may become engaged, traumatize, and even perforate the heart, commands attention. Early in my dissections, I was impressed that there were, in fact, three right atrial appendages. In addition to the (superior) right atrial appendage, two are frequently present in the inferior wall—one anterior to the inferior vena cava orifice and the second at the acute margin.

Specimen E: 1 and 2: The inferior view from three different angles: The inferomedial fossa (I.M.F.) has been termed the appendix auricularis posterior of His and the subeustachian sinus of Keith, which perhaps describes the opinion held by these two workers of this structure. Perhaps the word "fossa" better describes the appearance seen in the majority of specimens; although when the external surface is examined, a protuberance is usually seen—see the specimens on page 96.

Specimen F: 3 and 4: The transection has been carried out just above the acute margin passing through the A.V. membrane just below the posterior aortic annulus. The atria are attached to the A.V. membrane at the junction of its two divisions (R.F.T.). The atrial portion of the membranous septum (A.M.S.) is on the right, and the anterior leaflet of the mitral valve is on the left. In 3, the inferior segment is tilted to display the inferolateral fossa or appendage (I.L.F.). In 4, the inferior segment is rotated to display the inferomedial fossa, which is related to (a) the inferior vena cava posteriorly, (b) the supravalvular lamina anteriorly, and (c) the coronary sinus orifice on the left. Note the prominence of the crista terminalis (T.B.).

The Supravalvular Lamina

Specimen G: 5 and 6: The intact specimen is seen on page 88—2, where the mode of transection is indicated by an arrow. The transection passes steeply postero-inferiorly, anterior to the inferior vena cava, through the inferomedial and inferolateral fossae below, and the right atrial appendage above. In the upper segment, 5, the pectinate muscles are seen running towards the line of transection and in the lower segment, 6, they are seen terminating in the anterior vertical bundle (A.B.), the outline of which is delimited centrally by the thin supravalvular lamina (S.V.L.) (see 88—1, 2). The translucent inferomedial fossa (I.M.F.) is atrabecular, in contrast to the highly trabeculated inferolateral fossa or recess; re-examine 3 and 4 in this regard. In most specimens (92—6 is an exception), the anterior vertical bundle ends at the lateral boundary of the inferomedical fossa, as shown here; the thin inferomedial recess is then confluent with the thin supravalvular lamina.

In these specimens, both inferior fossae or appendages appear; often only one is present.

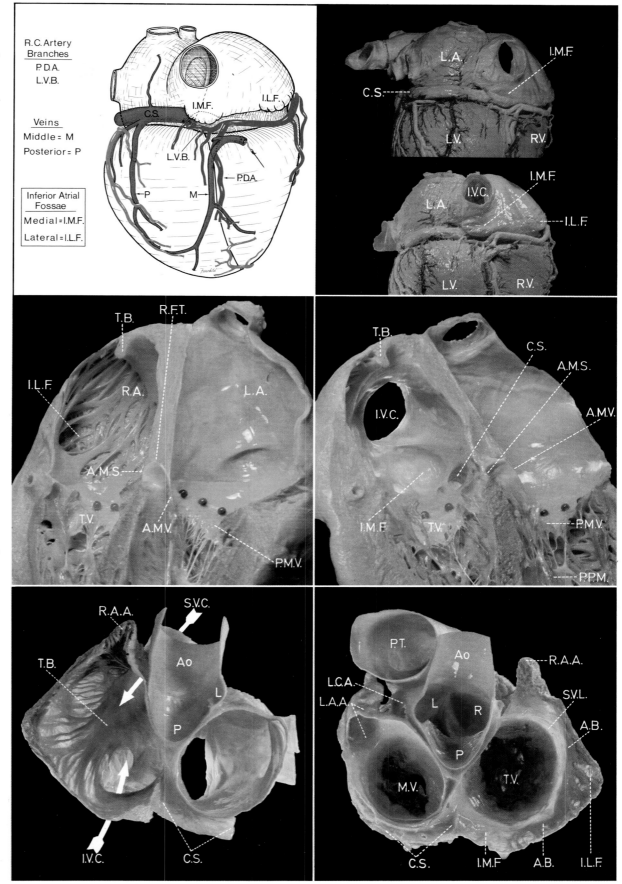

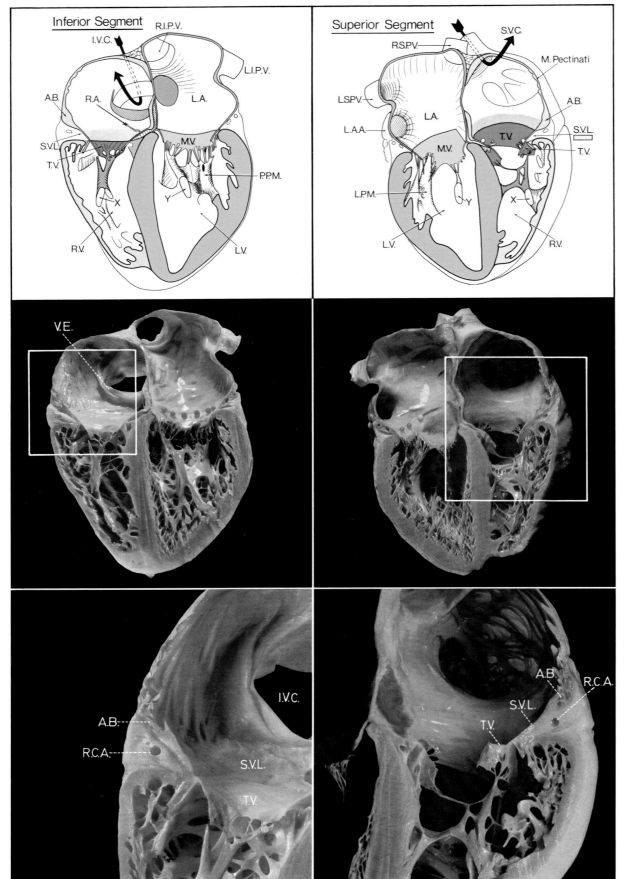

C. The Combined Attachments of the Right Atrium, Right Ventricle, and the Tricuspid Valve

I. The Supra-Ostial Lamina

The material on these two pages shows that a fibrous membrane exists between the tricupid ostium and the confluent supravalvular lamina of the right atrium and the tricuspid leaflets. To this membrane I have assigned the designation "supra-ostial lamina". This lamina and the tricuspid leaflets together may be termed the tricuspid membrane; note its similarity to the portion of the A.V. membrane formed by the subvalvular membrane and the posterior leaflet of the mitral valve.

Specimen A: 94—1–6 and 95—1 and 2:

1–4: The preliminary transection: The following structures are seen transected: (1) On the left, the obtuse margin—the lateral and posterior papillary muscles are in the superior and inferior segments, respectively. A posterior intermediate papillary muscle is seen with the posterior muscle. (2) The lateral wall of the left atrium midway between the superior and inferior pulmonary veins. The lateral left A.V. sulcus is seen in **2** and **4** and in an enlarged form on page **42—3**. (3) The inferior commissure of the mitral valve. (4) The posterior margin of the posterosuperior process of L.V., from which the apposed right atrial wall has been separated, as seen in all views on this page, with the exception of **5**. (5) The atrial septum through the upper portion of the fossa ovalis, as seen in **1** and **3**. (6) The inferior walls of the right chambers just below the acute margin.

5: An enlargement of the area indicated in **3** is seen with combined lighting. The extremity of the right ventricle at the tricuspid ostium is incurving, fragmented, and complex in comparison with its counterpart in the left ventricle. The pectinate muscles are seen terminating in the anterior vertical bundle (A.B.), which is labeled at the point of its cross section, and seen in the interior where it merges imperceptibly with the supravalvular lamina. All structures are labeled, with the exception of the one that is, in fact, the crux of this discussion—the connection between the right ventricle and the confluent supravalvular lamina (S.V.L.) and the inferior leaflet of the tricuspid valve (T.V.)—it is not defined in this photograph; although the wide seperation of the structures it joins is evident.

The Valvulo-Cameral Complex—in the Anterior Right A.V. Sulcus: This is seen in **94—6** and **95—1** and **2**.

6: The transection passes through the lower portion of **the anterior right A.V. sulcus**, i.e., above the area indicated in **4**. The same structures are now seen with surface lighting. Note the relation of the right coronary artery in the lower part of the anterior right sulcus.

1: The area of valvulo-cameral complex seen in **94—6** is shown in a larger scale (1.5:1).

2: Leaving the tricuspid leaflet undisturbed, a third transection has been made 3 cm superior to the level seen in **1**. A delicate membrane, the supraostial lamina (S.O.L.), extends between the supravalvular lamina-leaflet junction and the ostium of the right ventricle.

The Valvulo-Cameral Complex—in the Posterior Right A-V Sulcus: This will be demonstrated in three specimens. Note the absence of segmentation of the inferior wall of the right ventricle at the tricuspid ostium, and observe the similarity to its left ventricular counterpart. Three specimens are utilized to suggest that this simple pattern is typical.

Specimen B: 3: A retouched photograph of **4**. The supra-ostial lamina is disposed in the axis of the inferior wall of the right ventricle, paralleling the disposition of the elevated subvalvular segment of the A.V. membrane (see page 48). Note the small cardiac vein (V.P.).

Specimen C: 5: This specimen appears as **97—1–3**. The transection is just lateral to the orifice of the inferior vena cava. The anterior vertical bundle is not seen because of its more lateral termination.

Specimen D: 6: The same arrangement of the structures is seen. The supra-ostral membrane (S.O.L.) extends posterosuperiorly meeting the confluent supravalvular membrane and the tricuspid leaflet. Again the upper extremity of the right ventricle is non-fragmented in contrast to its appearance at a higher anterior level.

Comment: The relation of the right coronary artery to the supravalvular lamina is obvious in all the photographs; this lamina could easily be injured in the course of dissection of the artery. The fragile nature of the tricuspid valvulo-cameral complex should be remembered when tricuspid valve replacement is being carried out or, indeed, if plication of this valve is ever performed. Currently the latter operation is recommended by many workers in preference to valve replacement for the correction of tricuspid regurgitation associated with mitral valve disease. The surgeon is probably being deluded if he conceives of a ring into which he can place sutures and obtain a satisfactory base for either of the two surgical procedures. Indeed, the fragility of this connection, like that of the posterior leaflet of the mitral valve demands maximum care in the placement of the sutures in valve replacement and suggests the preference for the "subannular" placement of the prosthesis, particularly when the pressure in the right ventricle is elevated. If the seat of the prosthesis is placed above the leaflet remnant, which in the medical jargon of today is referred to as "supra-annular placement", the use of teflon pledgets to buttress the sutures appears mandatory.

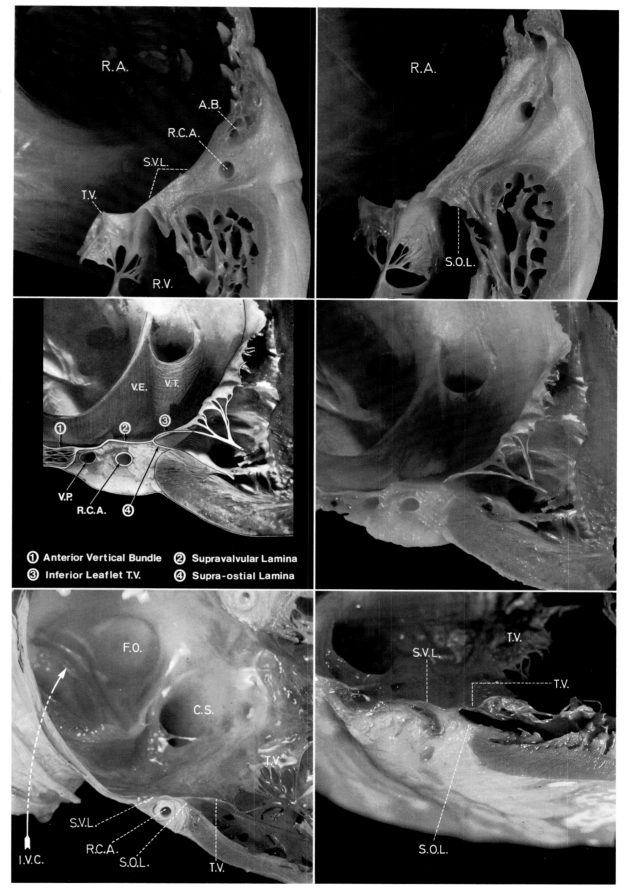

① Anterior Vertical Bundle　② Supravalvular Lamina
③ Inferior Leaflet T.V.　④ Supra-ostial Lamina

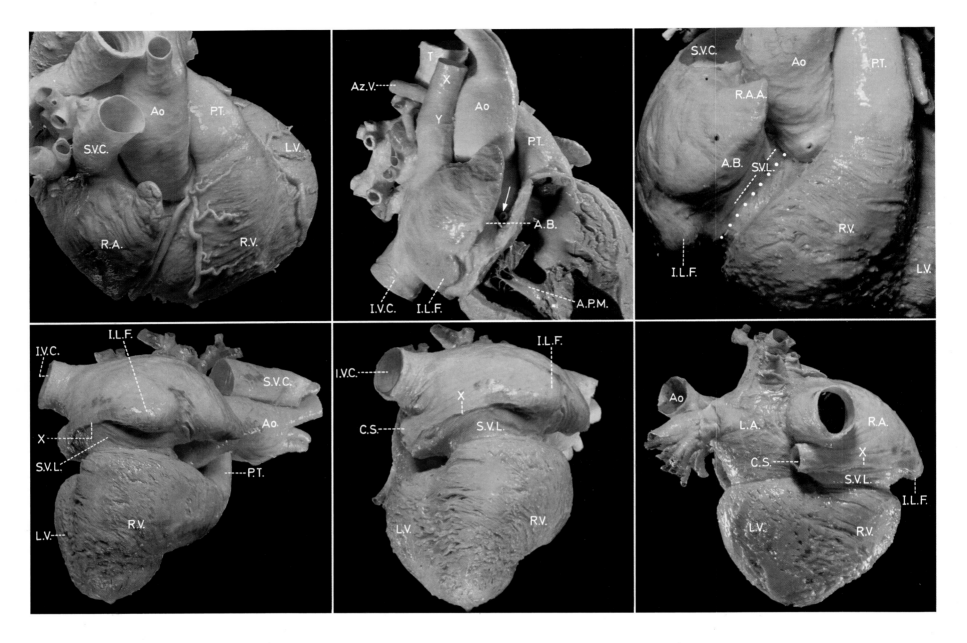

II. The Right Atrioventricular Sulcus

The right A.V. sulcus is divided into three parts—see the general comments on page 86 (1) **The posterior right A.V. sulcus** is related to the inferior walls of the right atrium and right ventricle. (2) **The anterior right A.V. sulcus** is above the acute margin and is related to the lateral wall of the right atrium. The anterior right A.V. sulcus exceeds the posterior in both width and depth. (3) **The right coronary fossa** is deep and expansive. The three walls of the right coronary fossa are (a) the posterolateral wall of the right ventricle, (b) the anteromedial wall of the right atrium, and (c) the aorta, which forms the medial wall. The walls of the fossa angle upward, roughly forming an inverted triangular pyramid; it is fat-filled and roofed by the pericardium and overlapped by the atrial appendage to a degree dependent on the size of the latter. In animals, anterior juxtaposition of the atrial appendages is common, and the envelopment then is complete.

Specimen A: 1: High R.A.O. view: Observe: (a) The anteromedial wall of the right atrium meets the left atrium at the middle of the posterior sinus; therefore, the fat in the right coronary fossa and the fat posterior to the aorta are continuous. (b) The right coronary artery arises in this deep fossa.

Specimen B: 2: R.A.O. view: Observe: (a) The potential height of the right coronary fossa—the arrow is directed to the origin of the right coronary artery. (b) The dimensions of the anterior right A.V. sulcus are, in this specimen, small in comparison with the next specimen. (c) A small inferolateral fossa or appendage (I.L.F.) of the right atrium is present.

Specimen C: 3–6: The terminal segment of the superior vena cava (S.V.C.) has been removed for an unrelated study. Note the disparity in length of the upper (X) and lower (Y) segments of this vessel in **2**.

3: Superior 330° view: The dotted line is at the "junction" of the atrial and ventricular walls. Observe: (a) The right coronary fossa is large. (b) A prominent ridge marks the course of the anterior vertical muscle bundle

(A.B.); a groove in this ridge forms the superior boundary of the inferolateral appendage (I.L.F.) of the right atrium. This groove is present in **2**.

In **4**, the **anterior and posterior right A.V. sulci** meet at the acute margin which extends between the inferolateral appendage (I.L.F.) and the apex. The posterior right A.V. sulcus is first examined at a 45° angle in **5**, then at a 90° angle in **6**, the inferior view. Observe: (a) The anterior sulcus is spacious and the posterior sulcus is shallow. (b) The pericardium has been divided at the line X—along this line the anterior vertical muscle bundle courses. The portion of the inferior wall of the right atrium formed by the supravalvular lamina (S.V.L.) meets the tricuspid membrane at an obtuse angle—also, see **94—4–6**. On page 63 examine the angle at the junction of the left atrium and the ventricle in the posterior left A.V. sulcus. (c) The inferolateral **appendage** is large in this specimen and small in **2**. (d) The posterior interventricular sulcus is not recognizable—this is the usual situation.

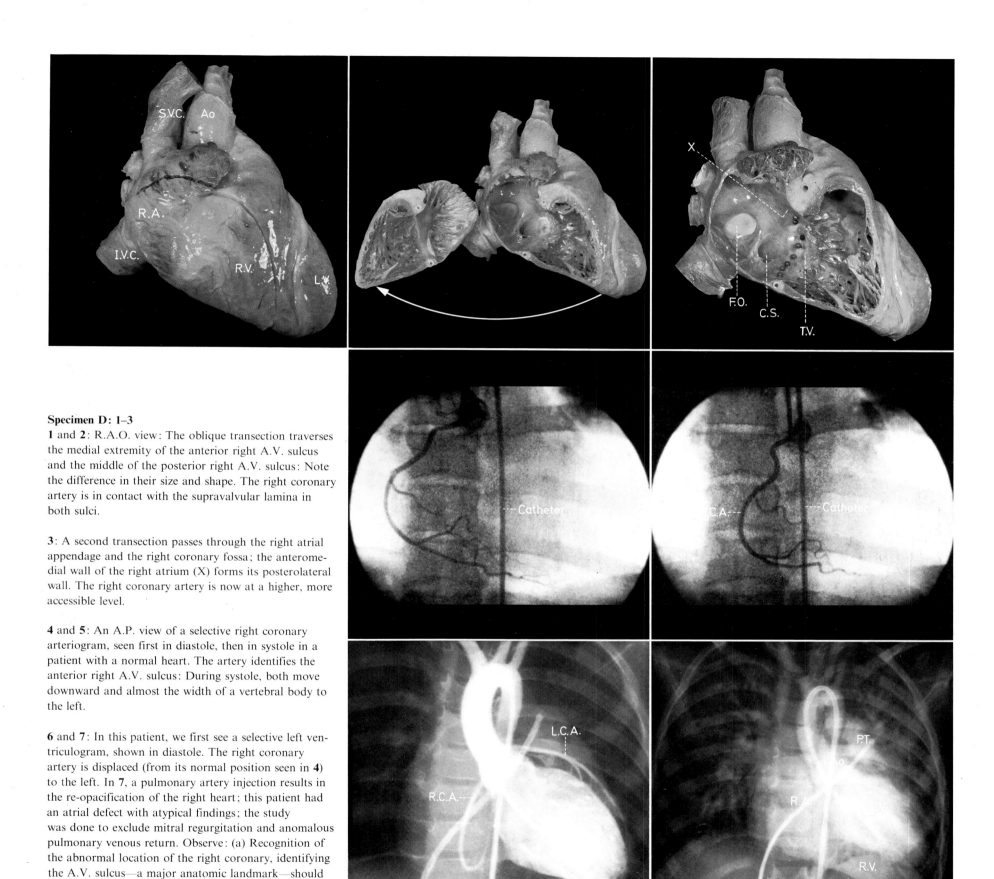

Specimen D: 1–3

1 and **2**: R.A.O. view: The oblique transection traverses the medial extremity of the anterior right A.V. sulcus and the middle of the posterior right A.V. sulcus: Note the difference in their size and shape. The right coronary artery is in contact with the supravalvular lamina in both sulci.

3: A second transection passes through the right atrial appendage and the right coronary fossa; the anteromedial wall of the right atrium (X) forms its posterolateral wall. The right coronary artery is now at a higher, more accessible level.

4 and **5**: An A.P. view of a selective right coronary arteriogram, seen first in diastole, then in systole in a patient with a normal heart. The artery identifies the anterior right A.V. sulcus: During systole, both move downward and almost the width of a vertebral body to the left.

6 and **7**: In this patient, we first see a selective left ventriculogram, shown in diastole. The right coronary artery is displaced (from its normal position seen in **4**) to the left. In **7**, a pulmonary artery injection results in the re-opacification of the right heart; this patient had an atrial defect with atypical findings; the study was done to exclude mitral regurgitation and anomalous pulmonary venous return. Observe: (a) Recognition of the abnormal location of the right coronary, identifying the A.V. sulcus—a major anatomic landmark—should alert the observer to the possibility of enlargement and counterclockwise rotation of the right heart; (b) the right ventricle extends below the left ventricle—see the comments (on page 33) regarding the terminology of its inferior wall.

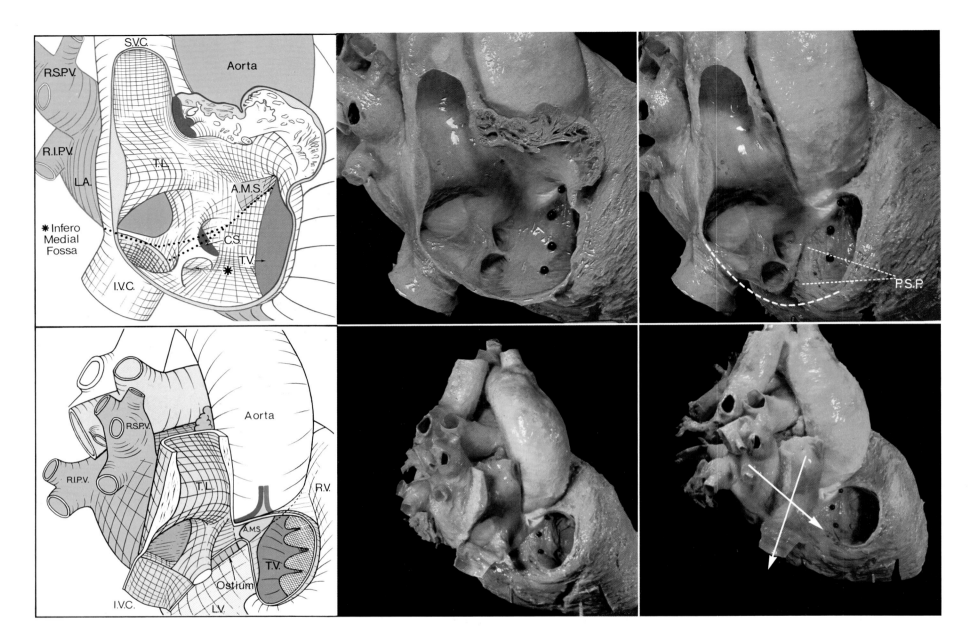

D. The Medial Wall of the Right Atrium

I. Its Subdivisions;
II. The Right Atrial Promontory

Specimen A: 1–6

1 and **2**: 300° view: The lateral wall, a part of the superior vena cava, and the lateral half of the posterior wall have been removed. The beads mark the attachment of the tricuspid valve to the A.V. unit. The membranous portion of the atrial septum and the membranous septum are transilluminated. In **1**, the upper and lower dotted lines represent the margin of atrial apposition and the ostium of L.V., respectively.

3: A 300° view: (1) The **anteromedial division of the medial wall** has been removed, disclosing its relation to the aorta and the posterolateral wall of the right ventricle. (2) The anterolateral portion of **the inferior wall** has been removed, disclosing its relation to the posterosuperior process of L.V. (P.S.P.). The lateral border of the inferior wall is indicated by the dashed line; the

medial and anterior borders are formed by left ventricular and tricuspid ostia, respectively.

Observe: (a) The noncavitary surfaces of **the anteromedial and posteromedial divisions of the medial wall** face in the directions indicated by their designations. Though highly contoured, their general axes form an angle of 135°. (b) **The junction of these two divisions** (seen in **3**) and the anterior wall of the antero-inferiorly directed superior vena cava form a straight line, which forms a part of the pathway followed by a catheter introduced from the left arm (see page 100); the line ends at the posterior border of the **membranous septum** and the nearby superomedial corner of the tricuspid valve. These facts explain the ease with which the valve and a defect in the septum may be transversed by a catheter when this superior route is used. (c) The degree of prominence of **the tuber of Lower** is increased by the muscles of the septal wall of the right atrium. This specimen is not unique; the development of cardiac muscles is as variable as that of the biceps brachii. (d) The **coronary sinus (C.S.)** is not provided with a valve. (e) The **anterior limbic muscle bundle**

lies in the antero-inferior margin of its fossa and terminates in the diminutive valve of the inferior vena cava. (f) Along the posterosuperior border of the fossa, the **posterior limbic bundle** extends to the orifice of the inferior vena cava. It is continuous above, with muscle fibers which course transversely and extend into the posterior atrial wall. These form a part of the "promontory" of Lower and may be separately termed **the bundle of Lower**.

4, **5**, and **6**: The specimen is now turned to 285° in **4** and **5**, then to 270° in **6**. The superior vena cava and lateral two-thirds of the inferior vena cava have been removed. The fat is removed from the upper portion of the posterior interatrial sulcus which, unlike the anterior, is easily recognizable. This is where the surgeon may separate the atria in order to incise the septal wall of the left atrium for the exposure of the mitral valve. Observe: (a) The muscles of the septal wall are well developed. (b) The arrows in **6** demonstrate the relation of the axis of the left atrium to the septal wall of the right atrium.

III. The Fossa Ovalis

Specimen B: 1: R.A.O. view: The line of the incision in this specimen passes through the axis of the left ventricle between the left and right aortic sinuses and through the midportion of the posterior aortic sinus. A large part of the lateral wall of L.V. has been removed (below the interrupted line), as has the wall posterior to the papillary muscles. Multiple small papillae comprise a posterior intermediate muscle that has been seen in **43—6**. Observe: (a) The septal muscles of the right atrium are thin—(1) a tuber of Lower (T.L.) is nevertheless present! (2) A fossa ovalis is barely recognizable due to its weak margination. (b) The muscles cover the septum with the exception of a membranous ellipse (Y) 8×5 mm in size which is 8 mm above the orifice of the inferior vena cava.

Specimen C: 2: 300° view: The scale is 1:1. Observe: (a) The membranous portion of the atrial septal wall, extending from the inferior vena cava almost to the superior vena cava (S.V.C.) orifice, is 32 mm in length and 20 mm in width. The lack of development of the muscle in its margins results in the virtual absence of a fossa ovalis.

Specimen D: 3–6: From the venae cavae, the transection passes obliquely to the left and anteriorly. The right segment of this specimen has been examined on page **88 (3–6)**. In **4**, the anteromedial wall has been removed. The beads represent the location of structures: yellow—right fibrous trigone; red—the ostium of L.V.; black—the attachment of the septal leaflet of the tricuspid valve. Observe: (a) In contradistinction to specimen A, the anterior limbic bundle (A.L.B.) is larger than the posterior (P.L.B.). (b) The axis of the strongly marginated fossa ovalis extends anterosuperiorly between the inferior vena cava and the posterior aortic sinus; its apogee is only 4.0 mm from the latter.* (c) In **6**, four muscle components are seen in the septal wall of the atrium: the bundle of Lower (L.B.), the posterior and anterior limbic bundles (P.L.B. and A.L.B.) and the precaval bundle (green)**. (d) In **5**, lighting is used to show the extension of the limbic muscle bundles (X) below the septal level. A small subseptal portion of the medial wall is present. If one examines specimens and clinical contrast studies, it becomes apparent that the inferior cavoatrial connection is not uncomplicated. It has long been known that muscle from both atria extends into their entering veins, so the observation that muscle extends below the septum does not warrant assigning a part to the atrium rather than to the vena cava. In spite of problems in terminology, drawing **6** demonstrates (and overstates) the fact that between the tubular vena cava and the septum, an obliquely disposed wall may be present. This wall may be perforated in transseptal left heart catheterization.

---

* The special designation apogee is apt: (1) Commonly, the axis of the greatest dimension of the fossa lies in the axis of the inferior vena cava, and a catheter passed from below will impinge on this point—the apogee of the fossa. (2) The apogee may be only 4 mm from the posterior aortic sinus. (3) A persisting probe patent foramen ovale will be found on its left side.

** Seen also in **98—1**.

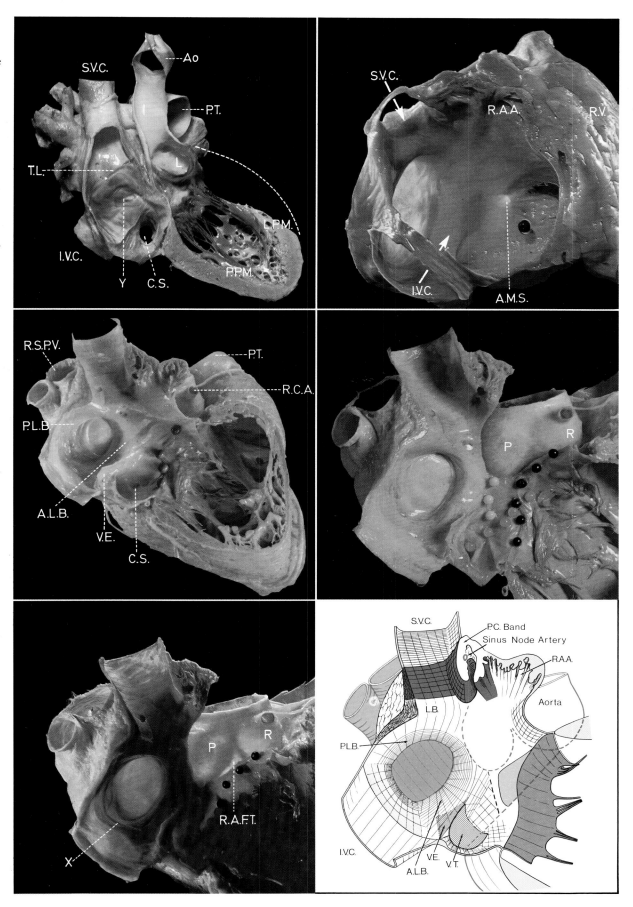

E. The Right Atrium and Cardiac Catheterization

When catheters (or pacemaker electrodes) are passed into the right heart for diagnostic or pacemaking purposes, the **superior route** may be chosen—a vein in the left (preferable) or the right arm is the site of introduction; if the **inferior route** is selected, a femoral vein—usually the right—is used for the entrance of the catheter or electrode. Even in small children, the percutaneous technique may be used. The relation of the anatomic features of the right atrium to the problem at hand is important in selecting the route.

The Superior Route —anatomic features: (a) **The superior vena cava:** (1) **Its lower segment** (as described on page 7) is directed inferiorly and anteromedially. (2) **The orifice** is above the septal wall. (3) **Its anterior wall** is above the superomedial corner of the tricuspid valve. These three anatomic features tend to direct the catheter into the right ventricle at the superomedial corner of the tricuspid valve in relation to the membranous septum; hence, defects in the latter are frequently transversed. This route was used in the early phase of catheterization, and the curved-tipped catheter could be passed without difficulty into the right ventricle and right pulmonary artery. (b) **The coronary sinus:** (1) **Its orifice** is located at the junction of the posteromedial and inferior walls. It is 10 mm postero-inferior to the membranous septum (which lies in the superior catheter pathway [v.s.]); hence, if the catheter tip at this point is directed posteriorly, the coronary sinus may be catheterized. (2) A **coronary sinus valve**, which may cover the orifice, is directed anterosuperiorly; hence, the superior route may be mandatory for coronary sinus catheterization (which is useful in the metabolic and hemodynamic study of the myocardial circulation). In the study of Wright, *et al.*, the valve was absent in approximately 25%; its greatest vertical dimension was under 4 mm in 40% and between 5 and 15 mm in 35% of the specimens. If coronary sinus catheterization is planned, review of prior coronary arteriograms should afford recognition of a prominent coronary sinus valve: During the venous phase, the efflux of contrast from the coronary sinus is directed in an anterosuperior jet-like manner—quite unlike its usual dispersion over the inferior wall of the right atrium—disclosing the presence of the prominent valve. (3) On page 191 attention is directed to the need for identification of the **pattern of the tributaries** of the coronary sinus in coronary sinus metabolic studies. (4) The **coronary sinus** itself may be inadvertently entered by a cardiac catheter or a pacemaker electrode. As it lies on the posterior wall of the heart, this event may be recognized by rotating the patient into a lateral view; however, the characteristic disposition of the sinus in a frontal plane should afford the "diagnosis". (c) The **fossae in the inferior wall** may be perforated by catheters passed from the superior route. The relation of the inferomedial fossa to the coronary orifice should be recalled when catheterization of the sinus is being performed. (d) The **valve of the inferior vena cava** may interfere with catheterization of the posteriorly located inferi-

or vena cava. Wright, Anson, and Cleveland demonstrated its variation in size in a study of 512 specimens. It was absent in 25%. Its greatest vertical dimension measured less than 8 mm in 55%; between 8 and 14 mm in 13%; between 15 and 20 mm in 6%; between 20 and 30 mm in 1%. (e) The **contour of the septal wall** is the major determinant in the catheterization of atrial septal defects. (1) A **sinus venosus defect**, lying on the upper slope of the septum just below the S.V.C. orifice, will be negotiated from above but, frequently, not when the inferior route is selected, especially if the septal wall is strongly contoured (see the specimen on page 98). (2) A **primum defect**, located just above the right fibrous trigone, is in the course of a catheter passed from the arm and will usually be transversed. (3) A **secundum defect** often is located in the inferior portion of the septal wall, the surface of which is directed inferiorly, posteriorly, and to the right. It faces the I.V.C. orifice; hence, catheters passed from below will (as an example of serendipity not skill) usually pass directly and without manipulation into the left atrium. Conversely, using the superior route (see page 98) catheter passage of this defect may not occur.

The Inferior Route —Anatomic Features: (a) The axis of the inferior vena cava is variable but, most often, is directed anterosuperiorly (as seen in **89—6**). (b) The orifice of the inferior vena cava is usually medial to that of the superior vena cava. It usually adjoins, but it is always adjacent to the atrial septum. (c) The coronary sinus is less easily catheterized from below. Prominent valves of this orifice and that of the inferior vena cava may make this impossible. (d) The compartments of the right atrial appendage may engage the catheter and perforation may result.* (e) A prominent I.V.C. valve may hinder catheterization of the right ventricle and the positioning of an electrode for His bundle recordings. (f) The characteristics of the atrial septum are of particular importance in catheterization of the left atrium using this route. A **probe patent foramen ovale** has been reported in the past in roughly 25% of normal adult hearts; however, in a recent paper, Schroeckstein, Wasenda, and Edwards have found an incidence of approximately 35%; it is apparent that its passage should be attempted before formal transseptal catheterization is performed: Recall that the location of the foramen at the apogee of the fossa ovalis is in line with the axes of the fossa ovalis and the inferior vena cava.** When the transseptal perforation technique is used, the Brockenbrough catheter needle unit (with the needle retracted) is first advanced into the superior vena cava, then with its tip directed to the left and posteriorly, i.e., against the septum, it is withdrawn until it "falls into" the fossa ovalis; through its membranous floor the needle is then passed. The fossa may be poorly marginated, even absent, rendering its identification difficult. Occasionally no membranous atrial septum exists; perforation of muscle is necessary (see page 99), and the performance of the study becomes more difficult. (g) The relation of the inferior vena cava to the **membranous septum**, located above the His bundle, should be noted in regard to recordings of the bundle which are usually carried out from below. Defects in this

septum also are easily catheterized from below in most instances.

At operation, the anatomy of the right atrium should not be ignored. Cannulae are passed through purse stringed areas of the lateral wall of the right atrium into the venae cavae to divert the venous return into the oxygenator. When the cannulae are being passed into the venae cavae, the smooth **posterior wall** of the sinus venarum should be followed. The precaval bundle, the compartments of the right atrial appendage above, the valve of the inferior vena cava and the inferomedial recess below will be engaged by an anteriorly directed catheter.

The anatomic features of the right atrium and their relation to catheterization and cannulation should be noted in the examination of the right heart in the next chapter.

---

* Strong muscle bundles joining the precaval and the upper end of the anterior vertical muscle bundle reduce the danger of appendageal perforation. The relative infrequency of perforation in the body of the atrium—between the pectinate muscles—is surprising.
** The utilization of the axes of the venae cavae requires lateral view examinations which are facilitated when biplane cineradiography is available.

Chapter 8: An Attitudinal Review of the Heart— An Introduction to Spatial Clinical Investigations

Introduction

Ultrasonography brings a new perspective in the study of physiology of the normal heart and affords greater comprehension of disease and its mechanisms. It has unfolded the epidemiology and pathophysiology of asymmetric septal hypertrophy and provides a safe and often superior technique for the determination of the type and degree of functional impairment of the heart. This technique, along with cardiac imaging with radio-pharmaceutical agents, is now added to cineradiographic and radiographic techniques, utilizing contrast agents, in the spatial study of cardiac structure and its abnormalities. This chapter is intended to provide an anatomic basis for this spatial examination. The four chambers will be examined in the four traditional radiographic planes; in some instances, the desirability of other examinations in either the horizontal or an elevated plane will also be indicated. Features, some of a nonradiographic nature, will be placed in summation. Before we commence this study, we will examine two separate features: (1) The two atria have been examined separately in Chapters 5 and 7. We will now examine transections to demonstrate the spatial disposition of each and the septum bet-

ween the two. (2) The mitral valve is a vital feature of left heart contrast studies; additive to the brief spatial examination on page 53, it will be seen here in two planes. Few structures can equal the anterior leaflet of the mitral valve in clinical interest and importance. The mode of its apposition to the posterior leaflet, and the line of flexion within the leaflet are important pathogenetic considerations. To the radiologist, the knowledge of the geometry of its planes is a prerequisite for his task. To the surgeon, the precise knowledge of the attachment of both leaflets brings sophistication and greater safety to the operation of valve replacement.

Technical Notes: (1) The material: Although 19 specimens will be used in this chapter, the examination of the right heart commencing on page 106 will consist essentially of dissection of a single specimen. (2) The right atrium is not attached, but apposed to the left atrium and has been removed without perforating either of the apposed walls. Such atrial separation is frequently possible when the membranous component in the foramen ovale is small. (When the atria are seperated, black cloth will usually be placed in the remaining chamber to effect the delimitation of the membraneous floor of the fossa ovalis—it will be denoted F.O.) This principle was, in part, used by some surgeons to correct atrial defects prior to the development of open techniques (Sondergaard). The statement that the two atria are only connected by the interatrial bundle, will often be found. However, when the separation is carried out through the septum, small scattering interatrial fibers will, in fact, require division; their disposition (in animals) has been described by Thomas (1959). (3) It is intended that the material in this work be used in conjunction with the study of the contrast examinations of patients. The greatest deficiency of the technique used here, the examination of the excised specimen, is found in the assessment of the axes of the inferior vena cava and the descending thoracic aorta. When a heart-lung preparation is employed, these vessels are the only structures seen which are not supported in the normal manner. Although it is apparent that a definitive statement regarding their anatomy depends on radiographic data, the quality of the information provided from excised material can be maximized if the following points are observed: (1) Both vessels are divided below the diaphragm which is included in the specimen. (2) The descending thoracic aorta is connected to the pericardium by mediastinal pleura and connective tissue— this is not divided prior to fixation. It is of interest that both structures and other vessels, e.g., the innominate artery, display a remarkable degree of configurational memory following perfusion fixation.

Before examining the pages on the mitral valve, turn to page 21 and observe the relation of the aortic sinuses to

the commissures of the valve. In frontal transections, different structures will be traversed in different specimens: On page 102, the frontal section traverses the commissures but not the aorta. On page 104, the commissures and the aortic annuli, 3 mm posterior to their nadir, are traversed. The differences in the structures sectioned depend on: (1) The shape and the axis of the ventricle—vertical and horizontal hearts are seen on 102 and 104, respectively. (2) The mode of attachment of the mitral valve: this is normal in the specimen on page 102; the length of the ostial attachments is reduced in the specimen on page 104.

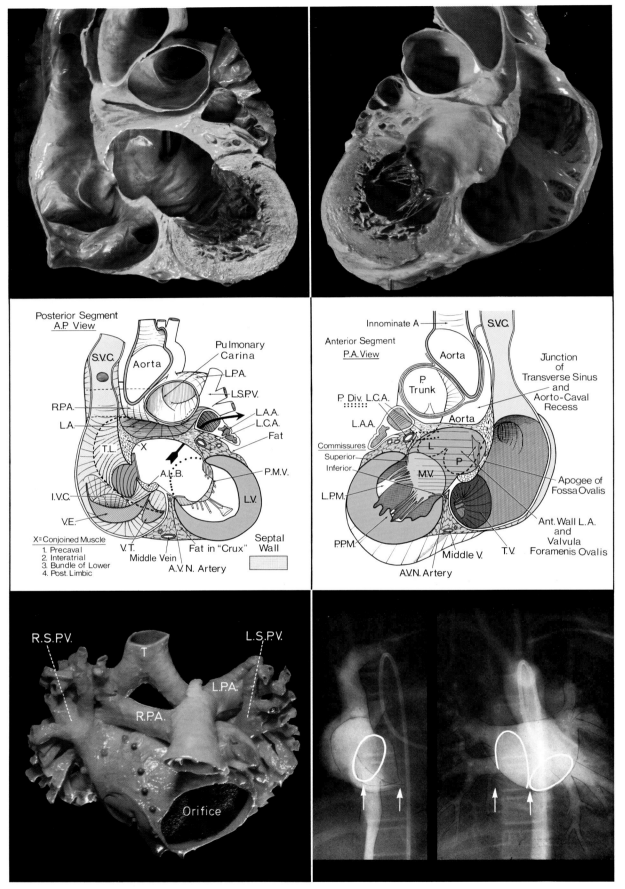

Posterior Segment
A.P. View

S.V.C.
Aorta
Pulmonary Carina
L.P.A.
L.S.P.V.
R.P.A.
L.A.
T.L.
L.A.A.
L.C.A.
Fat
X
A.L.B.
P.M.V.
I.V.C.
L.V.
V.E.

X=Conjoined Muscle
1. Precaval
2. Interatrial
3. Bundle of Lower
4. Post. Limbic

V.T.
Middle Vein
A.V.N. Artery
Fat in "Crux"
Septal Wall

Anterior Segment
P.A. View

Innominate A
S.V.C.
Aorta
P. Trunk
Junction of Transverse Sinus and Aorto-Caval Recess
P. Div. L.C.A.
L.A.A.
Aorta
Commissures
Superior
Inferior
L
P
M.V.
L.P.M.
Apogee of Fossa Ovalis
P.P.M.
Ant. Wall L.A. and Valvula Foramenis Ovalis
Middle V.
T.V.
A.V.N. Artery

R.S.P.V.
T
L.S.P.V.
L.P.A.
R.P.A.
Orifice

A. The Disposition of the Atria and the Atrial Septum
I. In the Frontal Plane

Specimen A: 1–4: The frontal transection passes through the commissures of the mitral valve. In **3** and **4**, the superior and anterior walls of the left atrium are red—its cross section and that of the septum and septal surface are grey. The fat in the crux and left coronary fossa is yellow—the single variance from the color code in this atlas.

(I.) The Right Atrium: (a) In a sagittal plane, the **sinus venarum** is disposed postero-inferiorly (pages 7 and 106); hence, this frontal transection, passing through the superior vena cava (S.V.C.), traverses the sinus venarum above and the body of the atrium below. (b) The **inferior wall** of the body is convex inferiorly and to the left; its medial portion is separated by the fat in the wedge-shaped crux from the left ventricle, the left atrium, and the inferior commissure of the mitral valve. The A.V. node artery is between the wall and the commissure. (c) In **1**, the inferior wall is retracted to display **the valve of the inferior vena cava** (V.E.), which is set at right angles to an A.P. view. (d) The **orifice of the coronary sinus** is near the median plane, underlying the nadir of the posterior aortic sinus. Its valve (V.T.) is oriented anterosuperiorly.

(II.) The Left Atrium: (a) Its **orifice** is indicated by the inverted dotted arc in **3**. (b) The attachment of the **anterior wall** to the A.V. membrane is seen in **2** and **4**. (c) The **superior wall** is separated by the transverse sinus of the pericardium from the overlying branching portion of the pulmonary trunk and right pulmonary artery. (d) The anterior wall of the appendage (L.A.A.) has been transected at its junction with the anterior, superior, and **left lateral** walls of the atrium. In the left coronary fossa, the posterior division (of L.C.A.) is anterior to the appendage. (e) A small, nonseptal portion of the **right lateral wall** appears at the apex of the crux—above the A.V. node.

(III.) The Atrial Septum: On this page the right and on the next page the left surface of the septum appears. (a) **The contour of the septal wall** results primarily from the wrapping of the right atrium around the left. A well-developed promontory of the right atrium (T.L.) is present. (b) **The fossa ovalis**: (1) Its **axis** is directed antero-superiorly; (2) **its apogee** is 3 mm from the posterior aortic sinus; (3) **its floor** is formed by the membranous valvula foraminis ovalis, a truncated ellipse, the upper border of which lies on the anterior wall of the left atrium (as seen in **2** and **4**)—a probe patent foramen ovale is present. (4) **Its marginal muscles** are in the line of transection; the anterior limbic band (A.L.B.) is below; the posterior limbic band is a part of the conjoined muscles (X) listed in 3.

Note: T.L. denotes the tuber of Lower.

Specimen B: 5: A.P. view of the left atrium which has been detached from specimen B, pages 124 and 125. The trachea and pulmonary trunk and their branches are in place. Observe: (a) **The upper part of the appositional surface of the left atrium faces to the right, superiorly and anteriorly.** (b) The line where the chamber has been detached from the A.V. membrane forms the orifice of the chamber.

102—6: A.P. view: The right and left atria appear in their diastolic phase. **The Right Atrium**: (a) The axis of the superior vena cava is directed slightly medially. (b) The axis of the inferior vena cava is staggered to the left of the axis of the superior; occasionally the two axes may be in line. (c) The inferior wall is marked by arrows; above it and to the right of the septum, **contrast extends to the median plane**; the coronary sinus orifice is here (see **1**). An ellipse marks the T.V. orifice.

The Left Atrium: The orifice is marked by an ellipse, the appositional area by a hoop. Like an inverted, wide-mouthed, earthen pot, this chamber extends to the right superiorly and posteriorly.

II. In the Horizontal Plane

Specimen C: 1–6: On the left, the horizontal transection passes through the superior commissure of the mitral valve (the leaflets are in diastole) and on the right, the upper portion of the large fossa ovalis. The beads identify the following: The attachments of the mitral valve = red; the tricuspid valve = green; the left fibrous trigone = yellow. The segments are in two vertical rows, and the views are attitudinal.

(I.) **The right atrium** in this plane roughly forms a right angled sector of a circle. Radii A and B are formed by the septal wall and the plane of the tricuspid ostium. The arc is formed by posterior and lateral walls—the point of division between the two is the terminal bundle which is best seen in **4**. In the upper segment, note the precaval bundle, the sagittal bundle and the compartments of the appendage. In the **inferior wall**, the anterior vertical bundle (A.B.) and the supravalvular lamina (S.V.L.) proceed to the crux (see **3** and **5**). The coronary sinus orifice (seen in **1** only) is near (usually to the left of) the median plane.

(II.) **Left Atrium**: (a) The five, poorly defined walls may be seen in **4**; the septal surface is largely in **3**. (b) This is the posterior chamber of the heart—note the contribution of the four chambers to the cardiac borders.

(III.) **The Atrial Septum**: The major portion of the **septal wall** is seen in the lower segment because the transection is high in the atrium; only the apogee of the fossa ovalis is in the upper segment. At all levels of transection, the atrial septum will be staggered to the left of the ventricular septum. The fossa ovalis is strongly margined by the limbic muscle bundles. The right atrium wraps around the left; hence, the major portion of its septal wall is on the opposite side of the septal surface of the left atrium and faces to the right and inferiorly. The membranous atrial septum is best seen in **5** (F.O.); its relations and those of the limbic bands (stipple) to the inferior vena cava and the coronary sinuses should be carefully noted in **1**. Other features: (a) Note the superior papillary muscle (S.P.M.) and the septal band (S.B.). (b) In diastole the anterior leaflet of the mitral valve swings anteriorly—see **5**. (c) Note the attachment of the posterolateral wall of the right ventricle to the A.V. membrane.

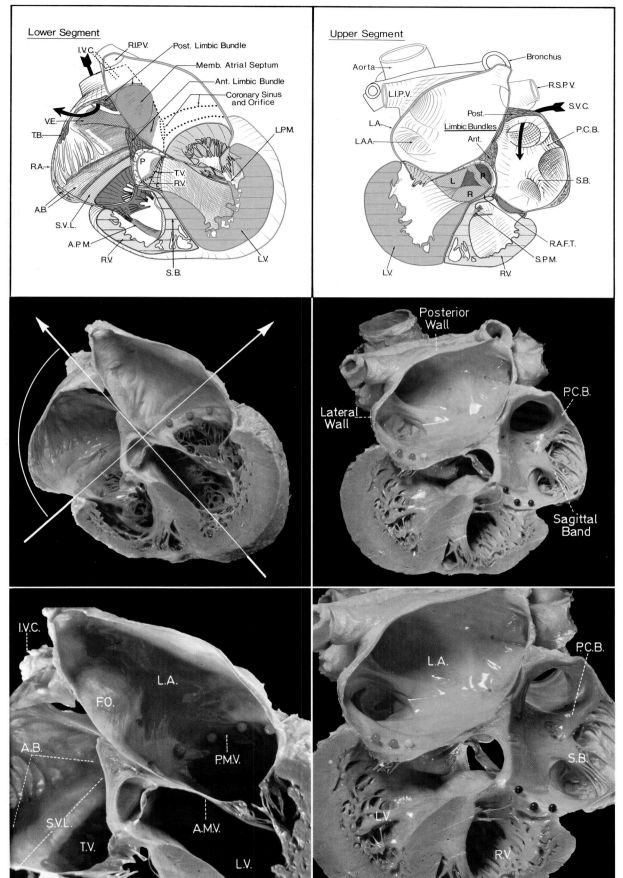

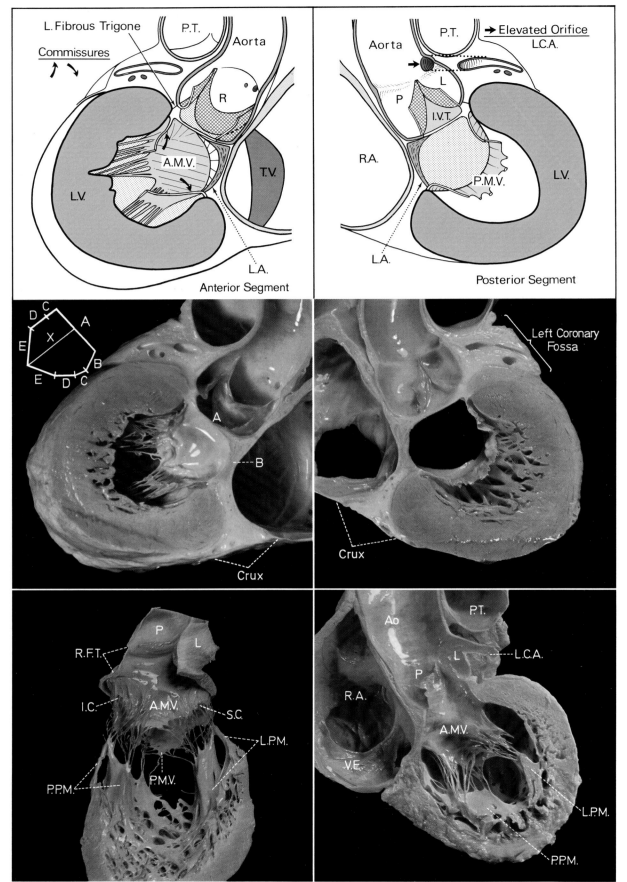

Anterior Segment

Posterior Segment

Left Coronary Fossa

Crux

Crux

B. The Disposition of the Anterior Leaflet of the Mitral Valve in the Frontal Plane

Specimen A: 1–4: The mitral leaflets are fixed in diastole. The frontal transection passes 3 mm posterior to the nadirs of the posterior and left aortic annuli and through the commissures of the mitral valve. The P.A. view of the anterior segment is seen in **1** and **3**; the A.P. view of the posterior segment appears in **2** and **4**. Observe: (a) In **1** and **3**, the transection passes through the left fibrous trigone, which is attached to the apex of the rounded ostial slope of the left ventricle. The superior commissure of the mitral valve is located 8 mm below the left fibrous trigone. (b) **The shape of the anterior leaflet of the mitral valve** is shown in the insert in **3**. (The shape is also shown in **10—2.**) The eight components of its borders and their lengths in this specimen are: (A)—The site of the left atrial attachment between the left and right fibrous trigones=28 mm. (B)—The attachment to the right fibrous trigone=10 mm. (C)—The attachment to the left and right sides of the ostium of L.V.=3 and 4 mm. (D)—The junction between the anterior and posterior leaflets—left=14 mm, right=10 mm. (E)—The free edge between the commissures and the apex=14 and 14 mm. X—the apex-base dimension=25 mm. Measurement (C) is unusual (a measurement of 10 mm is usual); this is associated with a reduction in the A.P. dimension of the outflow tract to 12.0 mm. (c) The lines of the largest attached margin (A) and the maximum depth (X) both meet the horizontal at an angle of approximately 45° and intersect at a 90° angle. (d) Below the posterior aortic sinus, note **the conjoined attachments of the left and right atria** to the right fibrous trigone. (e) The inferior wall of the right atrium, the nonseptal part of the right lateral wall of the left atrium (L.A.), and the posterosuperior process of L.V. form the walls of the fat-filled crux. (f) In **2** and **4**, the posterior leaflet is "attached" to the ostium of the ventricle. (g) The left coronary fossa is seen bisected: its roof=pulmonary trunk (P.T.); its floor=L.V.; its medial wall=the aorta. (h) Identification of the ostium of L.V. in all figures and dissections is a prime precept. The highest point of the ostium is seen (in **3**) at the left anterior fibrous trigone; the lowest point is seen (in **4**) just to left and posterior to the point of transsection—review page 18.

Specimen B: 5: A.P. nonattitudinal view. First examine early stages of the dissection of this specimen on **112—3** and **4**. Only the area of the anterior leaflet between the commissures and the apex is triangular: Note the eight borders.*

Specimen C: 6: **The anterior leaflet** is in mid-diastole. The transection is to the left of the posterior aortic nadir. Note the shape of the anterior leaflet—7 of the 8 boundaries described above can be seen. The axis of the greatest depth is at right angles to the annular axis.

The papillary muscles: Observe (1) their spatial disposition in **6** and (2) their relationship to the mitral and aortic valves—implied in **3** and evident in **6**. (3) The posterior muscle is flat and quadrangular.

* The leaflet forms a squat pentagon (page 26). See the eight components of its border: (a) The intervalvular is obscured on the left by the aortic valve. (b) The junctional (R.F.T.) is divided. (c) The two commissural, (d) the two ostial and (e) the free border(s) are all well seen.

The Disposition of the Mitral Valve in the Horizontal Plane

The mitral valve leaflets have been fixed in their systolic position. The plane of transection passes through the heart in a nearly horizontal plane; it is angled slightly posteriorly, superiorly, and to the right. The A.P. view of the inferior segment is seen following a rotation on its transverse axis of 45° in **1**, 75° in **2**, and 90° in **3** where the disposition of structures in the horizontal plane is seen. As the heart is rotated, the papillary muscles finally lie in a vertical plane; the lateral is not anterior to the posterior.

3 and **4**: Attitudinal views of the inferior and superior segments, with their drawings below in **5** and **6**: Observe (a) **The axis of the horizontally transected anterior leaflet in systole** and the axis of its hinge in both systole and diastole lie in a frontal plane. (b) **The left ventricular ostium** faces posteriorly, superiorly, and to the right. (c) If a line is directed midway between the septal and lateral walls, its axis is directed 45° to the right and posteriorly. **The axis of the papillary muscles** is angled 15° posteriorly to this axis. Hence, they will be seen en face, not at L.A.O. or 45° but at 60°. (d) Visually replace the upper segment over the lower—it is apparent that **the commissures of the mitral valve are in a frontal plane.** Their designations could appropriately be superior and inferior, and lateral and medial, but the addition of the words "anterior" and "posterior" incorrectly describe their spatial relationship. (e) The **membranous septum** and the right anterior fibrous trigone extend superiorly, to the right, and posteriorly. Their axis is angled inferiorly in relation to the axis of the muscular ventricular septum. The aorta normally overrides the latter; note the relation of the posterior aortic sinus to the muscular septum in **3** and **5**. This is normal—re-examine the specimen on page 103. (f) The line of section passes through the **sagittal muscle bundle** (S.B.), separating the atrial appendage into posterolateral (P.L.) and anteromedial (A.M.) compartments. The muscle bundle is poorly named—it extends to the right and anteriorly from its origin in the precaval bundle. (g) The axis of the right and left A.V. sulci are in the R.A.O.-L.P.O. plane. The expansive **right coronary fossa**, fat-filled and dominated by the right coronary artery, is seen between the right ventricle and aorta and the anteromedial wall of the right atrium. It is continuous with the fat posterior to the aorta. (h) The lowest portion of the transverse sinus of the pericardium is seen in relation to the posterior aortic sinus. (i) In photographs **2** and **3**, the superiorly directed, concave, upper margin of the membranous atrial septum is seen. During fixation, the perfusion pressure in the right atrium exceeded that of the left; hence, the superiorly directed convexity of the atrial septum seen here is artifactitious; however, this appearance may occur when a similar pressure gradient exists as a result of disease, e.g. isolated pulmonary stenosis.

Note: On these two pages, the crux and left coronary fossa are seen in one specimen (**104—1–4**) and the right coronary fossa in another (**105—1–6**).

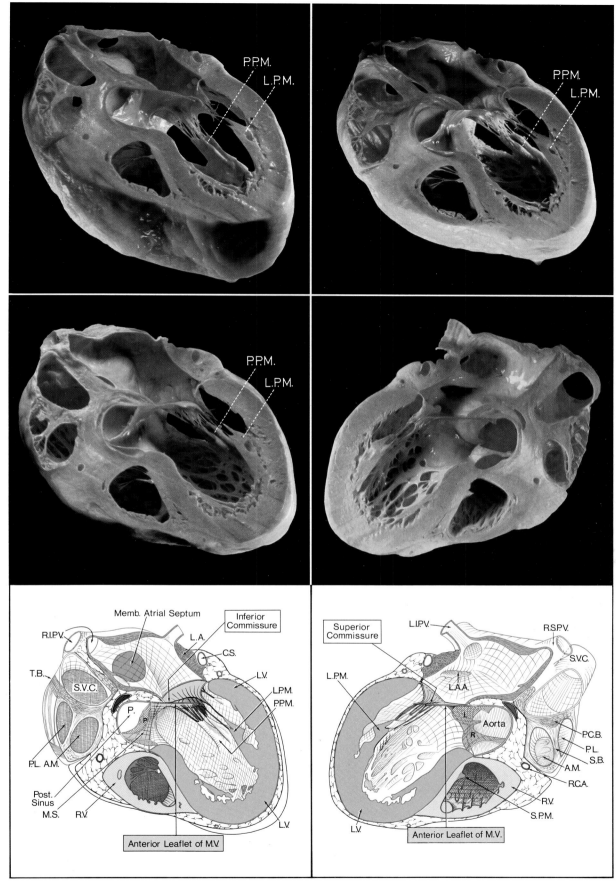

105

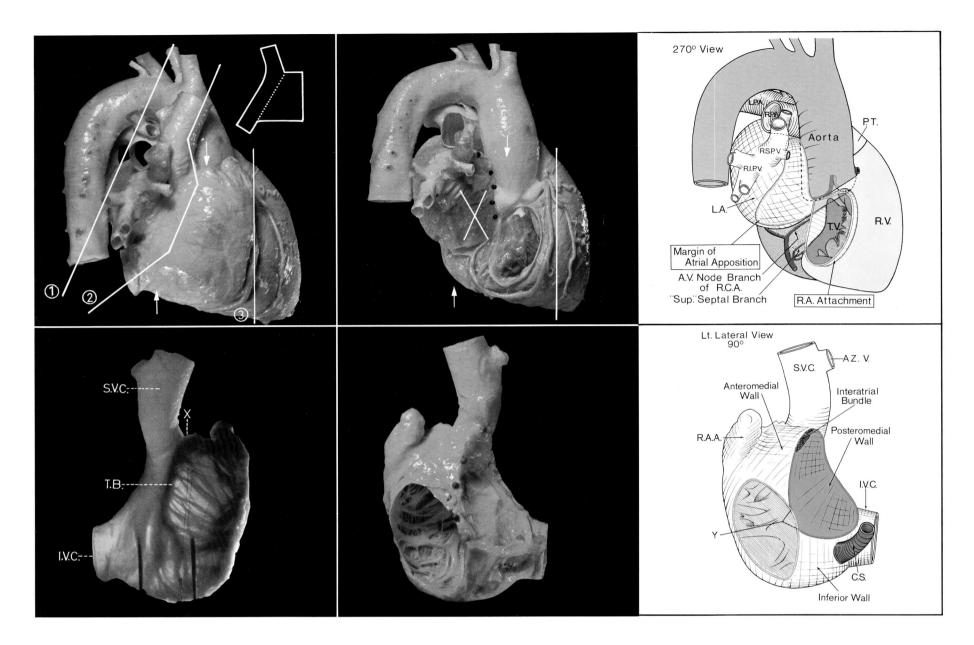

C. The Lateral Views—The Lateral Plane

I. The Right Heart in the Lateral Plane

With the exception of **107—3**, a single specimen will be seen on these two pages. All views will be right lateral with the exception of **5** and **6** and **107—5** and **6**, which are left lateral.

1: The intact specimen: The following are indicated by white lines: (1) The trachea and the right bronchial pathway; (2) The axes of the venae cavae and sinus venarum; (3) The anterior border of the right atrium. Arrows mark the cavo-atrial angles. Observe: (a) The upper segment of the superior vena cava parallels the tracheal axis. (b) The sinus venarum and the pulmonary veins parallel the bronchial axis. The upper and lower divisions of both veins are well seen. (c) the superior pulmonary vein is posteroinferior to the superior vena cava; the inferior vein posterosuperior to the inferior vena cava. (d) Note the distances between the angles and the anterior border of the right atrium: In this view, the outline of the body of the right atrium forms a trun-

cated right-angle triangle (see insert in **1**). Its greatest A.P. dimension is above the inferior wall.

2 and **3**: After removal of the right atrium: In **2**, the blue and red beads identify the anterior and posterior margins of apposition of the atria. The most anterior inferior red bead identifies the site of the A.V. node. The adjacent red and blue beads mark the ends of the right fibrous trigone. In **3**, the attachments of the right atrium to the tricuspid and A.V. membranes are shown, as is the triangular strip of right atrium between the two, which has been left in contact with the anterior extremity of the posterior superior process of the left ventricle; the latter is indicated by stipple. Observe: (a) The axes of the left atrium and the sinus venarum form the letter X. (b) The tricuspid ostium extends below the ostium of L.V. (c) The superior cavo-atrial angle: (1) It overlies the aorta. (2) It is directly above the superomedial angle of the tricuspid ostium. (3) It identifies the S.A. node; note the location of the proximal right coronary atery in **2** and visualize the course of a right sinus node artery in this view. The relation of the aortic an-

nuli at 270° can be plotted (page 108); hence, arteries from the left coronary artery to the node can also be visualized.

The Isolated Right Atrium: 4: 270° view: (a) The terminal muscle bundle (T.B.) descends from the superior cavo-atrial angle (X). In its upper course, it demarcates the posterior and lateral walls.

5 and **6**: 90° view: Observe: On page 103, three of the planes of the atrium are seen forming a right-angled sector of a circle. Here we can see that the sector angle varies at the different levels of the chamber. Above the tricuspid valve, the anteromedial wall and the septum form the radii of a sector of a circle with an obtuse sector angle; below, the radii are formed by the plane of the valve and the inferior wall. The attachment of the three walls (seen in this view) and the tricuspid ostium converge at the A.V. membrane (Y). The greatest transverse dimension of the chamber is found at the point of convergence. This point is located in a vertical line dropped from the superior cavo-atrial angle. Finally, visually replace the atrium in its bed in **2**.

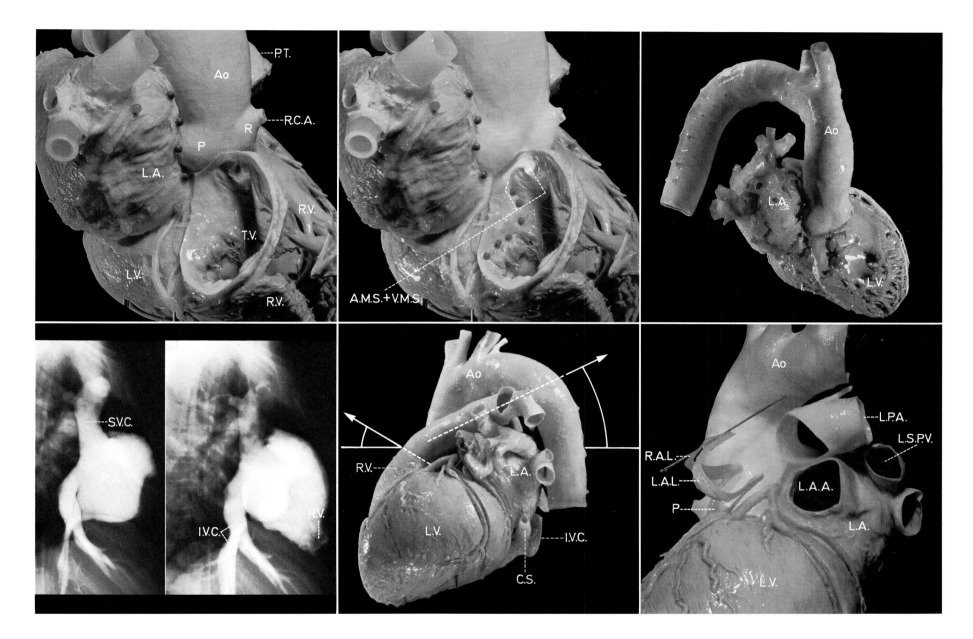

1 and **2**: With the exception of rims at the pulmonary and tricuspid ostia, the anterior and posterolateral walls of the right ventricle have been removed. Observe: (a) the conjoined attachments of the atria to the J-point of the A.V. membrane below the nadir of the posterior aortic sinus; (b) the location and relation of the bulging right and posterior aortic sinuses to the right ventricle and atrium; (c) the small red beads in **2** mark the line of muscular attachment of the septal leaflet of the tricuspid valve to the A.V. unit. The inverted U-shaped attachment of the leaflet to the A.V. membrane is seen above the latter. A 11.0-mm gap is present between the septal and anterosuperior leaflets. For three reasons this is relevant in tricuspid valve replacement. (1) The common A.V. bundle and R.B.B. run along the ostium of L.V. (2) The A.V. membrane here may be narrow. (3) The leaflet may be attached far posteriorly in relation to the His or common A.V. bundle. Therefore, as a result of needle injury, either the membranous septum could be perforated or heart block could result.

Specimen B: 3: The right heart has been removed. (a) The axis of the ascending aorta is vertical in this horizontal heart; these axes are independent of one another. (b) The left atrium continues the direction of L.V.

4: A right lateral view of a contrast study seen first in atrial diastole, then in systole: Observe: (a) The quadrangular outline of the body of the right atrium and compare with **106—1**. (b) In this view the inferior vena cava is always posterior to the superior vena cava; however, the axis of the inferior is variable—usually it and the axis of the superior form an obtuse angle; here the axes are virtually parallel. This is a vertical heart, which is an important factor affecting this relationship. (c) The inferior wall of the right ventricle extends well below the tricuspid valve.

Specimen A: 5 and **6**: Left lateral views: In **6**, the following have been removed: the free walls of the right ventricle; the atrial appendage; segments of the pulmonary trunk. pulmonary veins and aorta. Observe: (a) As seen here and in **1** and **2,** the infundibulum of the right ventricle extends above the left ventricle; the axis of the pulmonary ostium is an indicator of its size. (b) Note the axis of the pulmonary trunk and (c) the location of the pulmonary annuli.

Note: The isthmus of the aorta, a narrowing in its caliber, is seen just posterior to the subclavian artery in **3**. The aortic knob, (best seen on page 126) is (a) perpendicular to the plane of examination in the lateral view—and (b) posterior to the isthmus (in **3**) and posterior to the vertebral artery, which has an aortic origin in **5**. It is the highest part of the aortic arch.

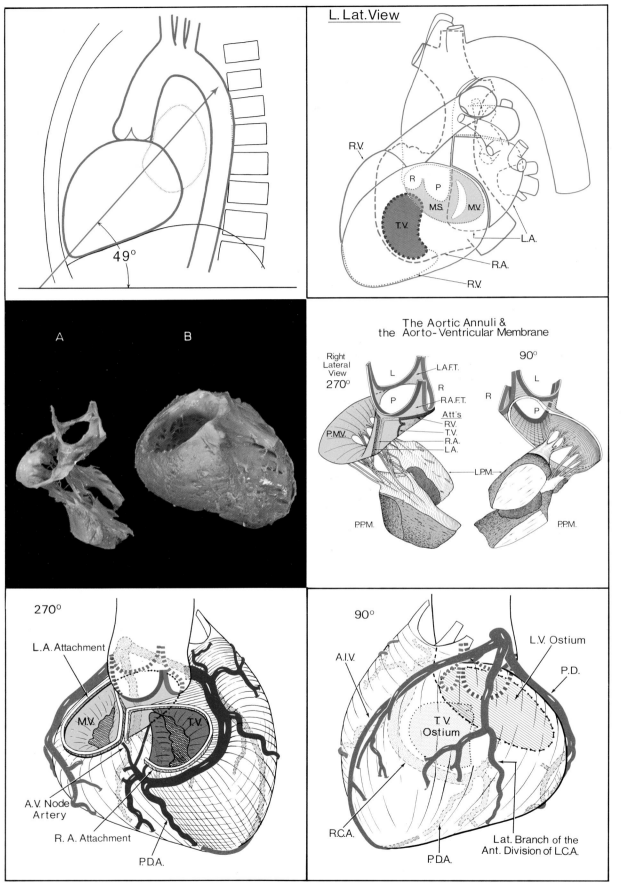

L. Lat. View

49°

R.V.

R

P

M.S.

M.V.

T.V.

L.A.

R.A.

R.V.

A

B

The Aortic Annuli &
the Aorto-Ventricular Membrane

Right
Lateral
View
270°

L

L.A.F.T.

R

P

R.A.F.T.

Att's
R.V.
T.V.
R.A.
L.A.

P.M.V.

L.P.M.

P.P.M.

90°

L

R

P

L.P.M.

P.P.M.

270°

L.A. Attachment

M.V.

T.V.

A.V. Node
Artery

R. A. Attachment

P.D.A.

90°

A.I.V.

L.V. Ostium

P.D.

T.V.
Ostium

R.C.A.

Lat. Branch of the
Ant. Division of L.C.A.

P.D.A.

II. The Left Heart in the Lateral Plane

(I). The Axis of the Left Ventricle

1: Left lateral view of a left ventriculogram: The axis of the ventricle, a line drawn midway between the upper and lower border, is elevated 49° above the horizontal plane.

Specimen A: 2: Left lateral view of a composite drawing of the progressive dissection seen on page 7. In this horizontal heart, the above axis measures 35°. The axis of the ventricle affects the orientation of the ostium of the left ventricle and the level of the aortic annuli.

(II.) The Spatial Dispostion and Relations of the Ostium of the Left Ventricle and the Aortic Annuli

Specimen B: 3–6

3: Right lateral view: This is the final stage of the dissection used for the composite drawings **5** and **6**.

A—the complex composed of the aortic annuli, A.V. membrane, and papillary muscles which has been removed from **B**—the isolated left ventricle—note its ostium.

4: The above complex is seen. Observe: (a) The aortic annuli are disposed from above downward in the following order: left, right, and posterior. This order is constant for all views. In the lateral views, the left is directly above the posterior and the right is anterior to both. How much easier it would be to describe these annuli by the spatially correct terms—the anterior and the right posterior and left posterior, rather than right, posterior and left. (b) Viewed from 270° the anterior division of the A.V. membrane meets the lateral plane at an angle of 120°. The attachments to it can be seen and examined in **5**.

5 and **6**: Observe: (a) The ostium of the left ventricle is identified in **5** by the attachment of the yellow A.V. membrane, the dotted line and the site of the attachment of the left and right aortic annuli; in **6**, it is identified by the lines disposed in its axis. (b) Re-examine the aortic annuli and their relations. (c) In the lateral view the mitral valve is located posteriorly in the heart. (d) In diastole, the anterior leaflet of the mitral valve is disposed in a frontal plane. (e) The anterior interventricular (A.I.V.) and posterior descending (P.D.A.) arteries identify the location of the interventricular grooves in this view. (f) In their upper courses, the right coronary and anterior interventricular arteries are superimposed. (g) The tricuspid ostium extends below the left ventricular ostium; therefore, branches of the related right coronary artery must pass superiorly if they are to be related to the latter. (h) The A.V. node artery passes to the right fibrous trigone—the posterior (or superior) septal passes to the apex of the posterior superior process, the anterior boundary of which is formed by the tricuspid ostium. Visualize the location of these landmarks in the left lateral view. (i) The large lateral branch of the anterior division of the left coronary atery (anterior descending) descends vertically across the lateral wall of the left ventricle, dividing it unequally into anterior and posterior parts.

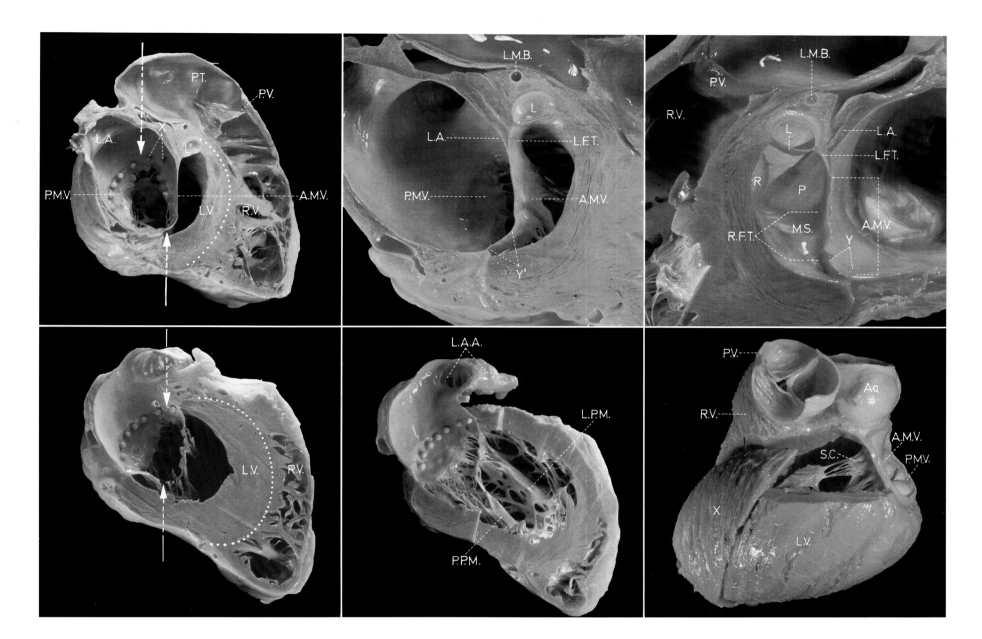

(III.) The Mitral Valve

Specimen C: 1–5: It is important to examine **79—3–6** which show drawings of the entirety of both segments of this 350-gram heart: The sagittal transection passes through the left aortic sinus and the anterior leaflet of the mitral valve. In **109—1–4**, the fat in the A.V. sulcus has not been removed as it has on page 79.

1: (a) The left segment is viewed from 240° to disclose the commissures of the mitral valve which are indicated by the vertical arrows; the inferior is anterior in this view—at 270° it underlies the superior. (b) Note the low attachment of the left atrium to the A.V. membrane—the intervalvular and left-fibrous trigones are confluent. (c) The leaflet (P.V.) attachment crosses the pulmonary ostium.

2: In this 270° view of the left segment, the scale is 1:1. (a) During diastole, the mobile segment of the anterior leaflet (of the mitral valve) swings anteriorly into the cav-ity of the ventricle; during systole, it returns to lie in the plane of the ostium of the ventricle. (b) The left main branch of the left coronary artery (L.M.B.) is in contact with the pulmonary trunk—a point to recall if a stenotic pulmonary valve is ever to be divided from below by a sharp instrument.

3: In this 90° view of the right segment, the scale is 1:1. Observe: (a) In the lateral plane of examination, through-out systole and diastole, the nonmobile segment of the anterior leaflet lies (obliquely) in a frontal plane. The in-tervalvular border, between the left and right fibrous tri-gones, and the junctional border, at the right fibrous tri-gone, are seen here. The ostial borders—the left (X in **1**) and the right (Y in **3**)—extend posteriorly. (b) The left aortic leaflet is directly above the posterior and both are posterior to the right aortic leaflet. (c) The (transillu-minated) membranous atrial septum is 6 mm posterior to the posterior aortic sinus. (d) In **2** and **3**, the trans-verse sinus of the pericardium separates the pulmonary trunk and the left atrium.

4: 270° view: A second sagittal transection has been made 16 mm to the left of the initial transection; it pas-ses just to the right of the superior commissure—see **1**. The attachment of the anterior leaflet to the left side of the ostium of L.V. is in the lamina removed. Observe: (a) the posterior location of the mitral valve in the ventricle; (b) the vertical disposition of the anterior leaflet; (c) the commissures are in a frontal plane.

5: An additional 10-mm lamina of the wall (of L.V.) has been removed to expose the cavity of L.V. Note the dis-position of the papillary muscles in this 270° view.

Specimen D: 6: Left lateral view with 45 ° elevation: Til-ting the x-ray tube will place the mitral valve orifice in profile. The degree of tilt will vary inversely with the axis of the ventricle—see the ostia in **108—1** and **2**. In addition, (a) note the high location of the discrete papil-lary muscle which provides attachment for the superior commissural chordae; a left lateral view appears in **44—5**; (b) incisions delimit the nonpapillary portion of the free wall of L.V., marked by the letter X.

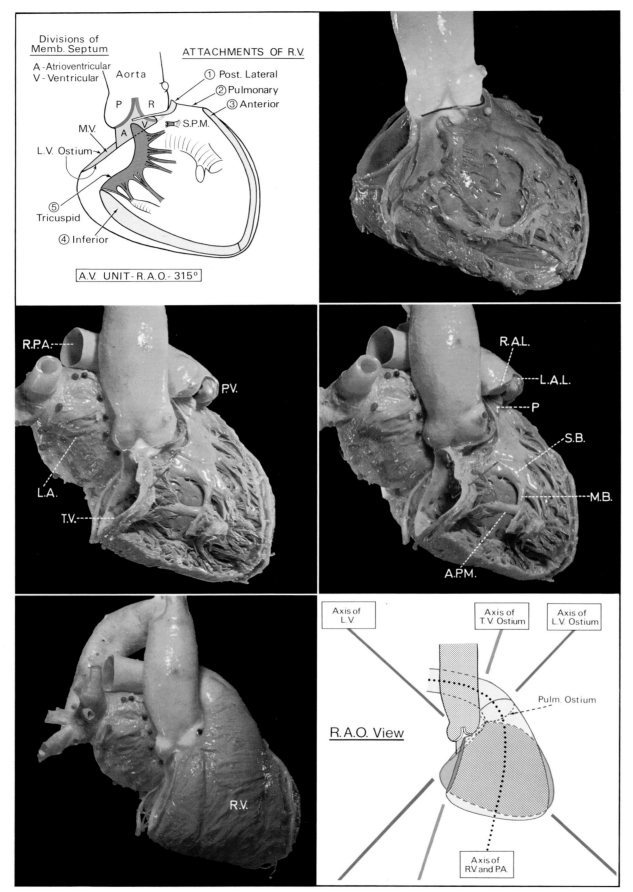

D. The Right Anterior Oblique View — The R.A.O.-L.P.O. Plane

I. The Right Heart

Specimen A: 110—1–6 and 111—1–4; A progressive dissection has been carried out; we will reassemble the parts.

Note: Unless otherwise indicated all views are R.A.O.

1: The aorto-ventricular unit—R.A.O. view (315°): Observe: (a) In the horizontal plane, the left ventricle is oriented in the L.A.O.-R.P.O. axis: the ostium is directed to the right, superiorly and posteriorly; in the R.A.O. view, the axis of L.V. (a line drawn midway between the upper and lower borders of the ventricle) and the horizontal form an angle of 45°: the ostium of the ventricle is almost closed and its axis crosses the left ventricular axis at a right angle. (b) The left ventricle is seen in its greatest dimension from this vantage point. (c) The five attachments of the R.V. to the unit are noted.

Note: This drawing should be used for orientation in the stages that follow.

2: 300° view of the A.V. unit: Observe: (a) The "opening" of the ostium of L.V. has increased—it will be open to its full extent at 225°. (b) The anterior division of the A.V. membrane is at a right angle to this plane of examination. (c) Note the club-shaped upper extremity of the septal leaflet of the tricuspid valve on the A.V. membrane. The small red beads indicate the muscular part of the line of attachment of the leaflet to the A.V. unit.

3 and **4**: The left atrium, the tricuspid rim, the inferior wall of R.V., and the pulmonary valve and trunk are in place. In **3**, the aortic sinuses and the membranous septum are transilluminated to display their location in relation to the aortic annuli and the ostium of L.V. in this view. In **4**, the relations of the posterior and right aortic sinuses and the pulmonary leaflets are seen.

5: The anterior and posterolateral walls are in place. Observe: (a) The right ventricle envelops the right aortic sinus. Re-examining **1–4**, we note the location of the superior papillary muscle (S.P.M.) below the nadir of the right aortic annulus. It marks the junction of the posterior walls of the sinus and infundibulum of the right ventricle.

6: (1) The axis of L.V. extends posterosuperiorly at an angle of 45°. (2) The axis of the ostium of L.V. crosses the axis of L.V. at a right angle. (3) The axis of the ascending aorta is vertical. (4) The axis of the right ventricle and the pulmonary trunk and the right pulmonary artery curves around the left ventricle and the aorta. (5) The tricuspid ostium, appearing almost closed from this vantage point, forms an angle of 25° with the axis of the left ventricular ostium and a 20° angle with the vertical. The angle formed by the intersection of these axes is relatively constant, although the angles of the axes vary— they are larger in a vertical heart and smaller in a horizontal heart as shown on the next page.

1 and **2**: The isolated right atrium. Observe: (a) The relations of the right atrium to the R.A.O.-L.P.O. plane of examination: (1) The axis of the plane of the tricuspid orifice is in the R.A.O.-L.P.O. axis; however, the plane is angled posteriorly on its vertex. (2) The highly contoured posteromedial wall meets the plane at a right angle. (3) The inferior wall is suspended in the plane of examination; its convexity faces inferiorly. (4) The anteromedial wall meets the plane at a 15° angle. Note: The convergence of these four planes occurs between the arrows in **2**. (b) In the horizontal plane, the right atrium forms a right-angled sector of a circle; the radii are formed by the valve orifice and the septum; the arc is formed by the posterior and lateral walls. (See the photographs **103—3** and **106—4–6**.) Therefore, in the R.A.O.-L.P.O. plane of examination, the greatest density in a contrast study will be adjacent to the tricuspid valve.

3 and **4**: The intact specimen is first viewed from R.A.O., then as a mirror image of L.P.O. in **4**. (a) The right atrium is in place; the lateral wall, forming the arc of the sector of the circle, is oblique to our plane of examination. (b) The ascending aorta and the branching portion of the arch lie almost in the same plane. The area of the aortic knob (X) crosses the plane of examination as seen in **4**. The aorta then descends almost parallel to the ascending aorta. (c) When we examine both photographs, the relation of the axes of the right and left ventricles and the elevation of the infundibulum above L.V. can be seen. (d) The right coronary artery and related A.V. sulcus mark the axis of the tricuspid ostium, which is deflected 20° posteriorly (v.s.). (e) As seen in **4**, the posterolateral radial artery (P.L.R.) descends almost vertically across L.V.—well separate from the ostium.* (f) In **4** and **110—5**, the proximal portions of pulmonary arteries are seen. Essentially, the axis of the left is directed toward us—the artery is seen end on and the axis of the right is horizontal and seen almost at a right angle.** (g) Compare the axes of the tricuspid ostium (in **3**) and the ostium of L.V. (marked by arrow in **4**).

Specimen B: 5 and **6**: A horizontal heart is seen before and after removal of the right heart. Observe: (a) The axis of the left ventricle is now only 35° above the horizontal; however, the axis of the ascending aorta is still in a vertical plane. (b) The vertical dimensions of both the right ventricle and the right atrium are markedly less than those in the main specimen just examined. The superior cavo-atrial angle and the pulmonary ostium are at the same level and the latter is scarcely above the left ventricle. (c) As a corollary to the shortening of the atrium, the superior vena cava is longer than normal (its lower segment is parallel and to the right of the ascending aorta in this, [as in all specimens] in this view). The ascending aorta and pulmonary trunk are similarly elongated. (d) The right coronary artery (and the tricuspid ostium) is angled only 12° posteriorly.

---

*   The posterolateral radial is one of the five modes of termination of the posterior division (the circumflex branch) of the left coronary artery described in Chapter XIV.
** As the left pulmonary artery continues, it descends vertically, bisecting the field of examination (see **4**).

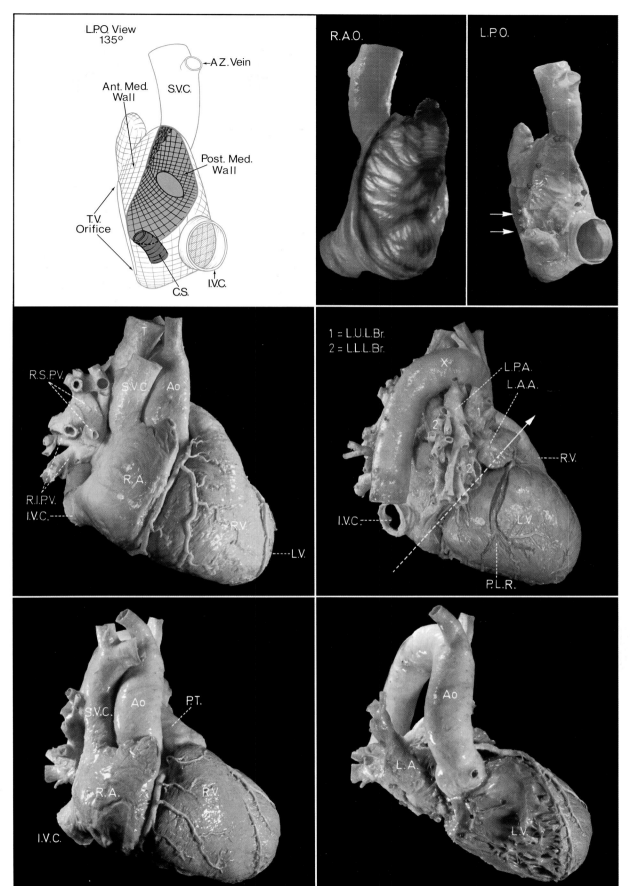

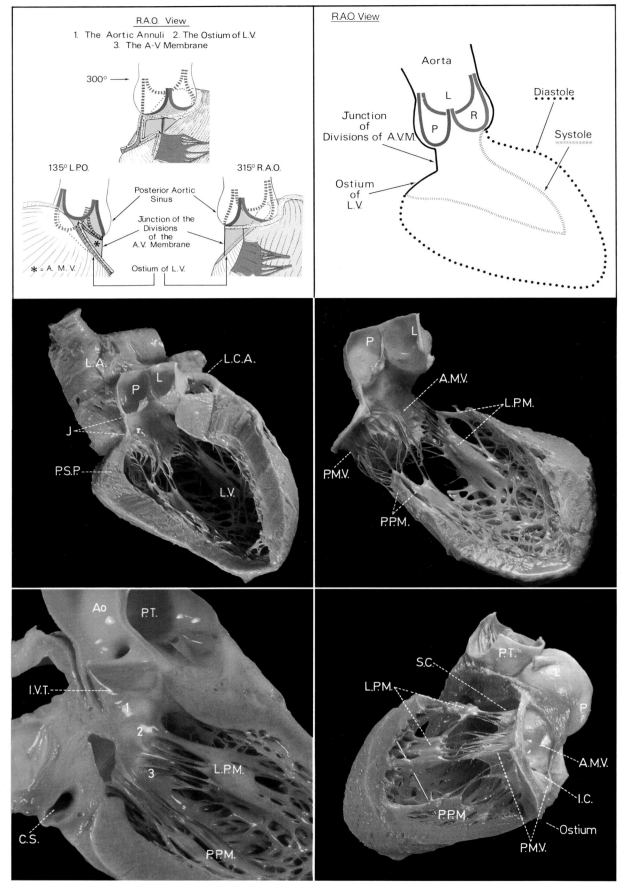

R.A.O. View
1. The Aortic Annuli 2. The Ostium of L.V.
3. The A-V Membrane

300° →

135° L.P.O.   315° R.A.O.

Posterior Aortic Sinus

Junction of the Divisions of the A.V. Membrane

* = A. M. V.   Ostium of L.V.

R.A.O. View

Aorta

Junction of Divisions of A.V.M.

Ostium of L.V.

Diastole

Systole

II. The Left Heart—R.A.O.-L.P.O. Plane

(I.) The Aortic Annuli, the A.V. Membrane, and the Ostium of L.V.

Specimen A: 1: At 300°: Observe: (a) The line of the posterior and right aortic annular commissure passes through the nadir of the left. (b) The anterior division of the A.V. membrane meets the plane of examination at a right angle. (c) The ostium of the ventricle is closing at 300° and is almost closed in the R.A.O.-R.P.O. plane. At 315°, a vertical incision (see **2—5** and **6**) through the nadir of the posterior annulus separates the A.V. membrane into its anterior and posterior divisions; their junction appears in an R.A.O. ventriculogram as a line extending from the nadir of the posterior annulus to the ostium of L.V. The planes of the anterior division and the anterior leaflet (A.M.V.) meet the R.A.O.-L.P.O. plane of examination at angles of 75° and 135°.

2: This drawing, made from a ventriculogram, shows these relationships in a patient. The aorta, junction of the divisions, and ostium, relatively constant in dimension, are indicated by a solid black line. During systole, the aortic sinuses increase in size, and a reduction in the size of the ostium of L.V. occurs; however, these changes are minor in comparison with those of the walls of the ventricle. The drawing is a composite of diastole and systole and, in one regard, is misleading; as the apex moves superiorly, the aorta moves inferiorly.

(II.) The Outline of the Cavity of the Left Ventricle

Specimen B: 3: R.A.O. view: We see the left segment of this specimen which has been divided by incisions. The upper part of one incision passes between the left and right aortic sinuses and proceeds to the apex. Observe: (a) The ostial slope is most prominent anteriorly under the nadir of the right annulus; however, in this plane of examination, it is seen intruding into the cavity of L.V. The indentation in a ventriculogram will be accentuated by systole (see **2**). From the apex, a second incision separates the posterior and septal walls and passes through the posterior superior process (P.S.P.). Between the latter and the posterior aortic sinus, the line (J) is formed by the junction of the divisions of the A.V. membrane. (b) The cavity of L.V. protrudes posteriorly in the area of the posterosuperior process of L.V. Posterior aneurysms often occur here.

(III.) The Relation of the Leaflets of the Mitral Valve to the Aortic Valve

4: The apical half of L.V. remains, affording insertion for the papillary muscles. The anterior leaflet of the mitral valve is in its diastolic position. Observe: (a) Its plane and its attachments are oriented at an angle of 135° to our plane of examination. (b) It is important in examining an R.A.O. ventriculogram to realize that this leaflet is almost entirely inferior to the aortic shaddow; what is more, so is over 50% of the posterior leaflet. The inferior and superior commissures of the mitral valve are approximately 10 mm postero-inferior to the junction of the divisions and the nadir of the left annulus, respectively. (Both are identifiable in a vertriculogram.) The posterior leaflet extends between the com-

missures attached to the ostium of L.V. (shown in **1**).
(c) Note the free border of the anterior leaflet—trace the segments of its attached border (see page 104).

(IV.) The Mitral Valve in Systole in the R.A.O.-L.P.O. Plane

Specimen C: 112—5: R.A.O. view: Here, not an incision as in **3**, but a transection has been carried out in the L.A.O.-R.P.O. plane. It passes further to the left; hence, the ostial slope of L.V. intrudes into the cavity to a lesser degree than in **3**. There are three planes of the anterior leaflet: (1) Only the intervalvular and junctional borders (the hinge of the valve) lie in a vertical plane, meeting the plane of examination at an angle of 135°. (2) The nonappositional and (3) the appositional segments lie in the plane of the ostium (pages 52 and 53) and perpendicular to the plane of the ostium.

Specimen D: 112—6: L.P.O. view: Observe: (a) Note the relation of the plane of the anterior leaflet to the plane of examination. (b) Note the location of both commissures and the posterior leaflet which is partially hidden by the ostium of L.V. Note the relation of the leaflets to the ostium of L.V. and to the aorta. (c) In the R.A.O. view, the obtuse margin is midway between the upper and lower borders of L.V. The lateral and posterior papillary muscles are located just above the obtuse and lower borders, respectively. The latter will frequently be well seen; the former will be obscured by contrast. Both muscles are seen in all four photographs.

(V). Cavity Outline and Prolapse of the Posterior Leaflet

Specimen C: 1–4: The left segment of this specimen has already been seen in **112—5**. The right and left segments are seen in **1** and **2**, with their drawings below. The scale of **3** and **4** is the same; in **2** it is larger. The line of transection has passed through the inferior commissure and the anterior leaflet of the mitral valve, just to the left of the junction of the anterior and posterior divisions of the A.V. membrane. Observe: (a) The normal protrusion of the cavity of the left ventricle between (1) the rounded, indenting ostial slope of L.V. and (2) the subvalvular segment of the A.V. membrane (X) and (3) the inferior commissure. It is important that this zone not be confused with prolapse of the posterior leaflet. (b) Muscularization of a chorda is seen at the upper arrow.

Specimen E: 5: An R.A.O. view in a different specimen, showing the subvalvular segment of the A.V. membrane, extending upward from the ostial slope of L.V., showing again this cul-de-sac which may be seen in a ventriculogram during systole.

6: Note the cul-de-sac in a normal cineventriculogram.

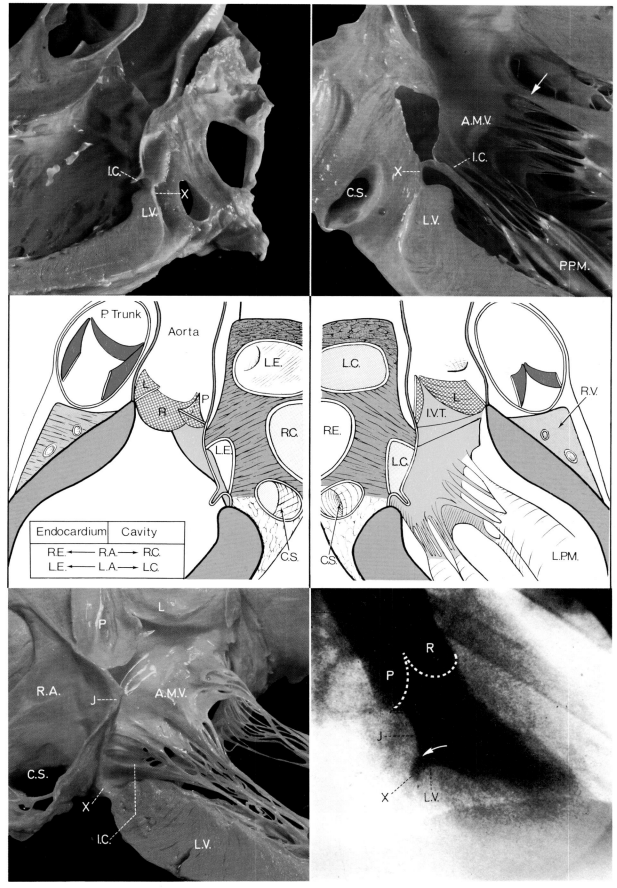

113

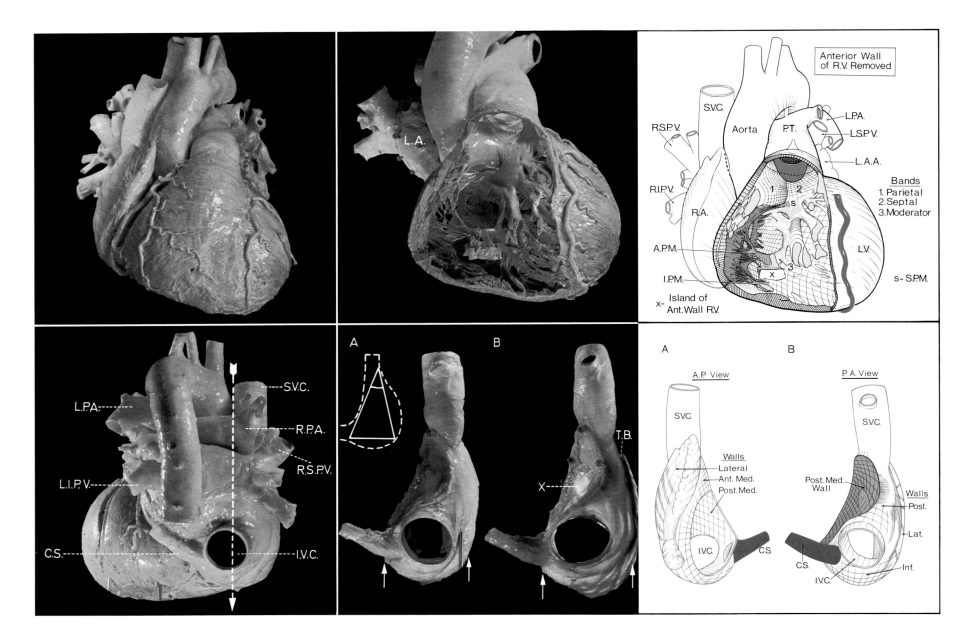

E. The Anteroposterior View—
The A.P. Plane

I. The Right Heart

Specimen A occupies these two pages. In **1**, the intact specimen, the aorta is anterior to a medial arc of the superior vena cava. In **2**, the following have been removed: (1) the right atrium (note the septal surface and axis of the left atrium); (2) the anterior wall of the right ventricle, with the exception of rims in relation to the tricuspid and the pulmonary ostia.

3 is the drawing of **2**, with the right atrium still in place. Observe: (a) The well-developed parietal band is disposed in the plane of the tricuspid valve, meeting the plane of examination at a 45° angle. It meets the septal bands along a vertical line extending upward to the posterior pulmonary leaflet. (b) The septal band has three stout fasciculi above, and its lower margin passes as the moderator band to the base of the anterior papillary muscle (A.P.M.). Note the location of the lower margin

in the sinus of the ventricle. (c) Note the location of the superior (S.P.M.) and inferior (I.P.M.) papillary muscles.

4: P.A. view: Examine this photograph along with the isolated right atrium seen in **5** and **6B**. Observe: (a) The right atrium wraps around the left atrium. (c) The inferior vena cava is largely medial to the superior vena cava as a result of this relationship. (c) The coronary sinus enters the junction of the medial and inferior walls of the right atrium; and in the A.P. plane, it is directly posterior to the ostium of L.V. as it courses in the posterior left A.V. sulcus. Its orifice is near the median plane. (d) The left atrium is the posterior chamber of the heart. (e) Re-examine the contrast study of a patient in **102—6** and note the medial extension of the contrast above the inferior wall of the right atrium.

5 and **6B**: P.A. view of the isolated right atrium. Observe: (a) The dark area of shadow in **5–A** delimits the septal or posteromedial wall. (b) The posterior wall in

5–B is between the septal wall and terminal bundle (T.B.). (c) The inferior wall extends between the arrows; note its inferiorly directed convexity. (d) In the separation of the atria, the membranous component of the septum (seen transilluminated [X]) remained with the right atrium; as seen on pages 107 and 110, the 'septal wall' of the left atrium is intact.* This may be inconsistent with embryologic concepts; however, I have observed it many times. It is possible to speculate that left atrial muscle develops on the left of the membranous component of the septum. (e) Note the appearance of the isolated right atrium seen in **5** and **6B**; visualize the chamber in **4**. Now re-apply the chamber as seen in **6A** to its bed in **2**. (f) In **5** and **6**, the long axis of the right atrium has been angled laterally on its vertex, resulting in an artifactitious disalignment of the venae cavae. Their true relationship is seen in **4**.

* Following separation of the right atrium from the left, cavitary and appositional surfaces may be described in both the postero-medial wall of the right atrium and right lateral wall of the left atrium. (See the index).

114—6: The isolated atrium: Observe: (a) In **one horizontal plane,** the right atrium forms a right-angled sector of a circle (see page 103). The two radii, formed by the tricuspid orifice (seen in **2** and **6A**), and the septal wall meet the plane of examination at angles of 135° and 45°; the chord of the arc of the sector is parallel to the plane of examination. The arc is formed by the lateral and posterior walls. (b) In the frontal plane, the chamber resembles a truncated, acute-angled triangle— the greatest transverse diameter roughly increases from above downward. (See insert in **5A**). It is greatest at the orifice of the coronary sinus. As a result of the contour of the atrial septum it is apparent that the angle of the sector of the circle will vary at the different horizontal levels. (c) Examine the lateral view of this specimen in **106—1:** the greatest dimension in a sagittal plane is also seen above the inferior wall. In angiocardiography, the degree of opacification will be greatest here. (d) The right atrial appendage is indepedent of these configurational considerations. It extends to the left and superiorly like a prow; inferiorly, it is continuous with the ridge in the lateral wall, which contains the anterior vertical muscle bundle.

1: A.P. view: The posterolateral wall of the right ventricle has been removed. In **2**, the 15° view, the chordae, passing from the superior papillary muscle to the anterosuperior leaflet of the tricuspid valve, have been removed, exposing the membranous septum. Observe: (a) The right aortic sinus bulges anteriorly. The overlying parietal band (seen in **114—2** and **3**) extends to the left and posteriorly at an angle to meet the septal band, which is directed posteromedially. The resulting cavity of the upper infundibulum resembles a wide-angled, triangular prism—two lateral faces of the prism are formed by the infundibular bands—one is formed by the anterior wall. (b) In the horizontal plane, the greatest dimension of the right ventricular cavity is just within the tricuspid orifice.

3 and **4:** The **pulmonary annuli** and their spatial orientation in this plane can be seen and the attachment of the posterior annulus to the A.V. unit can be noted. Observe the altitudinal disposition: like the aortic, the posterior is the lowest; however, the order of the **right** anterior and **left** anterior is the reverse of the order seen in the aortic annuli—the right anterior pulmonary annulus is the highest.

5 and **6:** We now end with **the aorto-ventricular unit**. In **5**, a black suture marks the right ventricular and right atrial attachments to the unit: Note the five attachments of the right ventricle as we move clockwise: (1) the superior or pulmonary, which extends from the left anterior fibrous trigone across L.V. to the anterior attachment; (2) the anterior; (3) the inferior; (4) the upper end of the posterior or the tricuspid is just below the right anterior fibrous trigone; (5) the posterolateral, which for a short distance is attached to the right aortic sinus—this is not rare—the right ventricle is attached to the aorto-ventricular unit and the aortic sinuses are a component of this unit; hence, the higher attachment should not surprise us. In this specimen the aorta constitutes a portion of the wall of the right ventricle!

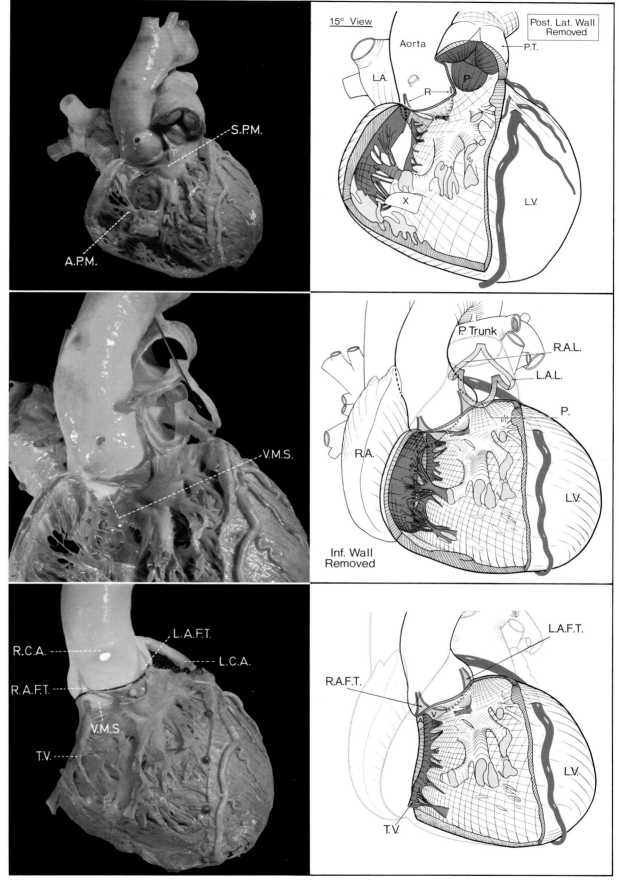

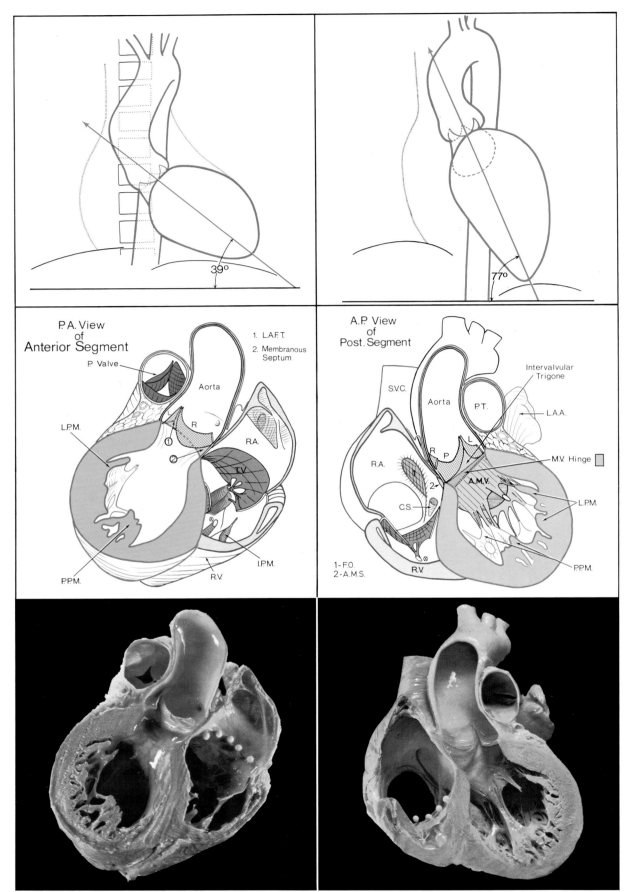

P.A. View
of
Anterior Segment

1. L.A.F.T.
2. Membranous Septum

P Valve

Aorta

LPM.

R

R.A.

T.V.

I.P.M.

P.P.M.

R.V.

A.P. View
of
Post. Segment

SVC.

Aorta

P.T.

Intervalvular Trigone

L.A.A.

R.A.

R

L

P

M.V. Hinge

2—

A.M.V.

C.S.

L.P.M.

1 - F.O.
2 - A.M.S.

R.V.

P.P.M.

39°

77°

II. The Left Heart—A.P.-P.A. Plane

1 and **2**: In determining the variable density of the contrast material in ventriculograms, the contour and dimensions of the cavity are the most important factors. One of the simpler features affecting these two factors is **the axis of the ventricle.** The cavity outline is shown here of ventriculograms of a horizontal and a vertical type of heart. In the specimen examined below, the axis of the ventricle in the frontal plane measures 60°. The axis is defined, herein, as a line drawn from the apex to the posterior and left aortic annular commissure. In **1**, the nadir of the posterior aortic annulus is precisely in the midline—often it is to the left.

Specimen A: 116—3–6 and 117—1–3
3–6: The plane of this vertical and almost frontal transection passes slightly obliquely, anteriorly and to the right; the left and right aortic leaflets and the membranous septum are transected. Observe: (a) **The lateral and posterior papillary muscles** (L.P.M. and P.P.M.) are inferior and extend anterior to the aortic valve. This transection passes through both; they could be termed superior and inferior—the use of the terms anterolateral and posteromedial should be questioned. (b) **The walls of the outflow tract of the ventricle are:** (1) **anterior**—the bulging ostial slope of the left ventricle, the left anterior and the right anterior fibrous trigones; (2) **left**—the ostial slope is less prominent, facing to the right and inferiorly; (3) **right**—the ostial slope recedes in prominence as it extends posteriorly. The membranous septum slopes upward and to the right, forming a portion of the outflow tract; (4) **posterior**—the intervalvular trigone and the hinge of the mitral valve (the mobile portion of the anterior leaflet is directed posteriorly during ventricular systole). (c) The anterior posterior measurements of the outflow tract may in adult females be only 10.0 mm. The percentage ratio of this measurements to the greatest A.P. dimension of the ventricle is usually not over 20%.

Comment: Subaortic stenosis of the membranous type is a relatively infrequent congenital malformation. At operation, when the outflow tract is examined through the opened aorta, the obstructing membrane, demilunar in shape, with the opening directed toward the right, is seen attached to the ostial slope of L.V. and to the anterior leaflet of the mitral valve. Care is taken to avoid injury to the latter. The membrane is usually easily removed with obliteration of the pressure gradient. The role of the mitral valve in asymmetric septal hypertrophy is more complex. Variations in the attachment of the anterior leaflet are not, as once thought, a mechanistic factor in this condition. As a result of configurational cavity changes, papillary muscle function is inappropriate allowing anterior motion of the anterior leaflet in systole—this results in outflow tract obstruction and, when the appositional tolerance of the mitral valve is exceeded, in mitral regurgitation. This would explain the benefit achieved by mitral valve replacement, as the sole procedure, in this disease.

Specimen A: 1–3

1: In the anterior segment of the same specimen, the septal wall slopes anteriorly and to the left as it extends inferiorly.

2: The posterior segment: Observe: (a) The hinge of the mitral valve is seen as a darkened strip below the posterior and left aortic leaflets; the axis of the hinge is depressed 40° below the horizontal. The nonappositional portion of the anterior leaflet is seen as a transilluminated area; the darkened area below is the appositional area, the major chordal attachment site. (b) Note the hemi-elliptic shape of the free margin of the anterior leaflet and its direction; the apex, which is free of chordae, points inferiorly and to the left at a right angle to the axis of the hinge; these axes are shown by the dotted lines. (c) The posterior leaflet and the related A.V. membrane are attached to the ostium far posteriorly: the greatest dimension of the inflow tract of the ventricle is formed by a horizontal line extended from this attachment anteriorly to the septal wall.* (d) In the fossa ovalis (F.O.) the transilluminated membranous component of the atrial septum is seen. Its axis extends anterosuperiorly. Its apogee is only 3.0 mm from the posterior aortic sinus. (e) The anterior leaflet billows anteriorly in diastole as shown in **2** and **3** and **116—6**. Visualize its obliquely inverted attachment—composed of intervalvular, junctional, and the two ostial segments. The shape of the free margin of the anterior leaflet is well shown in the detailed drawing **10—2**.

3: A retouched photograph has been made after excision of a large part of the ventricular walls, leaving a rim at the ostium and a portion of the inferior and lateral walls at the site of attachment of the two papillary muscles. This dissection demonstrates the great disparity in the anteroposterior dimensions of the inflow and outflow tracts of the left ventricle.

4: An A.P. ventriculogram: In an early phase of systole, the contrast is seen outlining the attachment of the posterior leaflet and the related A.V. membrane to the ostium of the left ventricle, the area just examined.

5: The left ventricle is seen in late diastole, then in late systole. The posterior and lateral papillary muscles may cause filling defects in the right and left borders of the ventricle in this view.

6: A drawing made of a supravalvular aortogram showing the disposition of the aortic annuli in this view.

On page 52 and 53, the mitral valve is seen in systole and diastole in the A.P., superior, and left lateral views. And on pages 104 and 105, the disposition of the valve is seen in the frontal and horizontal planes.

_____

* In the study of this photograph, orientation is facilitated by the use of **3** on this page and **116—4** and **6**. Below the anterior leaflet, the dotted line crosses the well-lit left atrial cavity and the dark left ventricular cavity.

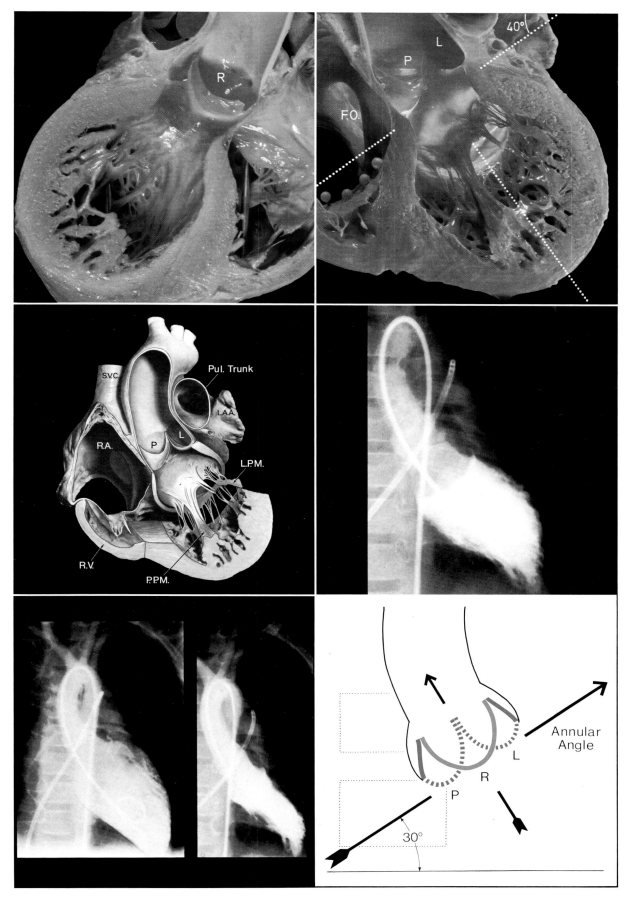

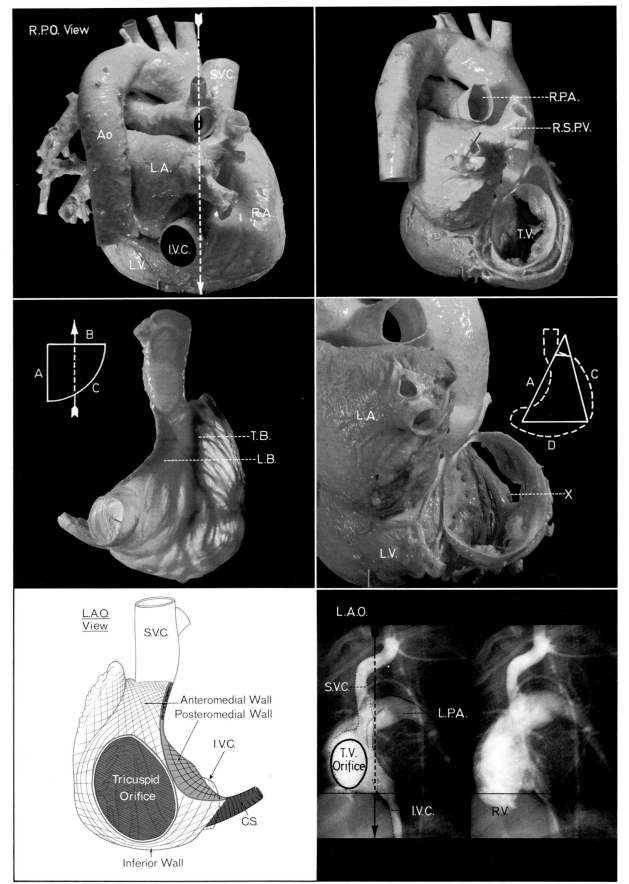

F. The Left Anterior Oblique View— The L.A.O.-R.P.O. Plane

I. The Right Heart

Specimen A: 118—1–5 and 119—1–4

In **1**, the intact specimen is seen—in **2**, the right atrium and a large part of the right pulmonary artery have been removed and the right inferior pulmonary vein has been retroverted to display the septal surface. Both **1** and **2** appear in the same scale. The isolated right atrium and the specimen, after removal of the right atrium and the walls of the right ventricle, are shown in larger scales in **3** and **4**. The L.A.O. view of the isolated right atrium and the L.A.O. view of an angiocardiogram taken following simultaneous injection into the left innominate vein and the inferior vena cava appear in **5** and **6**.

(I.) **The Right Atrium and the Atrial Septum:** (a) In the insert in **3**, the arrow represents the R.P.O.-L.A.O. axis of examination and its relation to the right-angled sector of a circle formed by the right atrium in a horizontal transection. These relations are: Radius B, the tricuspid orifice is at a right angle; Radius A, the septal wall is parallel; Arc C, the posterior and lateral walls are oblique. The **tricuspid orifice** is seen in **2**, **4**, and **5** and it can be deduced in **6**. **The septal wall of the right atrium:** its margins are seen in **3** and **5**; it presents a multitude of axes which form a spiral about the central axis of examination. Re-apply this surface to the septal surface of the left atrium seen in **2** and **4**. (b) The insert in **4** represents a cross section of the atrium in the L.P.O.-R.A.O. plane (which is at a right angle to the plane of examination)—again, the truncation of the triangle is above. A = septal wall; C = the lateral wall; D = the inferior wall. These facts determine the variable densities presented by the right atrium in this plane of examination. In both planes the greatest dimension of the chamber is lateral to the junction of the septal and inferior walls. (c) The inferior vena cava is staggered to the left of the superior—see the vertical lines in **1** and **6**. (d) The bundle of Lower (L.B.) extends into the posterior wall—see **3**.

(II.) **The Left Atrium** is directed superiorly and posteriorly. It is poorly seen in the L.A.O. view because the left ventricle and aorta overlap it—see **2**.

(III.) **The Right Ventricle:** (a) **The tricuspid valve:** (1) Over one-third of its orifice is inferior to the ostium of L.V. (2) The attachment of the septal leaflet to the A.V. unit is to the left of the septal margin (X) seen in **4**. (b) In late diastole, the **inferior wall** extends below the level of the right atrium when it is seen in late diastole—see **6**.

(IV.) **The Pulmonary Arteries:** The axes of their proximal portions are seen on page 125. The left is directed to 150°—hence, is seen here almost at a right angle—see **6** and **119—1**. The right is directed to 240°—hence, here at 225° it is seen almost on end—see **2**. It is also superimposed on the pulmonary trunk.

1: L.A.O. view of the intact specimen: The hemitubular configuration of the infundibulum can be seen. The anterior interventricular coronary artery (A.I.V.) identifies the anterior interventricular groove.

2: With the exception of rims below the pulmonary and tricuspid ostia, the anterior wall of the right ventricle has been removed. Observe: (a) The parietal band of the infundibulum (P.B.) extends above the tricuspid ostium and, like the latter, crosses our plane of examination at a right angle. It meets the septal band (S.B.) at a line dropped from the nadir of the posterior pulmonary leaflet. (b) To reach the anterior wall the septal band passes to the left and anteriorly, extending the septal margin to the right and reducing the dimension of the left half of the chamber. The band lies in the L.A.O.-R.P.O. plane.

3 and 4: The remainder of the walls of the right ventricle has been removed. (a) **Note the altitudinal order of the pulmonary annuli** described on page 115. (b) The greatest horizontal dimension of the right ventricle is on the inner surface of the plane of the tricuspid orifice—also see 118—4 and 81—6.

Specimen B: 5 and **6**—see also **108—3–6**
The I.V. grooves are identified by the corresponding arteries. These two drawings, along with **4**, can be examined together and the following noted: (a) **The tricuspid valve** is above the apex of the ventricle: The attachment of its septal leaflet is to the left of the septal margin (this is also shown in **4**): The lower third of the orifice or ostium is below the ostium of L.V. (b) The **inferior wall of R.V.** is between the acute margin, the inferior margin of the tricuspid ostium and the posterior I.V. groove. (c) The **posterior wall of L.V.** is crossed by the two posterior branches of the left coronary artery. In this plane of examination, these two walls (of R.V. and L.V.) extend posteriorly and superiorly at a varying angle, here approximately 45° (see page 194). (d) The axes of the ventricular (muscular) septum and atrial septum are deflected posteriorly on their vertices. The membranous septum is oblique to these axes and also curves around its own vertical axis. In **3** and **4**, only a small portion of the ventricular division of the membranous septum is visible from L.A.O.; in the R.P.O. view (**5**), the atrial portion (A.M.S.) faces posteriorly and to the right. (e) Examine the lateral view of this specimen on page 108 and note that the lateral branch of the anterior division (of the left coronary artery—L.C.A.) descends vertically midway between the anterior and posterior portions of **the lateral wall of L.V.**; hence, in the L.A.O. view, the artery identifies this line of division; therefore, the anterior half of the lateral wall extends obliquely between the anterior interventricular groove and the left border of L.V., while the posterior portion of the lateral wall of L.V. is disposed in the plane of examination (i). The knowledge of the location of **the ostium of L.V.** is the key in the differentiation of the related posterior division from branches of the lateral wall.

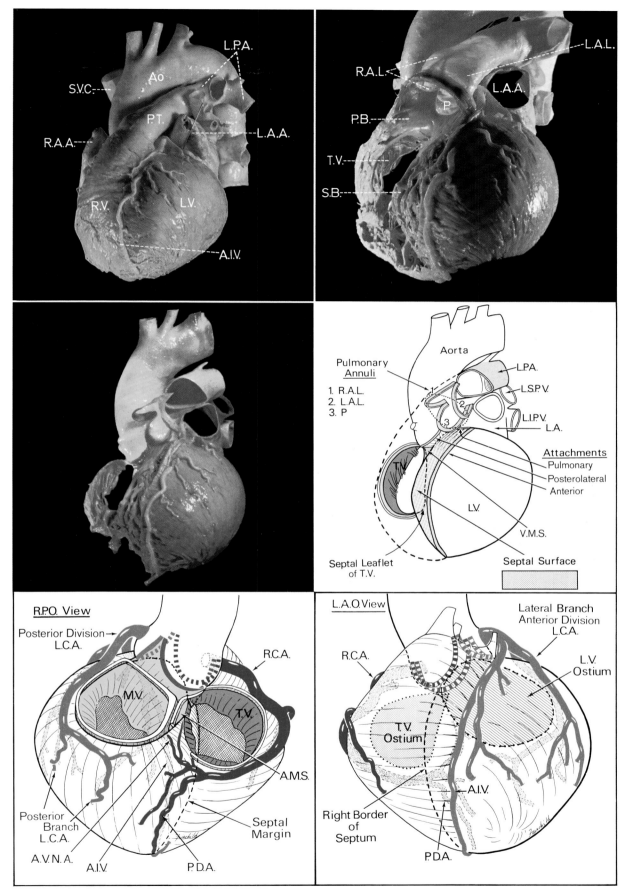

119

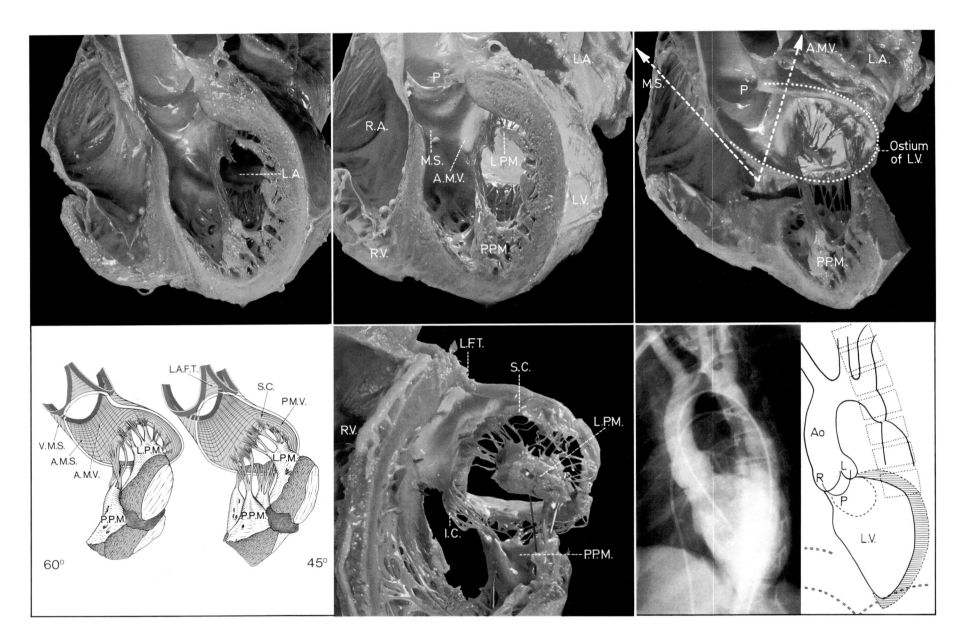

II. The Left Heart—L.A.O.-R.P.O. Plane

(I.) The Membranous Septum
Specimen A: 1–3
1 and **2**: L.A.O. view: A description of the mode of transection and the A.P. view of this specimen appears on pages 116 and 117. Here, the posterior segment has been rotated into the L.A.O.-R.P.O. plane of examination. The yellow bead in **2** marks the ostium below the posterior aortic leaflet. **3** is the 60° view: a larger scale view is seen on page 37—**2**. The ostium of L.V. is indicated by the horseshoe-shaped dotted line. Observe: (a) The **membranous septum** extends to the right and superiorly. The **anterior leaflet** of the mitral valve extends to the left and superiorly. The two structures meet at an angle of 60°, forming the junction of the A.V. membrane (see arrows in **3**). (b) The **posterior aortic leaflet** is set at a right angle to the plane of examination. (c) See the **ostium of the left ventricle** and the posterior leaflet of the mitral valve—re-examine **119**—**6** and observe the location of this vital landmark.

(II.) The Aortic Annuli
Specimen B: 4: The excised A.V. membrane and aortic annuli of a specimen (**108**—**3–6** and **119**—**5, 6**) show the location of the membranous septum and the aortic annuli for orientation purposes for the above photographs and for **5** and **6** on the next page. At 60°, the nadir of the posterior annulus is in the axis of the commissure of the other two annuli. At 45°, the commissure between the left and right is seen shifted posterior to the nadir. The membranous septum "curves around" an axis, sharply deflected posteriorly on its vertex. In all views, the order of the annular heights is constant—note the relation of the commissures. They also are constant—from above downward they are: left and right; left and posterior; and posterior and right.

(III.) The Papillary Muscles
Specimen C: 5: 60° view: The scale is 1.5:1. Only a slender rim of muscle remains at the ostium of L.V. Observe: (a) The papillary muscles are in a vertical plane. This photograph was taken to simulate the filling defects created by the muscles at angiocardiography. At 45°, the lateral papillary muscle is to the left of the posterior muscle; at 60°, it is above the posterior. This is seen in all four specimens on these two pages. (b) The superior commissure (S.C.) is 10.0 mm posterior to the left fibrous trigone (L.F.T.).

(IV.) The Axis of the Left Ventricle
6: A left ventriculogram of a patient with a coarctation of the aorta prior to operation. Catheters have been passed via the femoral route into the left pulmonary artery and the left ventricle. A catheter will frequently pass through the site of the coarctation, providing valuable pressure data which provide a base line for measurements carried out during operation and in the post-operative evaluation. The latter should be carried out routinely to determine the quality of the surgical repair. **The axis of the septum meets the vertical plane at a 25° angle.** The axis in the normal heart, seen on the next page, is approximately the same.

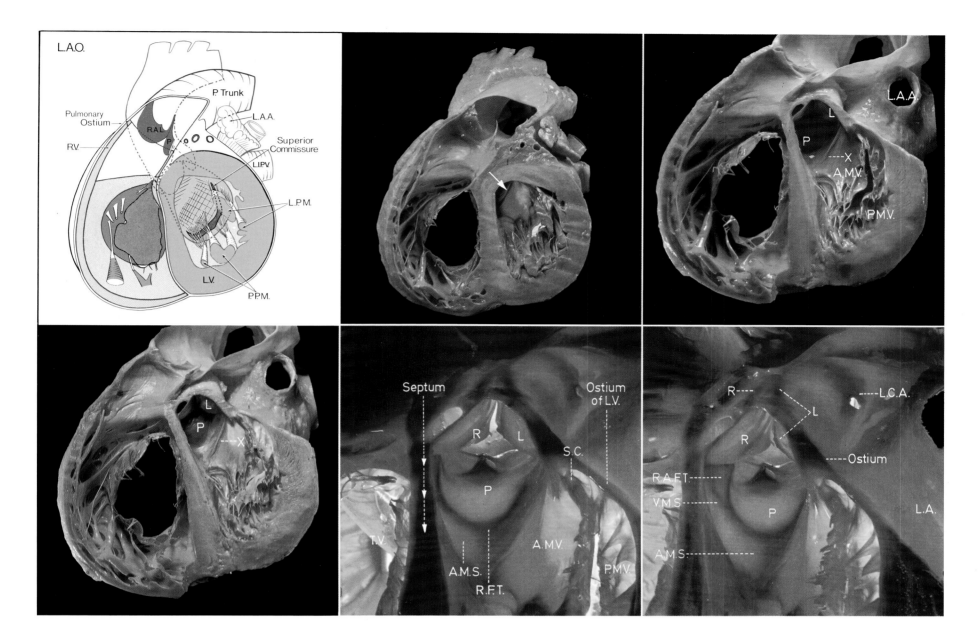

Specimen D: 1–6: The vertical transection passes in the R.A.O.-L.P.O. plane, i. e., at right angles to this plane of examination. The leaflets of the mitral valve are fixed in their systolic position. Photographs of both segments are seen on page 84. At this time we will examine the right posterior segment.

1 and 2: Observe: (a) The characteristic orientation of the axis of the collinear walls of L.V. and the aorta in this view—it intersects the axis of the infundibulum and pulmonary trunk—the two form the letter X.* (b) The characteristic disposition in this view of the papillary muscles—the posterior is to the right of the lateral. (c) The hinge of the mitral valve (marked by the arrow) is seen as a dark strip against the transilluminated anterior leaflet of the mitral valve. (d) In systole, the line of leaflet apposition forms a reverse C, concave superiorly, and to the right. The anterior leaflet, seen in systole, faces to the left and inferiorly.

3: Sufficient portions of the lateral and septal walls of the left ventricle have been removed to afford examina-

tion of the aortic valve, the outflow tract of the left ventricle and the mitral valve. An enlarged view is seen in **44—4**. Observe: (a) The muscular ventricular septum slopes to the right and superiorly. The aortic valve thus overrides its lower portion. (b) The ridge at the hinge (X) of the mitral valve, seen here and in **4**, extends from the left fibrous trigone to the ostial attachment of the right fibrous trigone. (c) The mitral leaflets are slightly separated to demonstrate the commissures. The nonmobile part of the anterior leaflet of the mitral valve meets the plane of examination at a 45° angle.

4: The mitral valve has been transilluminated. Observe: (a) In the right ventricle, the inferior ridge of the parietal band, separating the sinus and infundibulum, is directed towards the nadir of the right aortic sinus (which has been removed). Note the right aortic sinus-right ventricular cavity relationship: The right or inferior half is above the sinus, and the left or superior half is posterior to the infundibulum. (b) The posterior aortic leaflet is partially hidden; it will be seen in its entirety in **5**, the

60° view. (c) The ridge (X) produced at the line of the mitral valve hinge is seen.

5: 60° view: The aortic annuli, the pyramidal nodule on the posterior leaflet, and the nonmobile triangle of the anterior leaflet of the mitral valve can be seen as darkened areas. The junction of the divisions of the A.V. membrane is indicated by the line extending between the label R.F.T. and the posterior aortic annulus.

6: 75° view: At 60°, only the atrial portion of the membranous septum (A.M.S.) is visible. Now the ventricular portion (V.M.S.), which is tilted away from our view, and the right anterior fibrous trigone (R.A.F.T.) come into view.

---

* It must not be inferred that the axes of the infundibulum and pulmonary trunk are commonly collinear—see **79—3**.

G. An Introduction to Coronary Arteriography

The fundamental features and landmarks of the heart against which the arteries must be placed will be listed. The atria are set apart from this enumeration.

(1) **The left ventricle:** (a) **The ostium** may be divided into aortic and mitral parts. The mitral division is the important landmark to which the posterior division of the left coronary artery (v.i.) is related; it is divided into three parts, posterior, left lateral, and right lateral. (b) **The three borders** demarcate the three walls. The borders are: (1) The anterior I.V. sulcus and the pulmonary attachment (of the right ventricle to the A.V. unit). (2) The posterior I.V. sulcus and the tricuspid attachment. (3) The obtuse margin. (c) **The walls:** The septal wall is between (1) and (2). The posterior is between (2) and (3). The lateral is between (1) and (3). (d) **The axis of the ventricle:** This may be compared to the slant height of a cone in geometry. It passes from the apex to the ostium. The obtuse margin is an axial line. An axial line, placed midway between the borders of the lateral wall, will divide this wall into anterosuperior and postero-inferior parts. The lateral wall can also be divided vertically (by a lateral branch) into unequal parts—(see page 168 and 169).

2. **The right ventricle:** (a) **The two ostia**: The tricuspid ostium, divisible into four parts, superior, anterior, inferior and septal (page 84), constitutes the important relation and provides derivation for the first three divisions or segments of the right coronary artery. The attachment of the pulmonary ostium forms the anterior border of the left coronary fossa and defines the upper end of the anterior interventricular sulcus: as a logical consequence the retropulmonary and interventricular segments of the anterior division of the left coronary artery (v.i.) are derived. (b) **The three borders:** (1) The acute margin. (2) The anterior and (3) the posterior interventricular sulci. **The three walls:** (1) Posterolateral. (2) Anterior. (3) Inferior. (d) **The axis of the ventricle** is a line projected from the pulmonary ostium through the middle of the anterior and inferior walls to the posterior I.V. sulcus. The axis, like the right ventricle, wraps around the left ventricle.

The truncal characteristics of the right and left coronary arteries are different. The right frequently possesses a long main trunk which extends from origin to termination; however, bifurcation can occur, rarely anteriorly (**114—1**) but commonly posteriorly (**69—3**). The left main branch may be so short as to defy measurement—in this study, it bifurcated in 91% and trifurcated in 9%. The products of bifurcation are termed the anterior and posterior divisions, replacing the terms, left anterior descending and circumflex. It may appear quixotic and a mere attempt at innovation to replace these traditional terms; however, they have unfortunate connotations. In a current textbook, the following statement appears: "The anterior interventricular sulcus contains the left anterior descending coronary artery". A second textbook contains the following: "The left circumflex artery is found in the atrio-ventricular sulcus, between the atrium and left ventricle, until it ramifies posteriorly". The simplistic relegation of these vessels to the sulci hinders the student from perceiving their logical subdivisions, their actual course, and their contribution to the supply of the walls of the left ventricle. The terms anterior and posterior divisions indicate only the supply to the anterior and the posterior parts of the heart and invite **the elicitation of their four prime characteristics** (see page 133). When trifurcation occurs, the intermediate vessel is termed the lateral division; it descends in the lateral sector of the lateral wall of the left ventricle.

As a preview of the coronary arteries, we will carry out an exercise and relate the course of the right coronary artery and the divisions of the left to the anatomic features of the heart listed above.

The Right Coronary Artery

The right coronary artery may extend from its origin to the obtuse margin of the heart. Four subdivisions of the artery may then be described; the first three are related to the right ventricle, the fourth to the left ventricle. **In its relation to the right ventricle, two basic courses are found.**

I. In approximately 95% of instances, the trunk bends around the three nonseptal divisions of the tricuspid ostium: As a logical consequence of this course, three subdivisions of the artery may be recognized, the right superior, the right anterior, and the right inferior. These may be seen in a specimen (**201—6**) and in an arteriogram (**195—5**). In arteriograms, identification of these subdivisions directs attention to their spatial disposition in each of the different radiographic views.

II. In approximately 5% of hearts, the trunk proceeds across the anterior wall, the acute margin, and the inferior wall, and reaches the posterior interventricular groove. This diagonal course between the axis and the tricuspid ostium of the right ventricle may be termed the circummarginal.

The right coronary may be confined to the supply of the right ventricle. Its fourth subdivision, the left ventricular segment, exists when it extends beyond the posterior interventricular sulcus. Here again, two courses are seen: (1) In a majority, it parallels and proximates the ostium of the left ventricle. (2) In the minority of hearts, it lies below the ostium and meets the axis of the posterior wall of the left ventricle at an obtuse angle.

The Left Coronary Artery

I. The Anterior Division: From its origin, this artery extends 2–3 cm anterolaterally and often nearly horizontally in the left coronary fossa, posterior to the pulmonary trunk, before it reaches and descends the anterior interventricular sulcus. The anterior division may, therefore, be divided into **retropulmonary** and **interventricular** segments. Small branches supply a small contiguous area of the right ventricle. Large branches to the septal, the lateral, and less often the posterior walls of the ventricle may arise from either or both of these two segments. Precision in the identification of the origin of these branches is important in establishing their relationship to occlusive disease, which commonly occurs in the proximal 4.0 cm of the anterior division. For example, from the retropulmonary segment, the main septal and a large lateral wall branch may arise—an occlusive lesion proximal to either bears a poor prognosis. The traditional term invokes an inordinate association of the artery to the anterior interventricular sulcus and to the supply of a limited area of the adjoining walls.

II. The Posterior Division: Its termination and its relation to the ostium of the left ventricle are interrelated and three groups may be identified. The incidence in a study of 100 hearts is as follows: **Group A:** The division terminates as the posterior descending in 12% and the posterior branch in 23%. Hence, in 35%, the trunk is related to both the left lateral and the posterior segments of the ostium of L.V. **Group B:** In 52% of hearts, the division terminates, not by bending around the A.V. sulcus as the term circumflex implies, but as a large vessel that courses on the obtuse margin, often to reach the apex. Between its origin and the obtuse margin, its relationship to the lateral segment of the ostium of L.V. may not be a close one; furthermore through 80% of its course, the obtuse margin is its line of reference. **Group C:** Here the termination is either: (1) proximal to the obtuse margin and unrelated to the ostium—7%; (2) on the posterior wall, but its course is circum-marginal and well away from the ostium—6%. In conclusion, the trunk of the posterior division may be well-separated from the ostium of the left ventricle or be related to one or to two of the segments thereof. In the study of arteriograms, recognition of the lateral and posterior segments of the posterior division results in greater attention to their direction and the relation of this direction to the plane of examination.

III. The Lateral Division: When a vessel arises from the left main branch of a size similar to the anterior and posterior products of trifurcation, it should receive this designation. It may cross the lateral wall in a vertical direction or extend diagonally toward the apex.

Chapter 9: The Great Vessels and the Pericardium

Introduction

Knowledge of the origin and course of the great vessels is a prerequisite to the comprehension of the details of the pericardial reflections. In turn, the understanding of the aorta and pulmonary trunk and arteries is dependent upon the knowledge of the spatial disposition of the trachea and proximal bronchi. The relationship of the airway to the major pulmonary vessels has great clinical implications in the pathogenesis and diagnosis of cardiac disease. As an example of the former, in children, the bronchi are small in caliber and their cartilage not fully developed. The left upper lobe bronchus is between the left main pulmonary artery and the left superior pulmonary vein. The artery is both superior and posterior; the vein is anterior to the bronchus. In addition, not infrequently, a large branch of the pulmonary artery is located between the left superior pulmonary vein and the bronchus. In the presence of large left to right shunts in infants, the pulmonary artery is dilated and under increased pressure, as may be the pulmonary veins when left ventricular failure exists. The left upper lobe bronchus may be compressed—atelectasis results. Compressive vascular forces may be exerted on the left main bronchus itself; its relationships will be noted in this regard.

The **spatial disposition of the airway** is critical in a consideration of lung disease which results from aspiration of particulate material—usually while the patient is supine and asleep. This has been termed bronchial embolism. Four anatomic facts account for the greater incidence of aspiration into the right lung; as these are relevant to cardiac anatomy and diagnosis, they will be enumerated

here. (1) The lower end of the trachea is deflected slightly to the right. (2) The right main bronchus is larger in caliber than the left. (3) In a frontal plane, the right main bronchus is more in line with the trachea than is the left main bronchus. (4) In a sagittal plane, the trachea descends postero-inferiorly—the right main bronchus and the bronchus intermedius continue this course. The axis of the left main bronchus is deflected anteriorly by the left pulmonary artery. Consideration of the bronchial axes is important in the diagnosis of the left atrial enlargement and in the appreciation of the effects of the latter on the airway.

On the next pages we can note some interesting comparisons and contrasts between **the airway and the artery to the lungs.** (A) The trachea descends postero-inferiorly into the thorax; the pulmonary trunk ascends postero-superiorly into the thorax. (B) Both bifurcate at an angle of 90°. (The angle of bifurcation of the trachea varies with age, body habitus, position and phase of respiration. The radiologic study of Alair, *et al.,* showed that the angle in the living is usually considerably less than 90°.) (C) In the interior of both, a carina (L.=keel) results from this bifurcation. (D) The axes of both fail to bisect the angle of bifurcation but form angles of 30° and 60° with their branches. In the airway, the tracheal axis and the right bronchus form the smaller angle; in the arteries, we see the reverse—the left pulmonary artery and the axis of the trunk form the smaller angle. (E) When the airway and arteries are seen from a lateral view, the relationship of the structures to each other in the sagittal plane is defined. The pulmonary trunk extends posterosuperiorly and the trachea extends postero-inferiorly—both bifurcate at an angle of approximately 20°—the structures which were more in line in (D) are again more in line—i.e., the short proximal left pulmonary artery continues the course of the trunk and is above the level of the right main pulmonary artery; the right main bronchus is in line with the trachea and posterior to the left. (F) The left atrium is suspended below and between the inverted Y-shaped airway by four slings—the four pulmonary veins. Indeed, the upper wall of the left atrium is 2.5–5 cm below the tracheal bifurcation. Due to the axis of the atrium, the intervention of the right pulmonary artery and its own more posterior direction, the right bronchus is separate from the chamber. The left main bronchus and its upper lobe branch are directly posterior to the left superior pulmonary vein (**124—1** and **126—4–6**)—the bronchus crosses the termination of the vein. These facts should be recalled if the transbronchial technique is ever used for the determination of left atrial pressure; they are especially pertinent if the left atrial enlargement is not marked.

Edwards and Burchell stated (in 1960) that **in primary pulmonary hypertension,** the enlarged, tense left pulmonary artery may result in the following: (1) Deflect the aorta to the right and superiorly and accentuate its indentation of the trachea; (2) depress and indent the underlying left main bronchus. (These structures are seen in the next pages.) The right pulmonary artery, lying in the trough formed by the middle lobe bronchus and apical segmental bronchus of the right lower lobe (see **157—1** and **2**), may separate and compress both.

In left atrial enlargement: (1) The angle of tracheal bifurcation may be increased mainly due to elevation of the left main bronchus. In a very interesting article, Le Roux and Gotsman note that when a giant left atrium is present, "The left atrium can enlarge to the right, to the left, or both, in front of or behind the venous orifices …". The right bronchus may be more elevated than the left when the enlargement is directed to the right. Both bronchi may be elevated and the angle of tracheal bifurcation may be 180° (Edwards). However, it is the left, not the right bronchus that is compressed. (2) The left main bronchus may be deflected posteriorly to parallel or be posterior to the right. In a lateral x-ray of the chest, the relationship of the main bronchi may be assessed by noting the location of the upper lobe orifices. (3) The left main bronchus may be compressed by the enlarged atrium from below. The pulmonary artery, which is often coincidentally enlarged and under increased pressure, not only compresses, but resists the ascent of the bronchus: The right bronchus is free of this dual liability. Obstruction of the left main bronchus will be added to the already compromised respiratory system. Atelectasis of the left lung may even occur.

The axis of the pulmonary trunk has been examined in Chapter 6. On page 125, the axes of the proximal part of the right and left pulmonary arteries will be examined. It will be apparent that an elevated sagittal view is needed if the trunk and the main branches are to be studies in a definitive manner—see the article of Kattan. As may be surmised from Chapter 6, a steep angle may be required. In a horizontal plane examination, a lateral view of the trunk and perpendicular views of the branches are needed. It has long been good practice to use selective injection of each artery and lateral views to study the intrapulmonary branches. A single A.P. view, with injection in the trunk, is as unrefined as the use of a single A.P. bronchogram with bilateral filling in the study of bronchial disease.

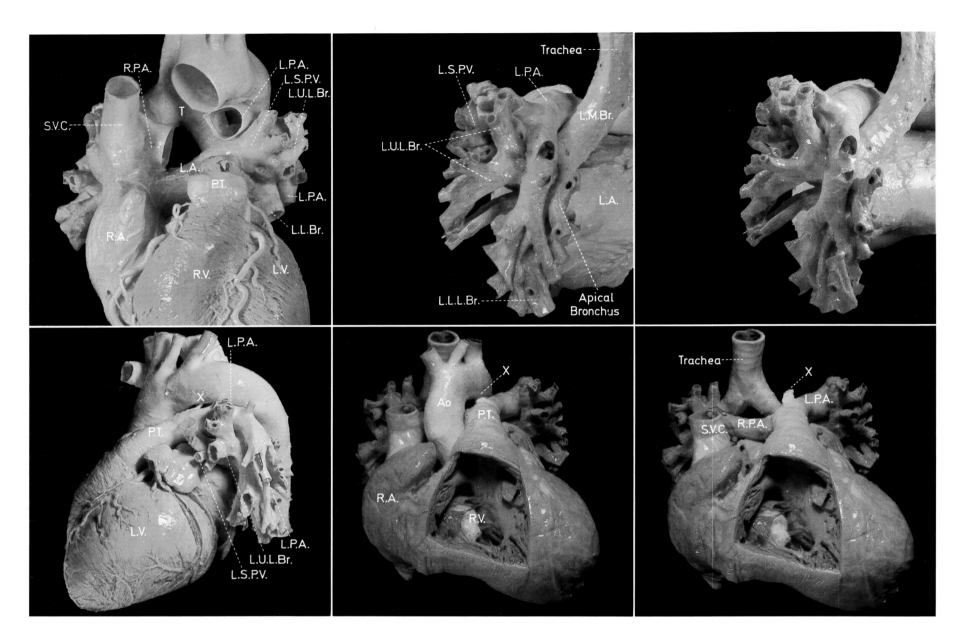

A. The Great Vessels

I. The Relations of the Pulmonary Arteries

Specimen A: 1: Superior A.P. view: The ascending aorta, the pulmonary trunk and the medial part of the right pulmonary artery have been removed. Observe: (a) The right pulmonary artery is anterior to the right bronchus and posterior to the superior vena cava and the right superior pulmonary vein. (b) The left pulmonary artery passes over the left main bronchus between the aorta and the upper lobe bronchus. In front of the latter is seen the superiorly directed upper division of the left superior pulmonary vein. (c) The tracheal bifurcation is 2.5 cm above the left atrium. (d) The relations of the bronchi to the left atrium have been discussed on page 123.

Specimen B: 2 and **3**: Nonattitudinal P.A. view with two modes of lighting: The left pulmonary artery winds above the left main (L.M.Br.) and left upper lobe bronchi (L.U.L.Br.) to reach the furrow between the latter and

the apical bronchus of the left lower lobe. It then descends on the posterolateral surface of the lower lobe bronchi. An enlarged left pulmonary artery may exert pressure on the left upper lobe bronchus from above and behind.

Specimen C: 4: The above relationships are seen in the left lateral view. The pulmonary trunk ascends superiorly at a 30° angle. The proximal left pulmonary artery continues its course; from its junction with the trunk the ligamentum arteriosum (X) arises. The left superior pulmonary vein (L.S.P.V.) is anterior to the upper lobe bronchus.

II. The Trachea, Pulmonary Trunk and Their Branches in the Frontal Plane

Specimen B: 5 and **6**: A.P. view before and after removal of the aorta: Observe: (a) **The tracheal bifurcation:** (1) is above the right pulmonary artery which lies on the superior wall of the left atrium; (2) is to the right of the median plane. (b) The axes of the left and right main

bronchi meet the tracheal axis at angles of 60° and 30° respectively and together form an angle of 90°—the right bronchus is more in line with the trachea than is the left. (c) The axis (in the frontal plane) of the right pulmonary artery is variable. Here it is slightly elevated; in **125—6** and **126—6**, it is depressed below the horizontal as it proceeds to the right. (d) The origin of the right pulmonary artery from the trunk is anterior to the left main bronchus—this is the site for ligation of the artery in right pneumonectomy—ligation to the right of the origin leaves a cul-de-sac in which a thrombus may develop and eventuate in lethal propagation into the left pulmonary artery. (e) If ligation of the left pulmonary is used, the ligature is placed on the right of the ligamentum arteriosum (X) (seen in **4, 5** and **6** and **125—2**).

Note: The term **pulmonary trunk**, used throughout this work, results in less confusion than "the pulmonary artery" (which divides into the right and left pulmonary arteries) and is preferred to "the common" or "the main pulmonary artery".

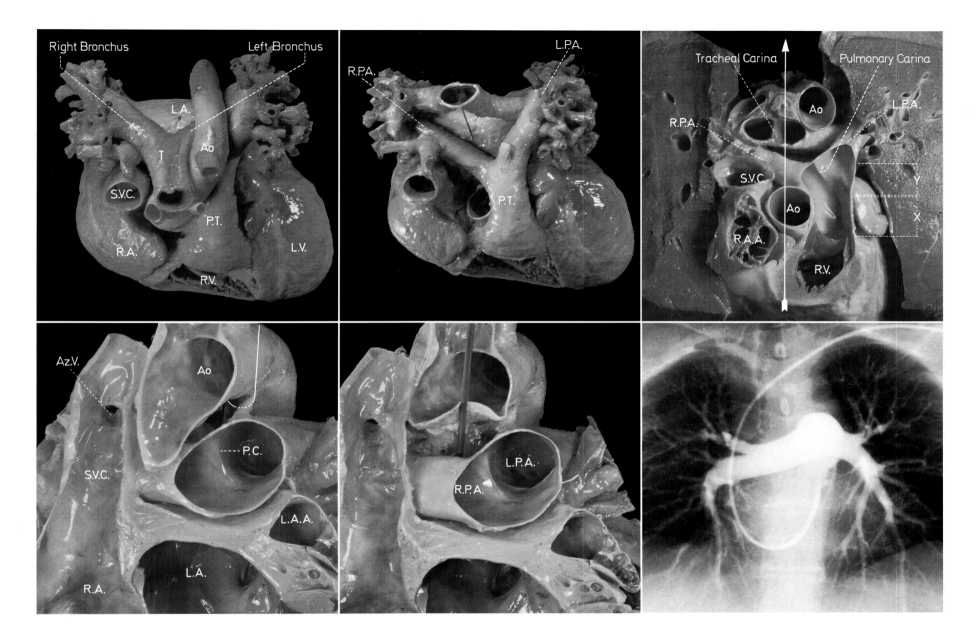

III. The Trachea, Pulmonary Trunk, and Their Branches in the Horizontal Plane

Specimen B: 1 and **2**: Superior view. In **2**, the aorta has been removed, and the trachea and bronchi have been swung posteriorly to expose the pulmonary trunk and the pulmonary arteries.

1: (a) The axis of the trachea is directed postero-inferiorly; (b) the tracheal bifurcation is deflected to the right by the aorta; (c) the right bronchus follows the plane of the trachea; (d) the left main bronchus is deflected anteriorly by the left pulmonary artery.

In **2**, (a) the pulmonary trunk is to the left of, and virtually parallels, the median plane. It bifurcates at an angle of 90°; its axis and that of the left pulmonary artery form an angle of 30°. Normally the axis of the right pulmonary artery is directed to 240°, the left to 150°. These axes are useful in planning the radiographic examination of these vessels (see comments on page 123). (b) The ligamentum arteriosum arises from the origin of the left pulmonary artery.

IV. The Pulmonary Carina

Specimen D: 3: Superior view of a horizontal transection: Observe: (a) The carina of the trachea is to the right of the median plane (arrow) and posterior to the right pulmonary artery. (b) The aorta is posterior to the left main bronchus and deflects it slightly anteriorly. (c) The pulmonary carina is anterior to the left main bronchus. (d) It is helpful to divide the pulmonary trunk into the nonbranching (X) and branching portions (Y) because the right pulmonary artery is given off essentially as a lateral branch of the trunk. Compare the His bundle; the left main bundle emerges as a "side" branch from the branching portion.

Specimen E: 4 and **5**: A.P. view of a frontal transection: (a) The pulmonary trunk has been transected through the anterior part of its branching portion, the posterior extent of which is demarcated from the left pulmonary artery by the pulmonary carina (P.C.). The axis of this carina is directed superiorly and to the right. When the transfemoral route is used, the catheter tends to enter the left pulmonary artery which is more in line with the

trunk than is the right; the catheter may become engaged by the pulmonary carina when it is directed into the right pulmonary artery. Pulmonary emboli may straddle the carina. (b) The superior vena cava has been divided at its origin—the azygos vein (Az.V.) marks the junction of the shorter upper and the longer lower segments (c) The posterior aortic wall has been elevated in **5**, displaying its relation to the right pulmonary artery. This is where a shunt between the two vessels may be created for the palliation of the tetralogy of Fallot (Waterston operation). (d) The white line shown in **4**, passing inferior to the ligamentum, indicates the left recurrent nerve which may be compressed between the aorta and an enlarged left pulmonary artery; the resulting vocal cord paralysis may disappear following correction of the cause of the enlargement of the artery.

6: Contrast has been injected into the pulmonary trunk; the prominent, superiorly directed convexity is produced by the branching portion of the pulmonary trunk in this A.P. view—superimposed upon the trunk is the proximal part of the left pulmonary artery.

125

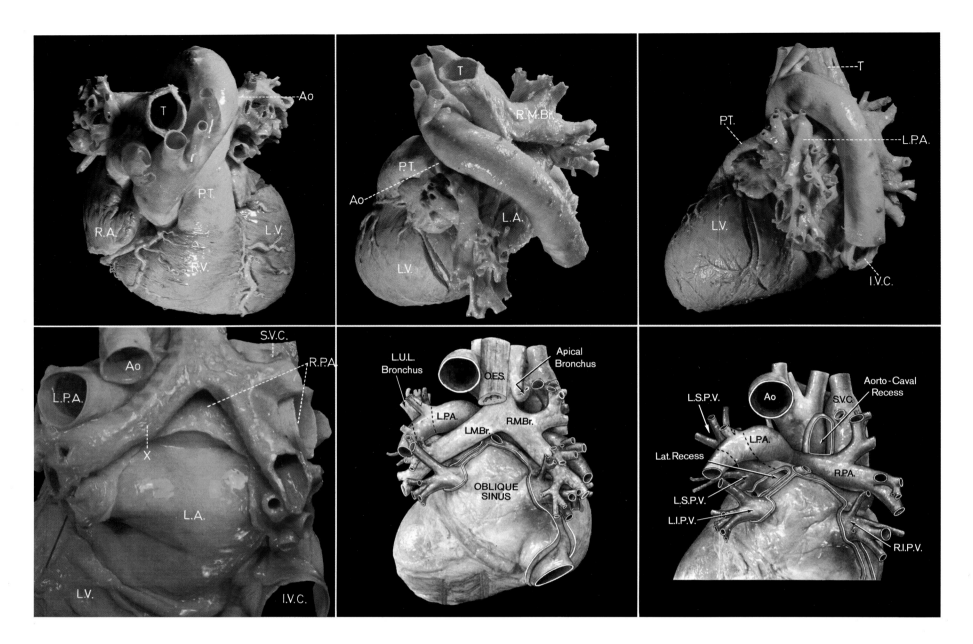

V. The Aortic Knob

Specimen A: 1–3. Views: **1**: Superior A.P. **2**: Superior L.P.O. **3**: L.P.O. The aortic knob, seen in a plain A.P. x-ray of the chest, is the portion of the aorta posterior to the subclavian artery which winds around the lateral aspect of the trachea, deflecting it to the left. Below the aortic knob is the left pulmonary artery as it courses in relation to the left main and upper lobe bronchi. The brachiocephalic arteries arise from a short segment of the aorta.

VI. The Airway and the Great Vessels

Specimen B: 4: P.A. view: Observe: (a) The **trachea** is 3 cm above the left atrium. (b) The angle of bifurcation of the trachea is variable. In this specimen, an angle of 90° is present. The main bronchi are directed at an angle of 30° to the right and 60° to the left of the tracheal axis. (c) The **descending thoracic aorta** is normally separated from the left main bronchus by fatty tissue. However, when the aorta is dilated, it comes in contact with

the bronchus; below the level of the resected aorta, the resulting indentation (X) is seen in the bronchus. (d) The **upper extremity of the pericardial reflection in the oblique sinus** is attached to the right pulmonary artery, which is located anteriorly between the tracheal bifurcation and the left atrium. In **5**, the reflection is to the left atrium.

Specimen C: 5 and **6**: The P.A. view: The specimen is seen before and after removal of the trachea and bronchi in order to demonstrate their relation to the vessels and the pericardium. Observe: (a) The angle of tracheal bifurcation exceeds 90°. (b) The left main bronchus is not in contact with the left atrium. The left upper lobe bronchus has been dislodged from its bed between the left superior pulmonary vein (L.S.P.V.) and the left pulmonary artery (L.P.A.). (c) The right pulmonary artery is anterior to the right bronchus.* (d) The **left lateral recess of the pericardium** (seen in **6**) is well developed. Note its proximity and anterior relation to the left main bronchus. Its proximity to the vestigial fold of the left

superior vena cava (Marshall) is indicated by the catheter which has perforated the pericardium in the concavity of the fold. (e) The posterior portion of the pericardium of **the aorto-caval recess** has been removed, displaying its attachment to the aorta, superior vena cava, and right pulmonary artery. The aorto-caval recess, located in relation to the vital lymphatic terminus, the paratracheal nodes, is a potential avenue in the pathogenesis of pericardial disease. (f) In **6**, the axis of the right pulmonary artery is depressed below the horizontal. (g) The main pulmonary artery to the right upper lobe arises posterior to the superior vena cava. (h) In **5**, note the bronchus to the apical segment of the right upper lobe—it originates from the trachea. In 1,000 bronchograms, this anomaly was seen by Leroux in 14: The tracheal origin of the entire upper lobe was found in 5. The tracheal origin is normal in many animals.

---

* The term, right bronchus, is used to denote the right main bronchus and the bronchus intermedius.

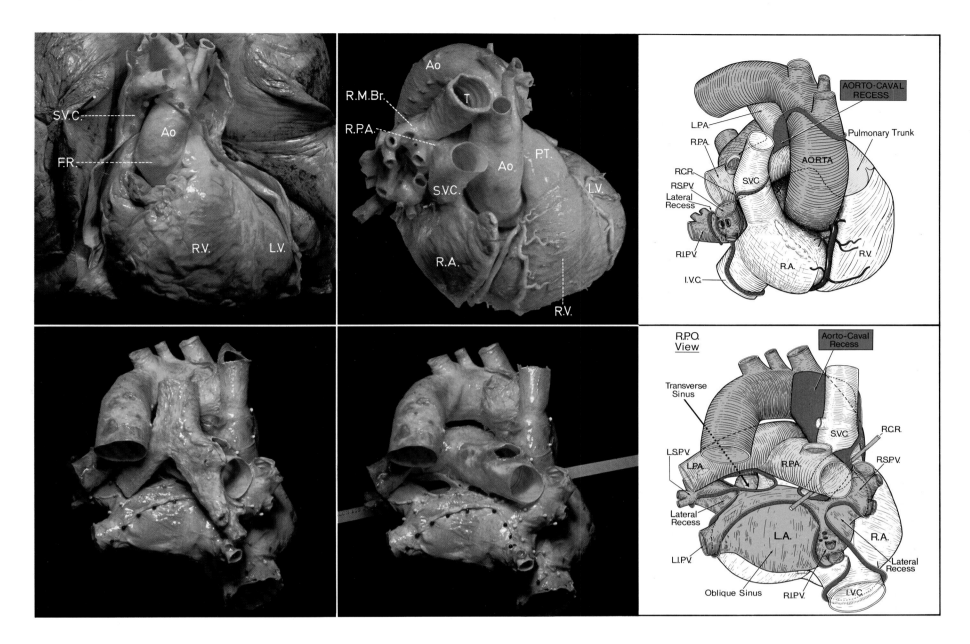

B. The Pericardium

I. The Aortocaval Recess

Specimen D: 1: Superior A.P. view: The red beads identify the attachment of the fibrous pericardium on the superior vena cava and the aorta. At the summit of this reflection, a finger can be passed posteriorly between the two vessels into the aortocaval recess. The right atrial appendage is everted, displaying the pericardial fold of Rindfleisch (F.R.) on the ascending aorta.

Specimen A: 2: Superior R.A.O. view: Observe: The deep aortocaval fossa is located between the superior vena cava, the aorta, and the trachea; its floor is formed by the right pulmonary artery; it is occupied by the important right paratracheal and anterior tracheal lymph nodes.

Specimen E: 3–6: Turn to page **158**—**5** and **6** for the left lateral view

3: The superior R.A.O. view. The aortocaval recess is located anteriorly in this fossa. Its wall of pericardium is attached to the right pulmonary artery, the superior

vena cava, and the aorta. It communicates inferiorly with the transverse sinus of the pericardium (X). The trachea projects postero-inferiorly into the thorax, bifurcating at an angle of 90°. The pulmonary trunk projects posterosuperiorly, bifurcating at an angle of 90°. See the trachea in **2**—visualize it in **3**.

4, **5**, and **6**: R.P.O. view before and after removal of the airway. Beads identify the pericardial divisions (page 132): black = posterior; yellow = lateral, except for the part in the fundus of the retrocaval recess which is red*. Observe, as we pass clockwise from above: (a) The attachments of the aortocaval recess and its relation to the fossa just described. (b) A probe has been directed posteriorly through the retrocaval recess (R.C.R.), perforating its posterior wall in order to demonstrate the proximity of the recess to both the right lateral recess and the oblique sinus. (c) From the lateral recess, the pericardial reflection descends onto the inferior vena cava, which it almost encircles; on reaching the oblique sinus, it is attached to the posterior surface of the right inferior pulmonary vein as it ascends to the

superior wall of the left atrium. It descends on the left, lying on the posterior surface of the left inferior pulmonary vein. Anteriorly, the reflection ascends into the well-developed left lateral recess, the uppermost reflection of which is almost in contact with the anterior reflection of the pericardium in the transverse sinus. In this heart, the pericardial recesses are well developed; the pulmonary veins could easily be encircled during an intrapericardial pneumonectomy, right or left.

In carcinoma of the lung, pneumonectomy is usually reserved for proximal lesions; therefore, the intrapericardial method should be used routinely. In an experience with over 200 such operations, I have found that a better cancer operation (on the right) is accomplished if the posterior wall of the aortocaval recess is incised at its vascular attachments and removed "en bloc" with the related mediastinal lymph nodes. As a corollary, in the resection of inflammatory disease violation of the recess exposes the pericardial cavity to contamination.

---

* In **5** a rod passes through the transverse sinus.

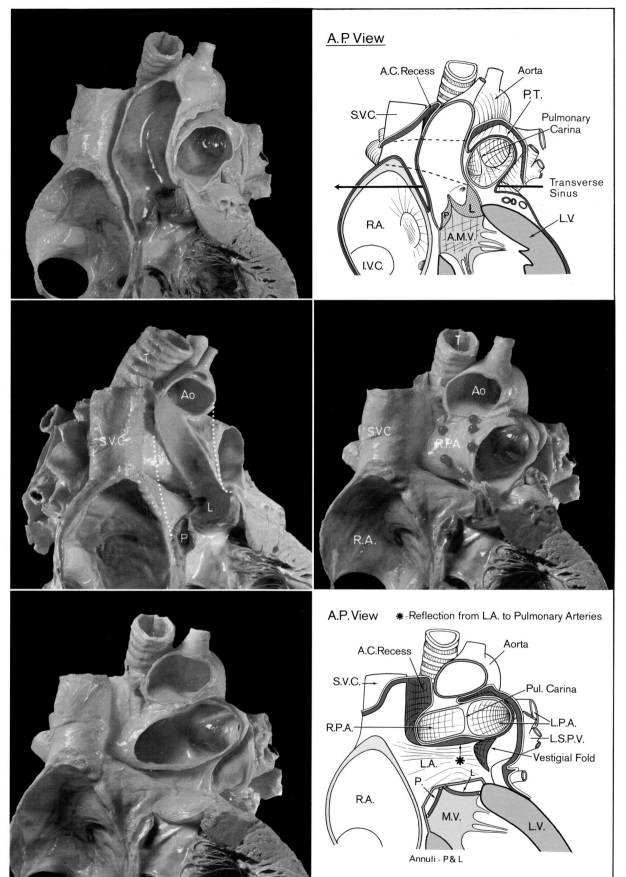

A.P. View

A.C. Recess
Aorta
P.T.
S.V.C.
Pulmonary Carina
Transverse Sinus
R.A.
P.
A.M.V.
L.V.
I.V.C.

T
Ao
S.V.C.
L
P

T
Ao
S.V.C.
R.P.A.
R.A.

A.P. View   *—Reflection from L.A. to Pulmonary Arteries

A.C. Recess
Aorta
S.V.C.
Pul. Carina
R.P.A.
L.P.A.
L.S.P.V.
Vestigial Fold
L.A.
*
L
R.A.
P.
M.V.
L.V.
Annuli - P & L

II. The Transverse Sinus

Specimen A: 1–6 and **129—1** and **2**. Examine the drawings and description of the dissection of this specimen on page **134—2–6**.

1 and 2: The A.P. view of the posterior segment is our starting point. Observe: (a) The pericardial reflection passes from the anteromedial wall of the right atrium onto the upper third of the posterior aortic sinus. (b) The reflection from the aorta to the superior vena cava forms the roof of the aortocaval recess.

3: R.A.O. view: The aortic wall, forming a part of the anterior wall of the transverse sinus and the aortocaval recess, is removed at the site of the pericardial reflection from the aorta to the atria, the pulmonary trunk, and the right pulmonary artery. The left posterior aortic wall has also been removed at the site of reflection of the pericardium from the pulmonary trunk to the aorta, disclosing the small recess between the right anterior aspect of the pulmonary trunk and the aorta. Inferiorly, the pericardium passes from the atria to the upper third of the aortic sinuses. It passes from the pulmonary trunk to the left aortic sinus in the left part of the transverse sinus. The rectangle of aortic wall, extending obliquely upwards from the left aortic sinus, is in direct contact with the pulmonary trunk below and, importantly, the origin of the right pulmonary artery above. If the aorta is encircled with a tape at operation, the dissection is made through this area; it should be carried inferiorly and to the right in order to avoid possible injury to the right pulmonary artery, which is posterior and above.

4: A.P. view: The spirally disposed rectangle of aorta has been removed: The beads indicate the pericardial reflection between the aorta and the trunk and the right pulmonary artery.

5: The anterior wall of the transverse sinus, composed of the nonbranching portion of the pulmonary trunk and adjoining ascending aorta, has been removed, displaying the posterior wall of the sinus which is formed by the adjoining anteromedial wall of the right and anterior wall of the left atrium. The branching portion of the trunk and the adjoining portions of the pulmonary arteries form the roof of the sinus; they are seen here and have been removed in **6**.

6: Note the reflection of the pericardium from the superior wall of the left atrium to the undersurface of the two pulmonary arteries in this specimen. The vestigial fold of the left superior vena cava (Marshall) is triangular in shape—its free border faces laterally—its upper border is attached to the inferior surface of the origin of the left pulmonary artery—its lower border is attached to the anterior surface of the termination of the left superior pulmonary vein. Healey reported that this structure may be attached to the pulmonary trunk or to the proximal portions of either pulmonary artery.

Specimen A, continued: 1: A.P. view: Use the drawing **128—6** for orientation of this photograph—the aorta and the pericardial "mesentery", between the left atrium and the pulmonary arteries, are present in the drawing and absent in the photograph. The red beads mark the reflection of the pericardium as it arcs over the superior vena cava and descends onto and crosses the left atrium. The black bead indicates the apex of the transilluminated triangular vestigial fold, again the upper and lower limbs of which are attached to the inferior surface of the left pulmonary artery and the termination of the left superior pulmonary vein.*

2: Superior view: Note the pericardial reflections forming the lateral recesses. The reflection on the left superior pulmonary vein meets the vestigial fold in a manner that corresponds to the reflections forming the retrocaval recess. In this specimen, the pulmonary artery does not, as it may, have an extrapericardial area of contact with the left atrium. Instead, a mesentery is present between the two which is formed by the fusion of the superior and posterior divisions (page 132); it forms a wall between the transverse and oblique sinuses. When the superior approach to the mitral valve is used, the pulmonary artery is displaced. The attachment of the pericardium between the latter and the left atrium may be a guide to the site of incision. The pulmonary artery crosses the left atrium just anterior to its summit, and the interatrial muscle bundle crosses the junction of the anterior and superior walls of the left atrium. The incision should be made above and posterior to the bundle, not through the unprotected area in the anterior wall of the left atrium.

Specimen B: 3–6: These photographs, with their underlying drawings, are the right and left "halves" of a specimen transected through the aorta and the left extremities of the posterior and right aortic leaflets.** Observe, in contrast to the preceding specimen: (a) The transverse sinus is less well developed. It is located above the level of the aortic sinuses. (b) The right pulmonary artery lies in direct contact with the left atrium. Also observe the left extremity of the aortocaval recess and the anterior and posterior reflections of the pericardium. Aortic stenosis in the adult most often results from the calcification of a malformed valve; when the antecedent is a stenotic valve, the valve orifice is often small and attempts have been made to enlarge it by incising the posterior aortic sinus and inserting an elliptical prosthetic cloth patch. Here we see where this procedure is carried out. Before the patch is sutured in place, the adjoining left atrial and aortic walls must be coapted by sutures—the incision is through the unprotected area of the atrium (U), hence, great care is necessary in this preliminary step if bleeding is to be avoided.

---

* The vestigial fold may be attached to the opposed surfaces of the right pulmonary artery and left atrium (**158—5**).
** The larger scale photographs (**54—5** and **6**, and **63—4**, **5**, and **6**) of this specimen should be reexamined at this time.

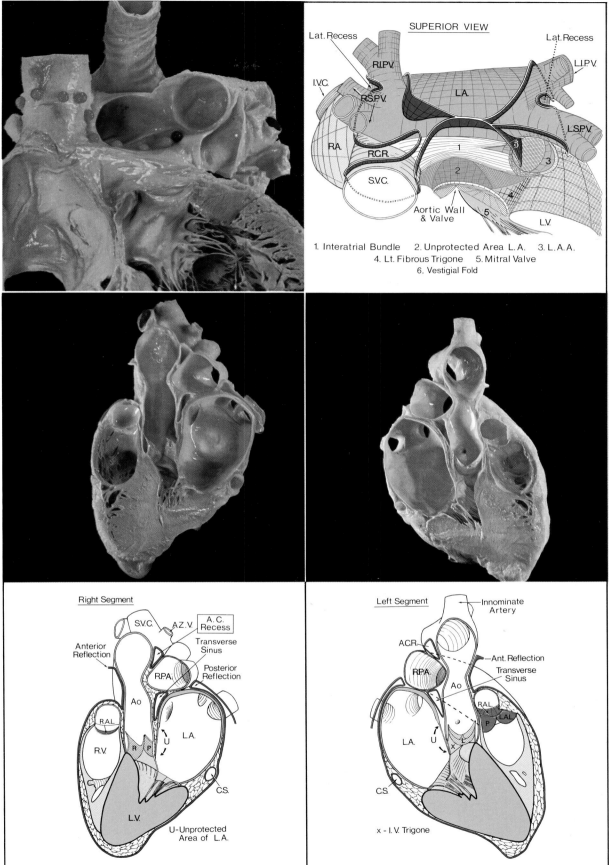

SUPERIOR VIEW

Lat. Recess — R.I.P.V. — Lat. Recess — L.I.P.V.
I.V.C. — R.S.P.V. — L.A. — L.S.P.V.
R.A. — R.C.R. — 1 — 3
S.V.C. — 2
Aortic Wall & Valve — 5 — 4 — L.V.

1. Interatrial Bundle 2. Unprotected Area L.A. 3. L.A.A.
4. Lt. Fibrous Trigone 5. Mitral Valve
6. Vestigial Fold

Right Segment
S.V.C. — A.Z.V. — A. C. Recess
Anterior Reflection — Transverse Sinus
R.P.A. — Posterior Reflection
Ao
R.A.L. — R — P — L.A.
R.V. — C.S.
L.V.
U-Unprotected Area of L.A.

Left Segment — Innominate Artery
A.C.R.
R.P.A. — Ant. Reflection
Ao — Transverse Sinus
R.A.L. — L.A.L.
L.A. — U — P
C.S. — x — L
x - I. V. Trigone

129

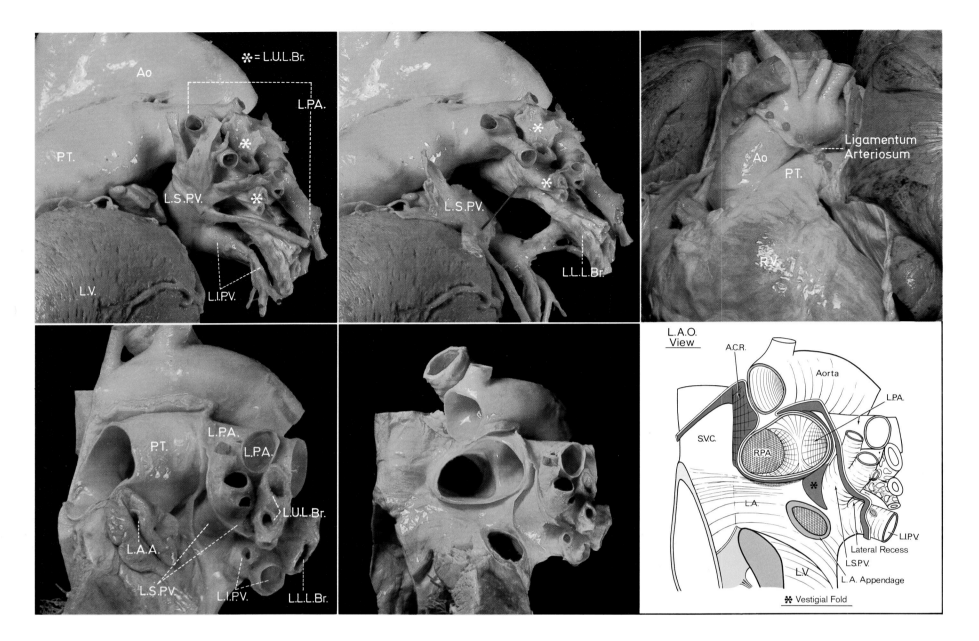

III. The Pericardial Reflections on the Sides of the Heart

Specimen A: 1 and **2**: A nonattitudinal L.A.O. view: In **2**, the left pulmonary veins are depressed. Observe: (a) The left upper lobe bronchus (L.U.L.Br.) is between the vein and the pulmonary artery. (b) On both sides, the pulmonary veins are superior and inferior and anterior and posterior to one another. (c) Arterial branches, larger than the one seen here, may pass anterior to the left upper lobe bronchus and add to the compressive vascular forces which may, in disease states, be exerted on the latter. The pericardial attachment to the vessels in this area will now be studied.

Specimen B: 3: A superior 15° view: The fibrous pericardial attachment (red beads) to the aorta and left pulmonary artery crosses the ligamentum arteriosum. A recess of pericardium covers the anterolateral aspect of the pulmonary end of a patent ductus arteriosus. During the operative obliteration or division of the ductus, the pericardium forming the recess (often termed the peri-

cardial lappet) is dissected from both the ductus arteriosus and the left pulmonary artery.

Specimen C: 4–6: This specimen was studied in the A.P. view on page 128.

4: Left lateral view: The left atrial appendage is folded on itself.

5 and **6**: L.A.O. view: The ascending aorta, the pulmonary trunk, and the proximal (intrapericardial) centimeter of the lateral wall of the left pulmonary artery have been removed, exposing the posterior wall of the transverse sinus. Observe: (a) The fibrous pericardium can now be traced inferiorly onto the pulmonary veins. (b) The lateral part of the proximal centimeter of the left pulmonary artery is intrapericardial—a ligature should be placed on the right side of the ligamentum arteriosum and include the pericardium anteroinferiorly.* Pneumonectomy is ordinarily only performed for malignant lesions of major bronchi; in order to be well proximal to the lesion I have frequently removed the lateral portion of the

pulmonary trunk, which is seen in the center of the photograph **4**. Ligation of the left pulmonary artery should never be used in cancer surgery; the ligature may slip off if a generous stump of artery is not left—in this stump, residual tumor may be found. Closure with continuous vascular suture beyond a clamp is secure and accomplished without difficulty. (c) On the left, the entrance to the transverse sinus is guarded by the vestigial fold and the left atrial appendage. (d) The left lateral recess of the pericardium is in contact with the lymph nodes found between the lingular and left lower lobe bronchi. (e) The recess formed by the vestigial fold corresponds to the retrocaval recess (on the right).

---

* Opening the pericardium is avoided in the treatment of inflammatory disease, which has become an uncommon indication for pneumonectomy.

Specimen D: 1: 240° view: **Specimen E: 2**, a nonattitudinal L.A.O. view. Note the superior vena cava/pulmonary artery relationship: Most often (see page 157) their lower margins are in a horizontal plane. The pericardium on the left side passes directly from S.V.C. to the artery. On the right side it is invaginated between the two posteriorly, forming the retrocaval recess. The right pulmonary veins (seen in **1**), like their left counterparts, are disposed in a posteroinferiorly directed axis. On both sides, a lateral recess extends between the two. In passing, note the following: (a) At 240°—the right pulmonary artery parallels and the left is perpendicular to the plane of examination. (b) The inferior wall of the pulmonary artery and the superior cavo-atrial angle (which marks the location of the sinus node, the terminus of the [right] sinus node artery R.S.A. in **2**) are in a horizontal plane.

Specimen F: 3—6: Views: **3** and **6**=270°; **4** and **5**=300°. In **3** the sino-atrial node is indicated by the dashed oval. In **4** two incisions have extended into the superior vena cava. The upper is just below the pericardial reflection; the lower, through the uppermost part of the atrium. These incisions are joined posteriorly at the site of the pericardial reflection onto the superior vena cava; the segment resulting has been removed. **5** and **6**: The upper division of the right superior pulmonary vein has been removed exposing the right pulmonary artery. Observe: (a) In **3**, the lower segment of the superior vena cava is directed antero-inferiorly; note the obliquity of the superior cavo-atrial junction. If a tape, used for the snare in caval cannulation, lies on the junction, the S.A. node may be injured. (b) The pericardial reflection passes from the superior vena cava to the right superior pulmonary vein where it forms a border of the entrance to the **retrocaval recess**; the anterior, posterior, and lateral walls of which are formed by the superior vena cava, the right pulmonary artery, and the right superior pulmonary vein. A posterior projection of the recess lies between the left atrium and the pulmonary artery. Note the proximity of the two pericardial reflections on the superior vena cava—the right lateral division in the retrocaval recess and the superior division in the transverse sinus: It is easier to place a tape through the extrapericardial area between the closest points of these reflections; however as mentioned, the tape may traumatize the sinus node. The tape should be placed at a higher level (indicated by the arrow in **5**), superior to the right pulmonary artery, i.e. 3 to 4 cm above the level of the node. (c) The inferior pulmonary veins are postero-inferior to the superior pulmonary veins—the **right lateral recess**, between the veins is postero-inferior to the retrocaval recess; its contact with the lymph node subterminus at the junction of the middle and lower lobe bronchi provides an avenue of spread of disease from the nodes to the pericardium. During middle lobectomy, usually performed for inflammatory disease, the recess should not be entered. The retouched photograph **6** emphasizes that the lateral recess extends posteriorly in the thorax.

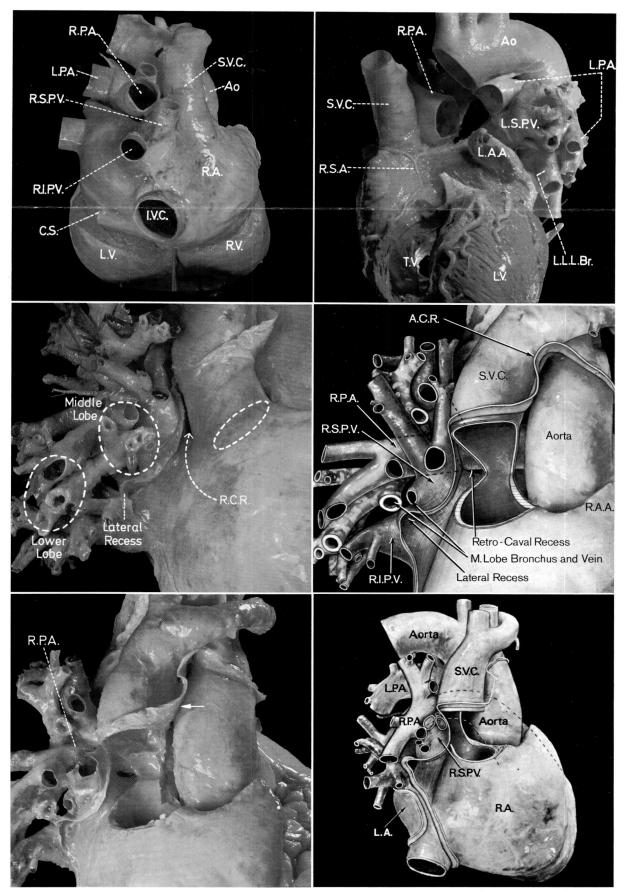

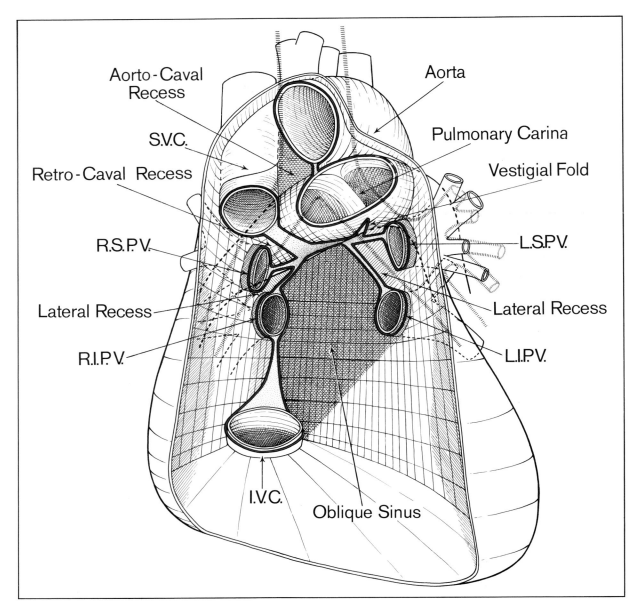

Aorto-Caval Recess

S.V.C.

Retro-Caval Recess

R.S.P.V.

Lateral Recess

R.I.P.V.

Aorta

Pulmonary Carina

Vestigial Fold

L.S.P.V.

Lateral Recess

L.I.P.V.

I.V.C.

Oblique Sinus

IV. The Summation of the Pericardial Reflections

1: A.P. view: An anterior window has been created in the fibrous pericardium. The heart has been removed after transection of (1) the branching portion of the pulmonary trunk (note the prominent carina and its obliquity) and the aorta anterior to the innominate artery, (2) the venae cavae and pulmonary veins at their atrial connections, and (3) the reflection between the left atrium and the right pulmonary artery. The serous pericardium (reflection) is colored green. The pulmonary veins are red. The left atrium is between the pulmonary veins and is inferior to the right pulmonary artery—it forms the anterior wall of the oblique sinus (delimited here by black cross hatch). Visualize the chamber in place when examining this drawing. The pericardial reflections may be grouped into the upper arterial reflection, in relation to the great vessels, and a lower continuous venous reflection, which is divisible into four divisions, posterior, right lateral, superior, and left lateral.

A: The Arterial Reflection: The visceral layer of the pericardium clothing the arteries meets the parietal layer at the lines of attachment of the fibrous pericardium, which descends across the superior vena cava on the right and across the aorta and left pulmonary on the left.

B: The Venous Reflection: (1) The **posterior division** extends between the anterior aspect of the inferior vena cava and the inferior margin of the left inferior pulmonary vein, forming the boundary of the oblique sinus. It is unindented. The reflection crosses the inferior pulmonary veins, but is separated from the superior pulmonary veins. Its summit may be attached to the left atrium or the right pulmonary artery—this is virtually its only variation. (2) The **right lateral division** extends between the anterior aspects of the venae cavae. In this specimen, prominent recesses—the lateral and retrocaval—are present. (3) The **left lateral division** extends between its junction with the posterior division (on the inferior aspect of the left inferior pulmonary vein) and the upper

end of the attachment of the vestigial fold to the left pulmonary artery. Two recesses are present. As on the right, the lateral recess is large—the recess of the vestigial fold is small in comparison with its counterpart, the retrocaval recess. (4) The **superior division** passes between the upper ends of the lateral divisions. Pericardium extends between the pulmonary artery (essentially the right) and the superior wall of the left atrium. When the posterior division is attached to the pulmonary artery, the two layers of pericardium in relation to it and the superior division may form a "mesentery" between the artery and the atrium which intervenes between the oblique and transverse sinuses. At other times, a wide area of the artery is not separated by pericardium from the left atrium. (See page 129.)

Recognition of the four divisions of the venous pericardial reflection is helpful in surgical operations. (a) In **left atriotomy** (see page 64) the adjacent parts of the right lateral and the superior divisions are divided when the superior vena cava is untethered. (b) In either a right or a left **intrapericardial pneumonectomy,** the posterior division and the related right or left division should first be identified by palpation. On the right side the two layers of serous pericardium between the inferior pulmonary vein and the inferior vena cava are first divided. The posterior division—unvarying in relation to the pulmonary veins—is identified by placing a finger in the oblique sinus. By means of bidigital palpation, the development of the two pericardial recesses (in relation to the pulmonary veins) can thus be determined. When the recesses are well developed—as in specimens shown in this chapter—division or ligation is easy. When the recesses are not well developed—and they may be virtually absent, particularly the lateral recess—careful attention to the location of the existing reflection is helpful. (c) **Venae cavae cannulation tapes:** The superior tape is placed at a site where much of the circumference of the vessels is extrapericardial (see **131—5**). The inferior tape is placed by penetrating the right lateral and posterior divisions of the reflection at the site of their maximal proximity—just below the right inferior pulmonary vein. (d) **Ligation of the right pulmonary artery:** In intrapericardial pneumonectomy, the specimen is removed along with the posterior wall of the aortocaval recess—note the relation of the inferior attachment of the wall to the superior (**131—1**) and posterior (**126—6**) divisions of the "venous reflection". When a mesentery is present beneath the artery (and the posterior division is therefore attached to the artery) only the posterosuperior part of the artery is extrapericardial—ligation within the pericardium is then facilitated. Knowledge of these relationships may be crucial if the need ever arises to control bleeding during the dissection of a matted hilum in pulmonary surgery—the pericardium may be entered and the artery occluded with a snare or a bulldog clamp.

Section III: The Coronary Arteries

General Remarks

This section is intended to provide an anatomic basis for the most urgent necessity in medicine today—the ability, in coronary artery disease, to quantitate the perfusion deficit and to assess the role of an involved branch in this deficit. If we are to study the natural history of the disease and determine the need for surgery and predict its results, such an exercise is necessary. In Chapter 3 the obtuse margin is redefined; it is readily identified in x-ray studies, and, along with the interventricular grooves it demarcates the three walls of the left ventricle—the arterial supply to each is assessed as part of the total quantitation. In Chapter 6 the crux, the key to clarification of arterial dominance and the supply of the posterior wall. has been studied. The clinician must be armed with the knowledge of the very wide variations in the number and size of branches and the various mode of branching which may be encountered. In this atlas over 75 hearts may be seen in the study of these variations. Following this study, the great imprecision of the division into "one", "two" and "three-vessel disease" will be apparent.

For many generations an orderly method has been used in the study of extracardiac arteries. Four fundamental facts are established: (1) the origin; (2) the mode of termination; (3) the course and relations and arterial subdivisions derived therefrom; and (4) the mode of branching and the precise area of supply of each of its branches. Replication of this elicitory approach will ease our task and bring order to our knowledge of anatomy—it will also prove salutary in our management of obliterative disease. The arrangement of this section effects concordance with this fundamental anatomic method and emphasizes its basic importance and utility. **The right and left coronary arteries will not be examined separately:** Their cardinal feature is the wide variation seen in their reciprocal development; one cannot be understood separately; **their origin,** found in Chapter 10, comprises an examination of their orifices and the mode of attachment of the left main branch and the proximal segment of the right to the aorta. The atrial arteries are placed in Chapter 11 to emphasize their importance and also their uniqueness—the origin of their main element, the sinus node artery, is often remote from its major area of supply. In Chapter 12, the study of the **branches** precedes the study of the **course and relations,** found in Chapter 13, because it affords description of their terminology. In most instances, in the specimens used in the exposition of the above subject matter, the **termination** of both arteries appears; however, the mode of termination of the posterior division of the left coronary artery (the circumflex branch) presents complexities of such degree and number, that Chapter 14 is devoted to its consideration.

Chapter 10: The Origin of the Coronary Arteries

Introduction

When a student examines the origin of the coronary arteries, three important features emerge: **I. The left main branch has wide variations in its spatial disposition**: In a horizontal plane, the axis may be anterior, transverse, or posterior: In a frontal plane, the axis may be superior, horizontal, or inferior. In any anatomic study, be it in a laboratory or a clinical setting, it is essential that both axes be defined. What is the clinical relevance of these axes? First, and most evident, they dictate the radiographic plane for the optimal examination of this vessel in which severe occlusive disease is not only common but life endangering—emergency bypass surgery is carried out in many centers. The second and conceivably more fundamental effect of these axes relates to the design of the coronary artery orifice—the axes are the major determinant of this design. **II. The right coronary artery displays a characteristic proximal segment**—it is 1.5 cm in length—which extends in a perpendicular manner from the right aortic sinus—a smooth orifice results. The left main branch, conversely, as a resultant of extremes in either of the two axes—and these extremes are not uncommon—may display a knife-like incisura at the inferior or one of its lateral margins. These orificial incisura are striking anatomic features. What is their significance: One may conjecture that they may be a factor in the following: (a) the production of turbulence downstream; (b) impaired flow due to skimming; (c) they may act like a flap valve—a parallel can be drawn with the angle of His in esophagogastric competence. This mechanism may reduce coronary flow when the pressure in the aorta rises and expands its walls—a possible explanation for the sudden, hitherto unexplained deaths during exercise in the absence of coronary atherosclerosis. **III.** Variations occur in the site of origin of coronary arteries. Any discussion of coronary arteries would be meager without consideration of these variations (the variation in termination—arteriocameral fistulae are not considered) which may be classified as congenital anomalies. This constitutes the only variance from the stated aim—the study of normal anatomy. These variations may accompany an otherwise normal heart therefore their inclusion is deemed appropriate—three reasons may be cited: (1) A surgeon may unwittingly divide a major arterial trunk (a) in an aortotomy when the orifice is elevated and in a cardiotomy when the trunk pursues an abnormal course as a consequence of translocation of its originating orifice. (b) A surgeon may also, during valve surgery, injure or occlude, by a suture, a major trunk when it pursues a unexpected or variant course—the so-called abnormal circumflex artery, the commonest translocation variation, is a good example. (2) A patient may be found to have a single or a translocated coronary artery following an otherwise normal hemodynamic and contrast study. What advice to the patient is appropriate? The study of Cheitlin, McAllister and deCastro (1974) invoked the flap valve mechanism (excerpts from a later article of these workers appears on page 150) and noted the marked disparity in the clinical significance of left versus right translocation. Translocation of the left is associated with sudden death, translocation of the right coronary is not—a similar marked disparity exists in the normal anatomy of two orifices. This work brings a new perspective into this clinical consideration. McAllister states that 7 patients have undergone operation because of the orificial consequence of the variation in the origin of the coronary arteries.

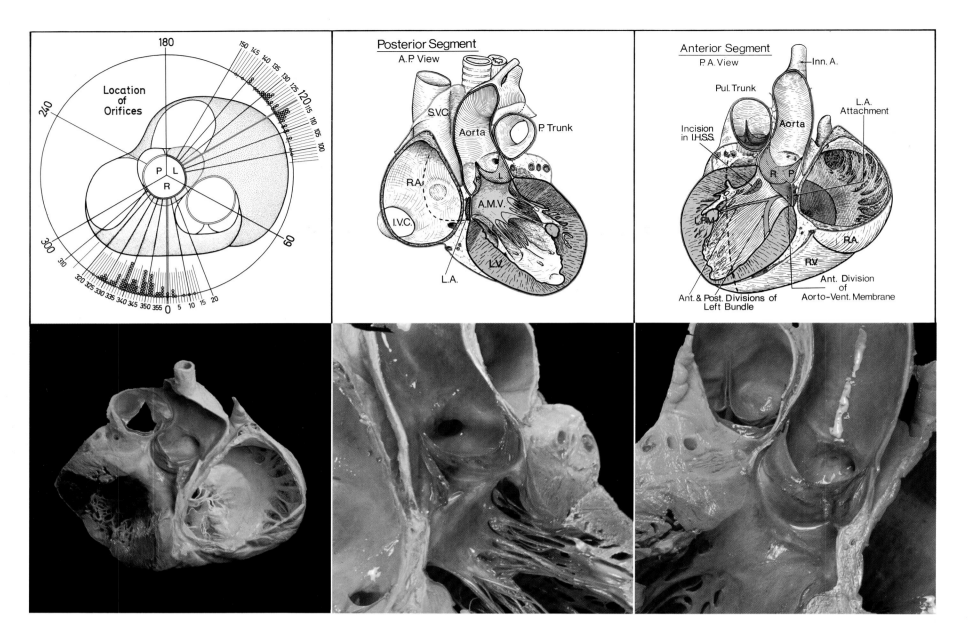

A. The Orifices—Their Location

I. The Location of the Orifices of the Coronary Arteries in the Horizontal Plane

1: Data from 50 hearts: The blue and red lines indicate the midpoints of the right and left aortic sinuses. The right coronary is destined to pass around the tricuspid ostium; hence, it would seem appropriate for its orifice to be located in the right half of the right aortic sinus—such is usually the case. The left coronary artery, which in the majority of instances supplies the anterior and left lateral part of the heart, would be anticipated to usually arise from the anterior (or lateral) half of the left aortic sinus; however, the orifice is located anterior and posterior to its midpoint in approximately equal numbers. The commonly seen posterior location is unrelated to either the relative dominance of the anterior and posterior divisions or the axis of the left main branch in the horizontal plane.

Specimen A: 2–6: Additional photographs of this specimen appear on page **19**—**3–6** and in **128**—**1–6** and **130**—**4–6**.

2 and **3**: The lines of the oblique incision are indicated. The incision passes through the right fibrous trigone, separating the two divisions of the A.V. membrane. Anteriorly, it passes between the left and right aortic sinuses. **4**: The anterior segment is viewed from above; visualize the descent of a cardiac catheter to the right coronary orifice.

In **5** and **6**, the posterior and anterior segments, the left and right orifices are seen in a scale slightly smaller than 1:1. The drawings **2** and **3** may be used for their orientation.

5: The Left Orifice: In an attempt to avoid the alteration of terminology in common clinical usage, I have used the term "left" rather than the longer, "left posterolateral", sinus and leaflet. Examination of **2**, an (attitudinal) A.P. view, shows that in this specimen the

orifice is located in the posterior half of the sinus; this is an example of the importance of the correct anatomic description of structures. The sinus has a posterior and a lateral half and this would be indicated by the term "posterolateral". The reader should constantly be aware that, in this work, the expedient, not only nondescriptive but misleading terms, left aortic sinus and posterior aortic sinus, are used, and be mindful that each sinus has a posterior and a lateral half.

In the A.P. view, the orifice is obscured by the left leaflet, so it is shown here (in **5**) from 330°. It is elliptical in shape, 5.4 mm in width, and located 10 and 17 mm from the posterior and right aortic leaflets.

6: P.A. view: **The right orifice** is 2.7 mm in width and 10 and 16 mm from the posterior and left leaflets, respectively—both the left and the right orifices are deviated towards the posterior sinus. Note the incomplete sinus rim related to the orifice. Reid suggests that the sinus rim ensures "that the coronary arteries are kept primed with blood during systole".

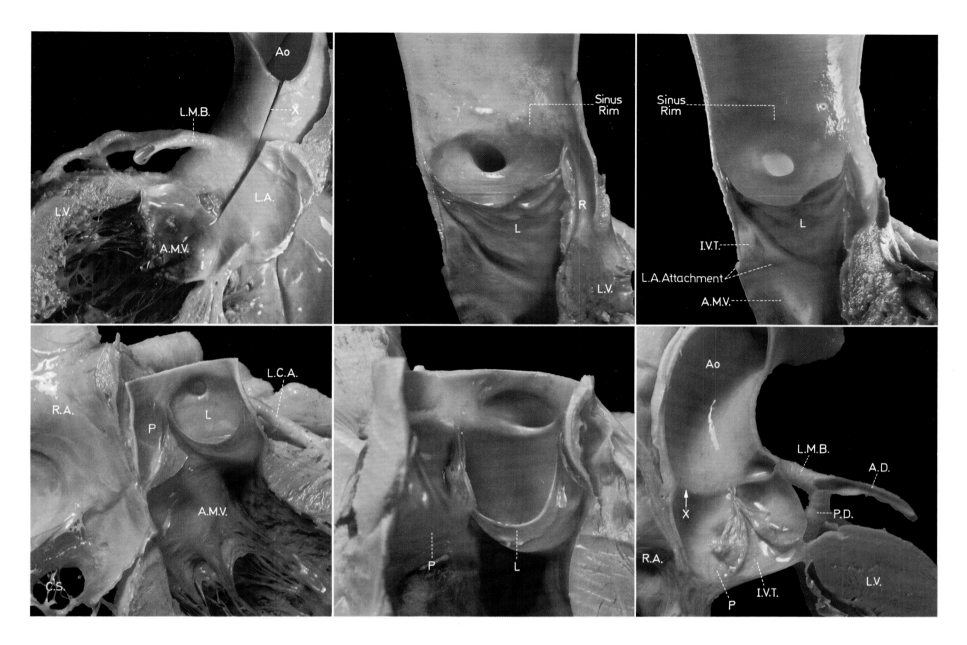

II. The Location of the Left Coronary Orifice in the Sagittal Plane

Specimen B: 1–3

1: P.A. view: This is the anterior segment, resulting from the frontal transection seen on page 102. Here, the left half of the anterior wall of the left atrium has been removed. Observe that the left main branch (L.M.B.) meets the surface of the aorta at an angle of 45°. The anterior segment is transected in the axis of the aortic bulb (see X) and the left segment resulting therefrom is seen next from a right lateral view.

2 and 3: The left coronary orifice is oval or elliptical, and a line joining the upper extremities of the left aortic leaflet passes through its midpoint. Note its relation to the left sinus rim. On page **23—4**, the normal relation of the orifice to the upper extremities of the annuli and the sinus rim is also shown. The sharp inferior margin of the orifice is seen as a density in **3**. This specimen demonstrates the usual location of the orifice in the

human heart. In **180—1** and **2**, examine an example of a left coronary orifice situated inferiorly in the sinus. Black *et al.*, in a valuable contribution on vascular injury following valve replacement, describe an instance of blockage of the right coronary orifice by an aortic valve prosthesis.

III. The Elevated Left Coronary Artery Orifice

Specimen C: 4:

On page **2—5** and **6**, both segments of this specimen are seen. On page **23—5** and **6**, re-examine the right segment—the right coronary orifice is located 6 mm above the right sinus rim. The tendency toward elevation is noted here in the left orifice, which is deflecting superiorly the left sinus rim in this R.A.O. view.

Specimen D: 5:

The left coronary orifice is located above the sinus rim. Note the prominent inferiorly located incisura in the orifice. It has been frequently stated that an elevated left coronary orifice does not occur. Instead, because of embryologic considerations,

origin from the pulmonary trunk would be the consequence. The degree of elevation, however, never approaches that seen in the right orifice, which we shall examine on the next page.

Specimen E: 6:

Following its initial frontal transection, this specimen is seen on page **104—1–4**. Here, the left coronary orifice is elevated above the left aortic sinus rim. The axis of the main branch is directed inferiorly. A sharp inferior incisura is produced at the orifice. It is accentuated by the sinus rim. Note the prominence of the posterior aortic sinus rim (X).

Comment: Reid stated, "The fleetest of animals, namely the dog and man, demonstrate the highest position of the coronary ostia". The height of the orifice affects the axes of the left main branch and the right proximal segment which, in turn, determine orifice characteristics.

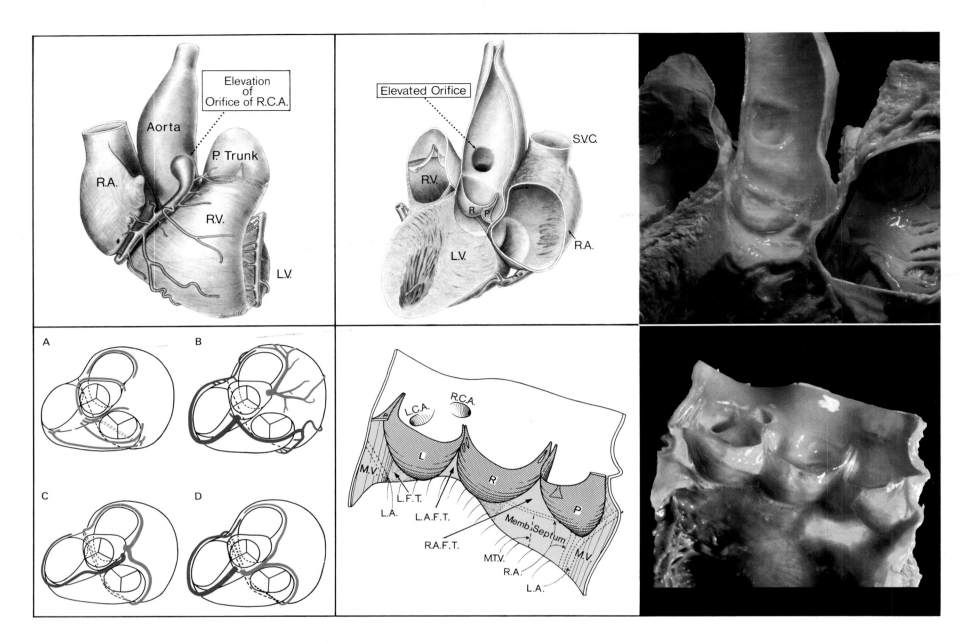

IV. The Elevated Right Coronary Artery Orifice

Specimen A: 1—3: In this specimen, the exterior view is seen in **1**; the interior view in **2** and **3**. The central area of **2** is shown in the photograph. The specimen had suffered from exposure to air and heat prior to its photography. The lower border of the 15-mm-wide funnel-like orifice is 12 mm above the right sinus rim. The presence of this relatively common anatomic variation has obvious clinical significance. (a) At operation, the right coronary artery may be injured by aortic clamping or even dissection or divided by an inferiorly located aortotomy. (b) It should always be recalled when difficulty is encountered in catheterizing the artery during selective arteriography. (c) Bellhouse *et al.* have suggested that, in the presence of an elevated orifice, the coronary flow may be impaired because of unfavorable mechanical factors, resulting in turbulence and skimming of blood. This variation can be cited as another reason why coronary arteriography is deemed essential prior to cardiac surgery in most instances.

V. The Extrasinal-Translocation of an Orifice

4-A: The **course of an anomalous artery** or branch may be: (1) preventricular (right), (2) preconal, (3) prepulmonary, (4) transseptal, (5) retropulmonary, (6) retro-aortic, and (7) retro-ostial.

4-B: A branch or division, e.g., the anterior interventricular, may be translocated.

4-C and **4-D**: The entire right or left coronary artery orifice may be translocated. In both examples, the course of the anomalous artery is retropulmonary.

Specimen B: 5 and **6**: **Translocation of the right coronary artery**: This specimen was from an autopsy on a patient presenting no history or other evidence of any cardiac disease apart from slight adherence between the right and left aortic leaflets. The right coronary artery originates from the left aortic sinus. The transilluminated membranous septum is seen below the barren right and posterior aortic sinuses.

Text for page 137

1: Translocation of the left coronary artery: In this instance, the orifice is located above that of the right, placing the translocated artery in jeopardy at aortotomy.

2: The translocated anterior interventricular branch may follow a varying course across the infundibulum or pulmonary trunk. This variation occurs not infrequently in association with the tetralogy of Fallot. This is particularly unfortunate because the artery, unless unusually low, would be spared by a transverse right ventriculotomy and in a patient with the tetralogy, a vertical incision may be mandatory to insert a patch to enlarge the infundibulum. It is, therefore, not surprising that a rather large number of deaths have resulted from the division of this artery in the correction of this malformation. Pre-operative coronary arteriography, using a supravalvular aortogram in small children or the selective technique in larger patients, would seem to be indicated.

Arteries may run intramurally across the right ventricle; hence, the awareness of the arterial variation and its identification at operation cannot be offered as a countermeasure.

3: Hackensellner has suggested that the primordiae for the coronary arteries are present in all six sinuses (aortic and pulmonary) and normally, development only occurs in the left and right aortic sinuses.

4: (a) **Accessory coronary arteries** associated with normally perfused hearts have been reported in 13 patients (Chinn). The numbers in relation to the pulmonary sinuses indicate the origin of the accessory arteries. (b) It is an interesting fact that **translocation of coronary arteries to the posterior sinus** in a normal heart is unrecorded in humans*. It has been seen in deer in New York State (Bishop) and in the wildebeest in Africa (Wallach). I have studied 48 hearts of deer from northern Michigan, and none demonstrated this finding. (c) and (d) are taken from the studies of Edwards on the location of coronary arteries in **transposition of the great vessels.** (R = Right Coronary Artery; A = Anterior and P = Posterior Divisions of Left Coronary Artery). In a later study, Shaher and Puddu have reported the findings of the Toronto group in this condition.

5: The theory of Abrikossoff has been used to explain the variations seen in the anomalous origin of the coronary artery from the pulmonary trunk. The number (1) and the solid line indicate the normal division of the truncus arteriosus and the resulting normal disposition shown in the next drawing. The other lines and their numbers indicate abnormal modes of truncal division in this drawing; the resulting abnormalities are likewise indicated in the next drawing.

6: (1) The normal development is seen. (2) The origin of both coronary arteries from the pulmonary sinuses is incompatible with life for more than a few weeks; when the pulmonary artery pressure falls, myocardial infarction and death ensue. (3) This represents the common abnormality seen. The duration of life depends on the degree of development of collaterals from the right coronary artery. Operative correction has been accomplished by (a) ligation of the anomalous artery at its pulmonary origin, which interrupts the "steal" of blood from the coronary circulation, or (b) by interposing a vein graft between the aorta and the distal end of the anomalous artery, following its division and proximal closure. (4) When the right coronary arises from a pulmonary sinus, usually no disease results. (5) When the adjacent left aortic and posterior pulmonary primordiae fuse (Hackensellner—see 3) or the primitive left is split (Abrikossoff), as shown here, an arterial branch connects the left coronary artery and the pulmonary sinus, resulting in a steal phenomenon. Although surgical correction is simple, the relevance of the lesion to symptoms is not easily established.

---

* McAllister (1975) has observed 7 hearts with double translocation—the right coronary artery from the posterior aortic sinus—the left from the right aortic sinus.

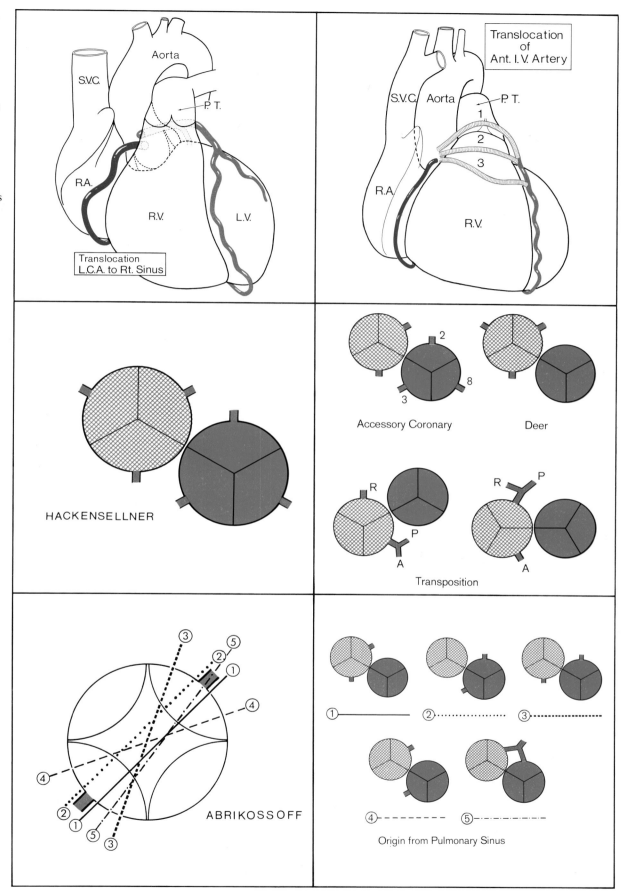

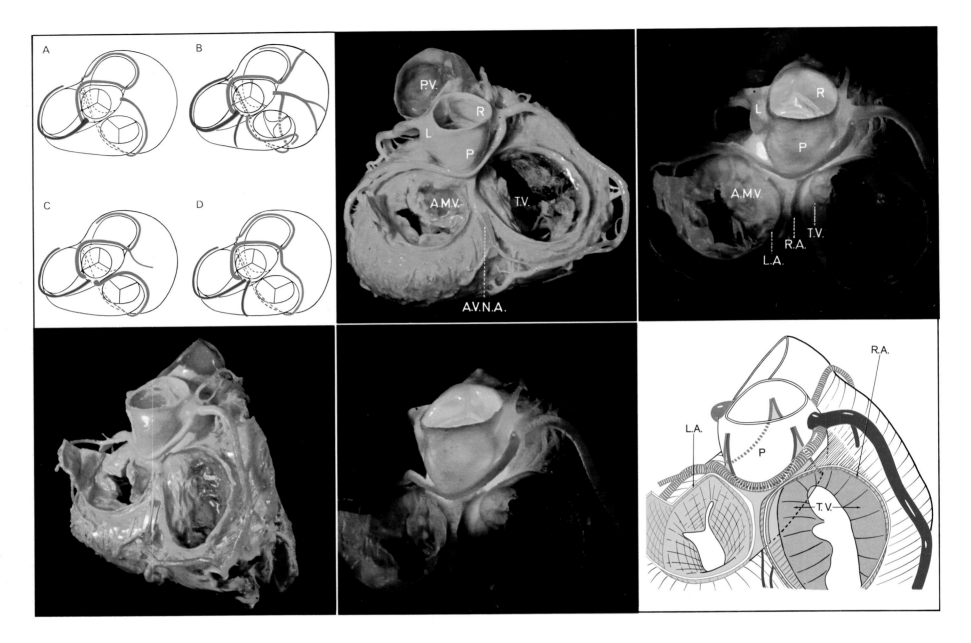

VI. The Anomalous "Circumflex" Coronary Artery

Translocation of the posterior division of the left coronary artery to the right aortic sinus is, in the traditional terminology, "the anomalous circumflex coronary artery": It is one of the most common coronary artery anomalies and has great clinical significance. It may exist alone or be associated with other variations.

In 1-A, the abnormality is seen in its simple form. It may arise from a separate orifice, as shown below. **1-B:** The specimen described herein: An associated abnormality of the anterior interventricular branch is present (see page 183). **1-C:** Translocation of both divisions of the left coronary artery is present. **1-D:** The retroaortic course of the left coronary artery, associated with two separate right coronary artery orifices, is depicted. C and D are reported cases wherein both coronary arteries arise from a single sinus. These variations should not be confused with the variation, the single coronary artery—they are examples of translocation.

2: The specimen is seen from the (near) right posterior oblique view (240°) with 45° of elevation. The anomalous vessel arises with the right coronary artery from the right aortic sinus. It first courses just above the attachments of the tricuspid valve and the right atrium to the aorto-ventricular membrane. It then winds around the bottom of the posterior aortic sinus and continues across the intervalvular trigone and the left fibrous trigone to terminate on the lateral wall of the left ventricle.

In **3**, the specimen is seen from the same vantage point: It is transilluminated to emphasize the relations between the artery and the aortic annuli.

4, 5 and **6:** The specimen is viewed attitudinally from a near right lateral position. The relations of the vessel to the aortic annuli and the tricuspid valve are seen. In this part of its course the artery could be injured by a deeply placed suture during replacement of either the aortic or tricuspid valves or in the placement of a patch to close a primum type of atrial septal defect. The occurrence of

this arterial variation is an additional reason why coronary arteriography is a vital prelude to most cardiac operations.

This statement, which will be repeated on other pages, will probably not go unchallenged. The occurrence of anomalies of the coronary arteries is the lesser reason for the advocacy of this policy. In the recent past, an axiom of the management of chest disease dictated the invariable exclusion of its dominant disease, tuberculosis. Today, in the Western world, coronary artery disease is the dominant disease of the heart, and its exclusion prior to the surgical correction of acquired disease in adults seems necessary: This has been my practice. This policy is contingent on a low risk in the use of coronary arteriography: Again, in my opinion and experience, this is possible if every care is observed in its performance: Some examples of the measures which I have used for many years are: (1) The injection of a total body dose of heparin (100 units per kilogram body weight) into the artery when it is entered by the needle and before a guide wire or catheter is introduced; (2) in

an attempt to minimize deposition of platelet masses
and their dangerous embolization, (teflon-coated) guide
wires are handled with scrupulous care and removed
from the catheter before it reaches the origin of the brachiocephalic arteries; (3) the procedure should be con-
ducted with dispatch—if ever prolonged to one hour,
additional heparin is given. It is of interest that an
"anomalous circumflex coronary artery" is found in
approximately 1% of all hearts (Ogden)—the risk of
arteriography is very much less.

The specimen has interest apart from the topic of discussion. (a) The anterosuperior and septal leaflets of the
tricuspid valve form a continuous broad sheet which
extends far posteriorly to gain attachment to the A.V.
membrane only 5 mm from the junction of its divisions
(the right fibrous trigone). The atrial portion of the
membranous septum is, therefore, small. (b) The posterior aortic annulus is located high above the left ventricular ostium. The membranous septum as a whole is
therefore large.

---

1 and **2**, R.P.O. view: The anomalous artery and the
anterosuperior segment of the attachment of the left
atrium to the aorto-ventricular membrane are coterminous. This indicates the danger of injury to this artery
during mitral valve replacement. Myocardial infarction
and death have also been reported from entrapment of
the vessel between the seats of the two prosthesis following combined aortic and mitral valve replacement.

3 and **4**: An elevated L.P.O. view: The anomalous vessel, which is striped, is seen passing onto the lateral
wall of the left ventricle, with a smaller branch passing
to the left atrium and the posterior wall of the left
ventricle. The large anomalous septal branch, passing
anteriorly into the muscle behind the lateral third of the
posterior pulmonary sinus, can be seen. In passing, note
the large left fibrous trigone (L.F.T.), which is confluent
with the intervalvular trigone (I.V.T.). This is a site
where annular subvalvular aneurysms can occur in relation to the aortic annuli (see page 15). Also, we can see
in the photograph the relation of the left anterior
fibrous trigone (L.A.F.T.) to the posterior pulmonary
sinus. Peer into the aorta, and note the single orifice for
the right coronary and the anomalous circumflex coronary arteries. A better view is seen in photograph **5**.
In coronary arteriography, it would be possible to
catheterize the right coronary artery only, and miss the
presence of the anomalous artery, implying either an unrecognized separate orifice of the posterior division or
occlusion at the origin of this division.

6: A.P. view: The anterior wall of the right ventricle has
been removed. Note the transilluminated ventricular
portion of the membranous septum (V.M.S.). Above
and to the left, the transilluminated posterior pulmonary
leaflet is seen. Below the latter, the anomalous septal
artery is seen commencing its course. The further course
and significance of this artery will be seen on page 183.

Note: The reader is urged to examine the beautiful and
anatomically informative arteriogram of the anomalous
circumflex artery on pages 114 and 115 of the monograph of Baltaxe, Amplatz and Levin.

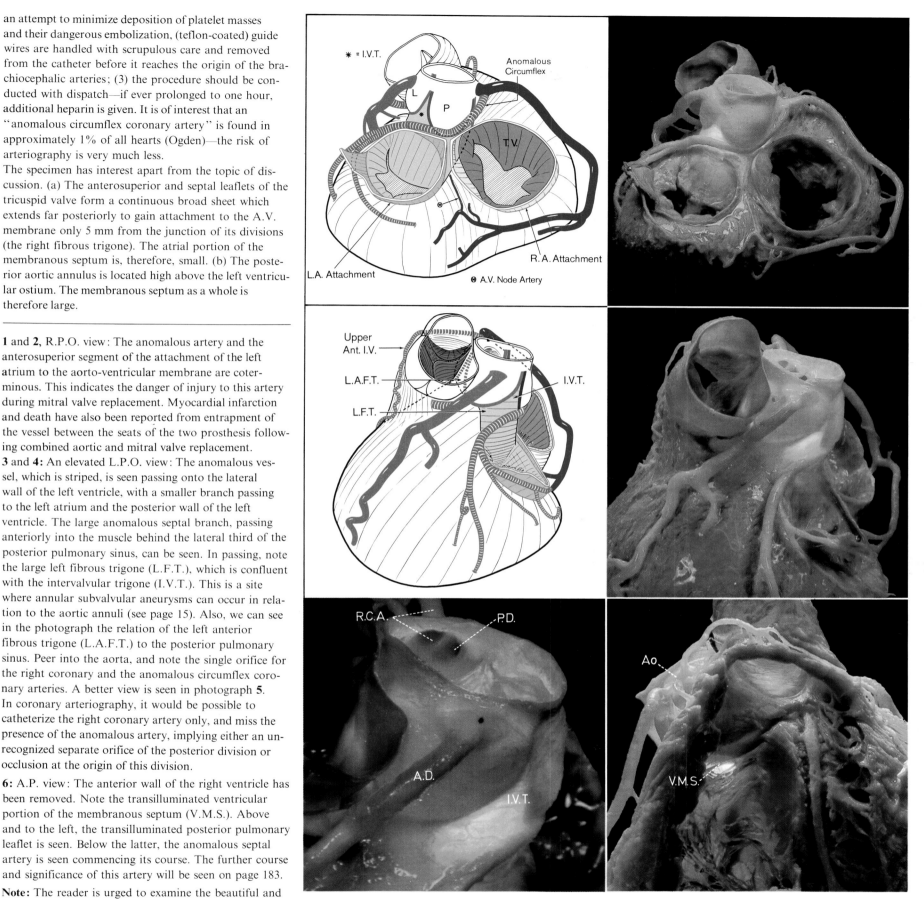

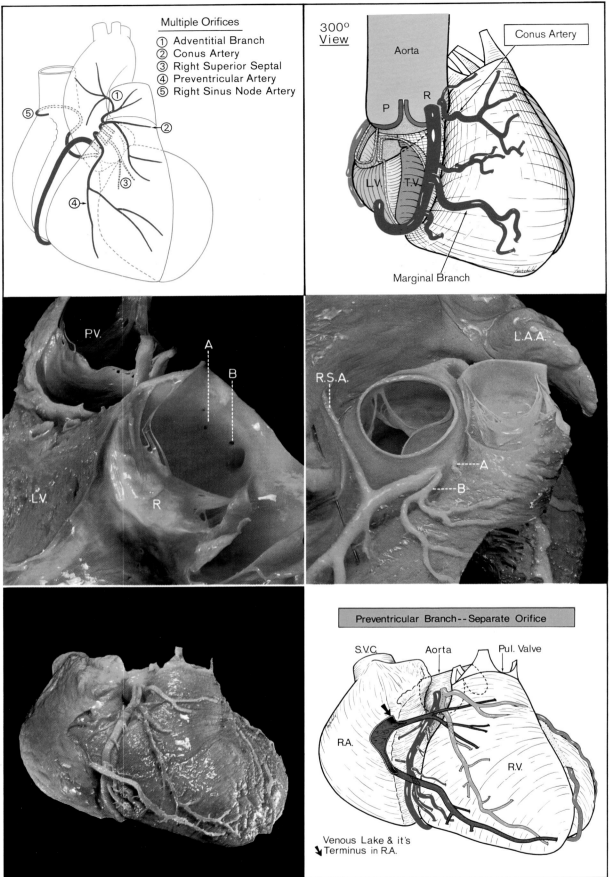

Multiple Orifices
① Adventitial Branch
② Conus Artery
③ Right Superior Septal
④ Preventricular Artery
⑤ Right Sinus Node Artery

300° View

Conus Artery

Aorta

Marginal Branch

P.V.

A

B

L.V.

R

L.A.A.

R.S.A.

A

B

Preventricular Branch-- Separate Orifice

S.V.C. Aorta Pul. Valve

R.A.

R.V.

Venous Lake & it's
↓ Terminus in R.A.

B. The Orifices: Variations in Number

I. Multiple Orifices in the Right Aortic Sinus

Findings in 100 hearts

Number of orifices	Number of hearts
1	47
2	48
3	4
4	1

This study was done in 1967, on previously prosected specimens. The left coronary orifice was solitary in all 100 hearts. In 53%, multiple orifices for the right coronary artery were present. In the 48 examples of a double orifice, the secondary branches involved were—the conus artery (43), preventricular (2), adventitial (2), and right sinus node (1). In the total material, the conus artery was present in 48% of the specimens.

1: Listed are arteries which may arise from a secondary orifice in the right aortic sinus.

Specimen A: 2: A conus artery is seen. It is, by convention, defined as a branch to the infundibulum (or conus) arising from a separate orifice. It is to be differentiated from a **conus branch** of the right coronary artery.

Specimen B: 3 and 4: This specimen is seen following perfusion fixation. It is not included in the above table.
3: P.A. view: The right aortic sinus shows the presence of three small orifices to the left of the main orifice.
4: Superior R.A.O. view: The secondary orifice (B) supplies a large conus artery. The other two secondary branches (one of which [A] is seen in the center of the photograph) supply the posterolateral wall of the right ventricle.

Specimen C: 5 and 6: A photograph and drawing of a specimen showing the presence of a large preventricular branch (orange), which supplies much of the anterior wall of the right ventricle: It arises as a separate orifice and gives off a large conus branch. In the earlier series of 100 hearts, four demonstrated large preventricular branches. Three other examples, in hemodynamically fixed material, are shown in this text. The artery supplies much of the free wall of the right ventricle and could be injured by a ventriculotomy. It is important not to assume that a second coronary orifice in the right aortic sinus is necessarily that of a conus artery. A secondary orifice may pose a problem in cannulation coincident to aortic valve operation. It may be large enough to be of physiologic significance, but not large enough to cannulate with ease and without trauma. Apart from this topic, note the two anterior cardiac veins. They vary in number; most often four are present. They may cross the A.V. sulcus either superficially or deep to the artery. Most often, they drain directly into the right atrium as seen here. A "small cardiac vein" may contribute to or constitute their mode of drainage.

II. Multiple Proximal Branches of the Right Coronary Artery

Specimen D: 1 and **2**: All of the left and the anterior portion of the right aortic sinus (pink) have been removed. In this specimen, a conal branch and two branches to the posterolateral wall of the right ventricle arise from the proximal few millimeters of the right coronary artery. A fourth branch (R.S.S.) is directed inferiorly to the attachment of the right aortic annulus to the left ventricular ostium. This branch indicates the course of a right superior septal artery. (See the classification and description of the septal arteries on page 172.) Note the relative proximity of the right coronary artery to the right bundle branch of the conduction system, which is located under the membranous septum (yellow). Selective catheterization of the right coronary artery will usually fail to identify a separate orifice in the right coronary sinus*. Conversely, a catheter may pass into one of the several branches that emerge from the right coronary artery just beyond its orifice; a hyperselective injection may result and obstruction of the main right coronary might be suspected. Occlusive disease of the right coronary artery frequently occurs at, or commences at, the junction of the **proximal** and the **continuing** segments. The conal branch may arise from either segment—i.e., above or below the occlusion—the site of origin of a branch will be determinative of its role in collateral circulation. Great emphasis has been placed on the protective role of the conus artery which has been termed the Third Coronary Artery. This is an appealing concept, and although conal arteries are seen in approximately 50% of human hearts, they are usually small in size; hence, in my opinion their importance in effecting collateral circulation has been exaggerated. It has been stressed that injection in the right aortic sinus will not only identify a conus artery, but obviate the development of spasm of the main artery which is relatively common. It is essential that good definition of the right coronary be accomplished and the selective technique, in most hands, is preferable.

III. The Short Left Main Branch

Specimen E: 3–6: The specimen will be examined first (in **3**) from a superior left lateral view, then (in **4**) from a "posterior" view (210°). The left atrium has been removed—black cloth is in the right atrium. The left main branch measures 2 mm from the margins of the orifice to its bifurcation. After transection, a right-angle examination of the left and right aortic sinuses will be seen in **5** and **6**, respectively.

5: In the transected specimen, the left aortic sinus is seen from the R.A.O. view: It is apparent that hyperselective catheterization of either the anterior (A.D.) or posterior division (P.D.) could result.

6: The right aortic sinus is shown: The main right orifice is only 5 mm from the right and posterior annular commisure. To its left, two small separate orifices can be seen (with difficulty).

* In the laboratory, injection into the right trunk results in filling of the conus artery and efflux from its orifice (Fulton).

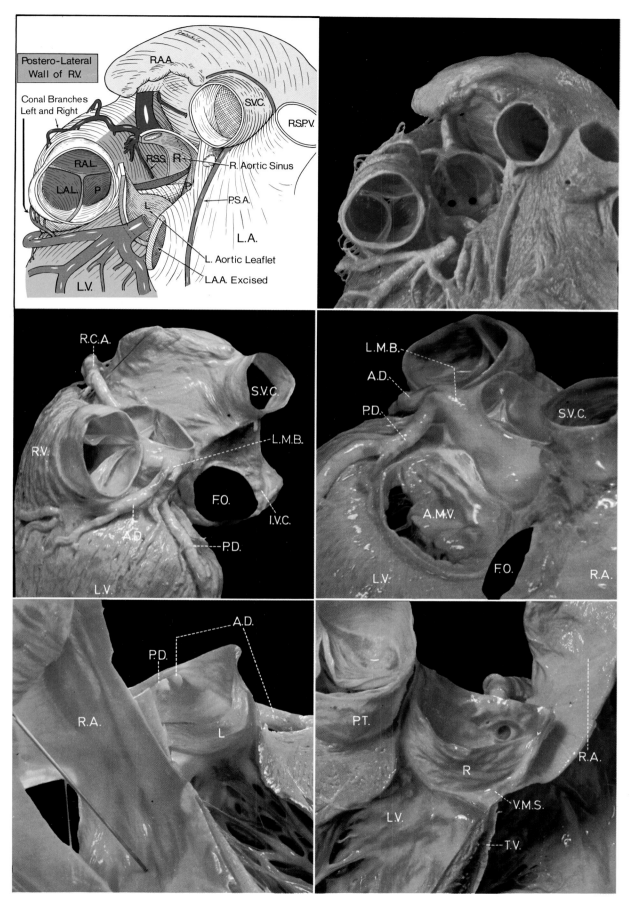

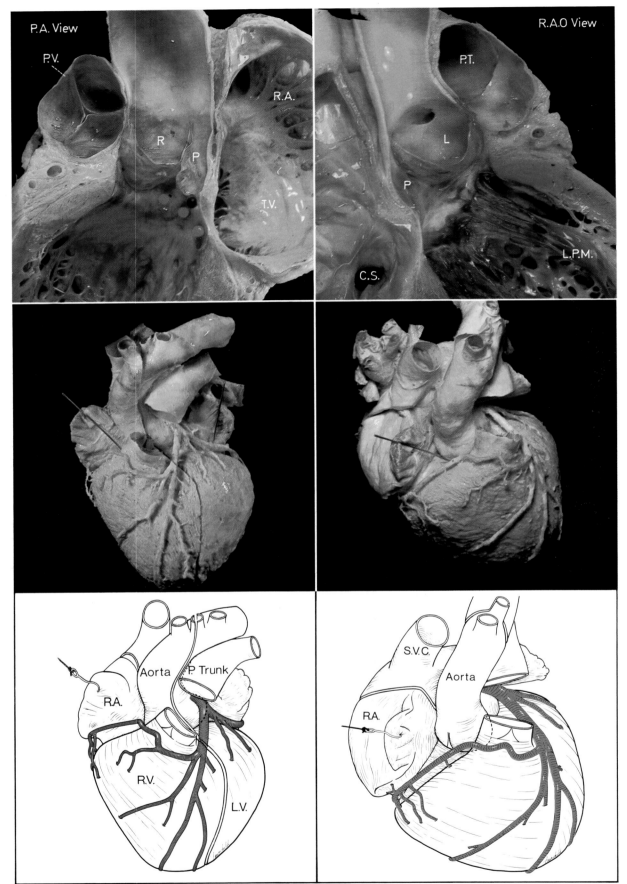

P.A. View

P.V.

R.A.

R

P

T.V.

R.A.O View

P.T.

L

P

C.S.

L.P.M.

Aorta   P. Trunk

R.A.

R.V.

L.V.

S.V.C.

Aorta

R.A.

IV. The Single Coronary Artery

A single coronary artery has a single orifice and is to be differentiated from translocation of both divisions of the left coronary to the right aortic sinus. The condition was first described by Thebesius in 1716, and it appears to be relatively uncommon, particularly in otherwise normal hearts. (It is seen in association with congenital malformations, e.g., the tetralogy of Fallot, ventricular septal defects, and bicuspid aortic valves.) In 1971 Hillestad and Eie collected 85 and reported 3 new cases. In 1966, Gasul, Arcilla and Lev opined that the condition was much commoner than the number of reported cases would indicate.

When the condition is identified, three major clinical implications exist. (a) A patient with this variation is in greater jeopardy following the development of coronary occlusive disease because of the reduction in the possible avenues for the development of collateral circulation. (b) The anomalous course of its branches has resulted in a significant number of deaths in connection with cardiac incisions, especially in the complete repair of tetralogy of Fallot. The dangers inherent in the retro-aortic course of coronary artery branches have already been described on page 138. (c) The frequent coexistence of a bicuspid aortic valve, which is less evident than other associated malformations, may eventuate in calcific aortic stenosis in the fifth or sixth decade of life.

The source of the specimen seen in **142—1–6** and **143—1** was an adult accident victim with no history of cardiac disease. On external examination the heart appeared normal; it was fixed and bisected for study. Only then was the variation noted. The incisions passed between the left and right and through the midpoint of the posterior aortic leaflet. In **1** we see the P.A. view of the right anterior segment and in **2** the R.A.O. view of the left posterior segment. The red beads in **1** identify the upper border of the ostium of the left ventricle. The right aortic sinus is devoid of an orifice, the single artery arising from the left sinus. The course of this single coronary artery is shown in photographs **3** and **4** where the segments are apposed. Their related drawings are below. The inferior view is on the opposite page (**143—1**). The variation from the normal course of arterial branches consists of (a) the presence of a large vessel running obliquely across the anterior wall of the right ventricle inferiorly, simulating the course of a preventricular branch of a normal left coronary, and (b) a larger branch crossing the infundibulum and reaching the anterior right A.V. sulcus, whence its course simulates that of a normal right coronary artery. If this single coronary artery was associated with the tetralogy of Fallot, it is apparent that the branch crossing the infundibulum would be divided if the necessity arose to insert an outflow patch during the operative correction of this malformation*. This tragedy may be avoided by (a) preoperative coronary artery mapping and (b) the appropriate use of a valve containing conduit to bypass the obstruction.

In the next topic of examination, we will study the effect of the axis of the left main branch on the orifice characteristics; in this specimen, the axis is directed inferiorly and anteriorly in relation to the aortic wall—as a result (in **2**), a sharp incisura is seen at the anterior and inferior margin of the orifice. The incisura is formed by the acute junction of the aortic and coronary artery walls.

1: The inferior view of the specimen just examined shows the single coronary artery continuing to the acute margin, after giving off a large posterior descending branch.

2: The single left coronary artery: 2-A: This example would be classified by Smith as Type 1, presenting a pattern of a "hyperdominant" left coronary artery. **2-B: This is a diagram of the specimen we have just examined,** with the branch presenting an anomalous course over the infundibulum of the right ventricle. **2-C:** Here the anomalous branch courses over the sinus of the ventricle. These represent various anatomic configurations presented by a single left coronary artery which are described in the literature.

3 and **4: The single right coronary artery** presents a much wider variety in the course of the anomalous branches. These drawings are derived from reported cases.
The anomalous courses demonstrated are as follows: D, preventricular; E, transseptal; F, retropulmonary. The anomalous vessels replace the entire left coronary artery in the first two instances and the anterior division in the third instance.

4: In G, the retro-aortic course is followed by the vessel supplying the two divisions to the left ventricle. In H, the anterior division courses over the anterior wall of the right ventricle, and the posterior division passes in a retro-aortic location. In I, the anterior division passes in a preventricular course, and the posterior division of the left coronary artery is replaced by a "hyperdominant" right coronary artery which courses behind the tricuspid and the left ventricular ostia.

5: An L.A.O. view of a drawing made of an arteriographic study in a patient with a pattern which approximates that of a single right coronary artery. Only a small twig arises from the left coronary sinus. The coronary sinus and the interventricular veins are shown to demonstrate their utility in the identification of the branches of a single coronary artery. The main anomalous course here is the preconal. The cineangiogram was kindly made available by Dr. C. Schmidt of Milwaukee.

6: The coronary sinus locates the posterior portion of the ostium of the left ventricle in all views except R.A.O. In the latter, it is seen 10 mm posterosuperior to the ostium. The interventricular veins are more variable, less easily seen at arteriography and identify, with comparatively less precision, the respective interventricular grooves.

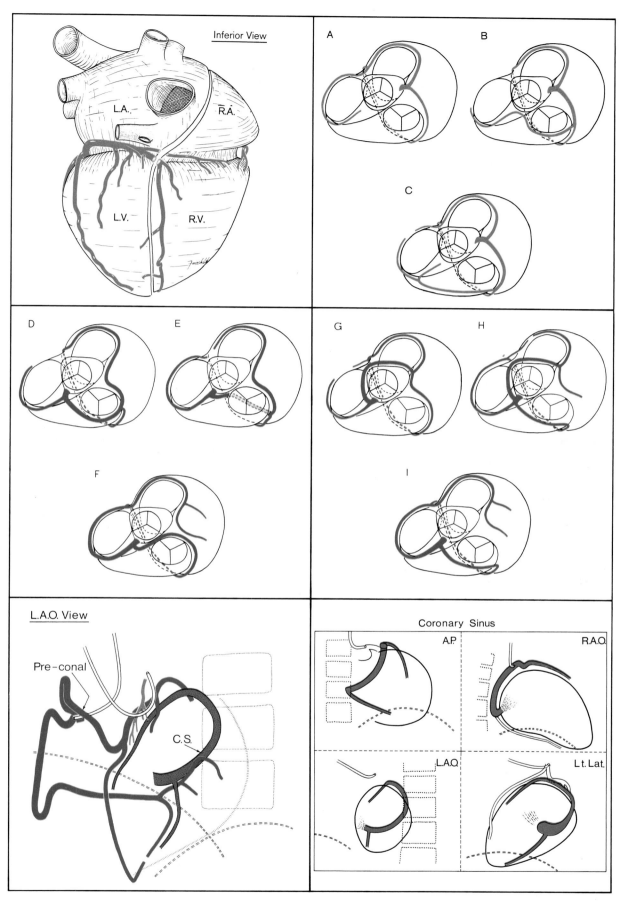

---

* See the articles by Friedman, Gádboys, Kirklin, Longnecker and their respective colleagues.

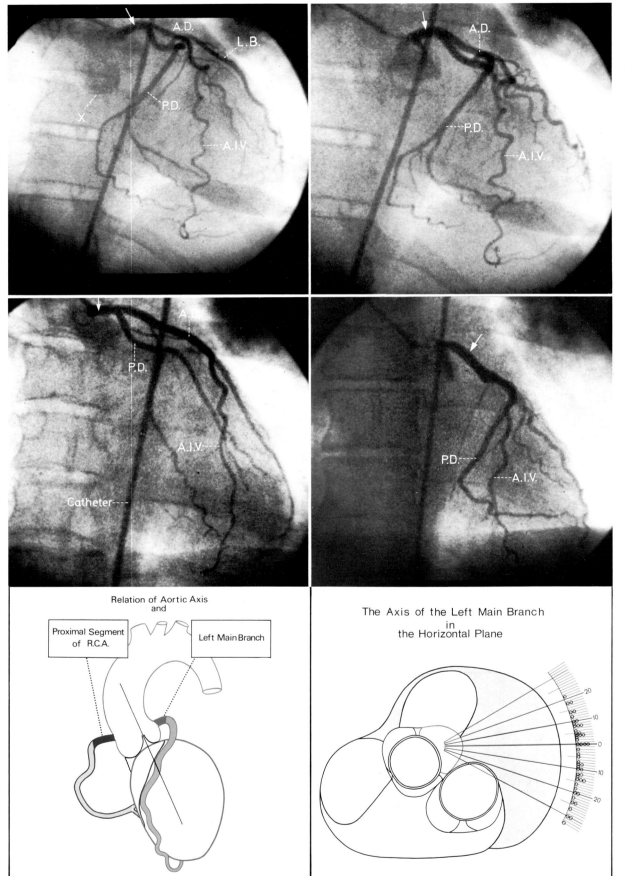

C. The Left Main Branch and the Proximal Segment of the Right Coronary Artery

I. The Axes of the Left Main Branch and the Proximal Segment of the Right Coronary Artery

Note: In this and the following five pages, the left main branch is marked by a short arrow.

The Left Main Branch in the Frontal Plane

1 and **2:** An A.P. view of a selective left arteriogram in end-diastole and end-systole: Observe: (a) In this instance, the left main branch is not straight; it presents a superiorly directly convexity. (b) **Its axis is directed superiorly 30° above the horizontal in diastole** and 20° in systole. In passing, also observe: (c) The motion of arterial branches provides some indication of the function of the portions of the ventricular wall to which they are related. (d) The motion of the posterior division (P.D.) is more evident than the motion of the anterior division (A.D.) — the anterior interventricular artery (A.I.V.) is accordionized, but its spatial location is relatively unchanged. (e) A lateral branch of the posterior division (L.B.) runs along the left lateral border of the ventricle in this view. (f) The nadir of the posterior aortic sinus (X) is to the left of the median plane — recall its relationship to the coronary sinus (page 91).

3: In a second patient, an A.P. view in end-diastole is seen. **The left main branch is disposed horizontally** in the frontal plane.

4: In this third patient, in end-systole, the axis of **the left main branch is depressed 35° below the horizontal**. It is almost parallel with the lateral wall of the left aortic sinus. The proximal portions of the divisions are superimposed on each other.
Before leaving the arteriograms of these three patients, note the variations in the relation of the anterior interventricular branch to the left cardiac border.

The Relation of the Axes of the Left Main Branch and the Proximal Segment of the Right Coronary Artery to the Axis of the Aortic Blood Flow.

5: Variations are seen in the axis of the ascending aorta. Hence, the axes of the left main branch and the proximal segment of the right, when observed in a single plane, do not necessarily reflect their relation to the axis of the aorta. This relationship is important in determining the configuration of the orifice of the left coronary artery.

The Axis of the Left Main Branch in the Horizontal Plane

6: This is measured, not from the center of the left aortic sinus, but from the site of its orifice. The anteriorly directed axis predominates. The axes in these 50 specimens varied from 21° posterior, to 33° anterior to lines passing transversely through the respective orifices. These axes should not be confused with the variations in the location (in the horizontal plane) of the orifice of the coronary artery in its sinus of origin (seen on page 134). The location of the orifice may affect but does not determine the axis of the left main branch.

144

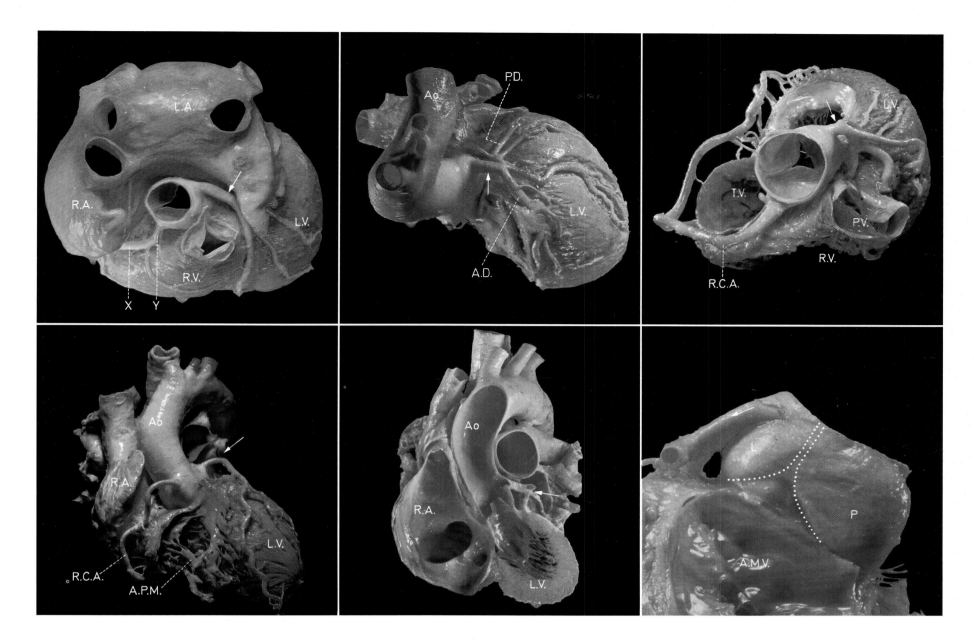

The Axis of the Left Main Branch in the Horizontal Plane

The superior view of three specimens will be seen in **1–3**. The characteristic of the right coronary artery origin will also be noted.

Specimen A: 1: The anterior axis: Observe: (a) The axis of the left main branch is 30° anterior to a transverse line. (b) The proximal segment of the right coronary artery extends anteriorly and to the right, forming at its origin a right angle with the right aortic sinus wall. (c) An obtuse angle is formed by the junction of the **proximal** (Y) and **continuing** (X) segments of the right coronary artery.

Specimen B: 2: The transverse axis: The right heart has been removed. The 18 mm-long left main branch lies in a transverse disposition. Several important additional features are displayed by this specimen and it will be examined in detail on page 180. At this time, note that the anterior (A.D.) and posterior divisions (P.D.) form an angle of 180°.

Specimen C: 3: The posterior axis: This is seen in the presence of a diminutive posterior division of the left coronary artery, demonstrating a lack of relationship between the relative development of the divisions of the left coronary artery and the axis of its main trunk. The right coronary artery projects from the right sinus at right angles to its surface in both the horizontal and vertical planes.

Obliterative disease of the left main branch is, unfortunately, not uncommon; in the performance of coronary arteriography, an assessment of its axis should be made and an additional examination may be made at a right angle to the axis.

The Axis of the Left Main Branch in the Frontal Plane

Specimen D: 4: The superior axis: A.P. view: The anterior wall of the right ventricle has been removed. The left main branch extends from the surface of the left aortic sinus at a right angle. The right coronary artery demonstrates its characteristic proximal segment.

Specimen E: 5: A near horizontal axis: A.P. view: The posterior segment is seen following a frontal transection which passes through the nadirs of the left and posterior aortic annuli. The left main branch is depressed only 10° below the horizontal plane; however, the axes of the left main branch and the aortic bulb form an angle of 55° — a sharp incisura at the inferior aspect of the orifice results.

Specimen F: 6: The inferior axis: P.A. view: Observe: (a) The left main branch (18 mm in length) is directed 25° below the horizontal, lying in contact with and virtually paralleling the lateral wall of the left aortic sinus. This results in a knife-like incisura in the inferior portion of the orifice. This is a P.A. view! The left aortic sinus is smaller than the posterior which, in turn, is smaller than the right.

Note: A description of the left main branch should include the axis in both the horizontal plane (anterior, transverse, or posterior) and the frontal plane (superior, horizontal, or inferior).

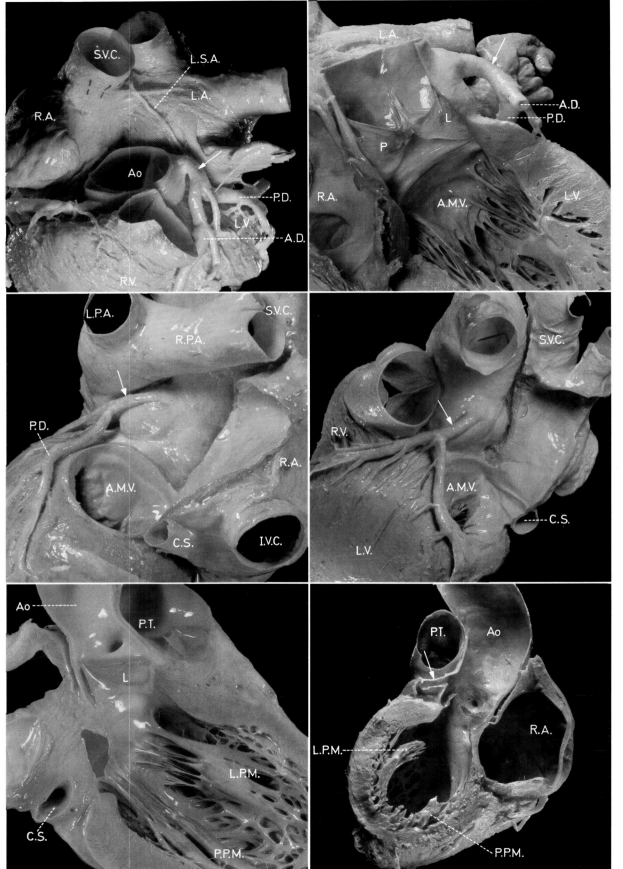

II. The Configuration of the Left Main Branch

Specimen A: 1: A superior left anterior view: The left main branch may demonstrate a straight linear disposition. In this specimen, the vessel emerges from the left aortic sinus at a right angle, then bends at a right angle before descending to its bifurcation.

Specimen B: 2: An A.P. view of the left and posterior aortic leaflets and sinuses: The left main branch is convex superiorly and to the left. Its proximal portion emerges from the sinus at a 45° angle; its distal portion is directed more inferiorly. These two specimens indicate the need for care in measuring the angle of the attachment of the left main branch to the aorta. In an arteriographic study, the proximal portion may not be opacified and only the inferiorly directed segment may be seen, providing misinformation about the axis of the left main branch and the characteristics of its orifice which are determined by the degree of angularity of the adjacent arterial and aortic walls. This can be avoided if care is observed in positioning the catheter just beyond the orifice and utilizing adequate pressure in the injection of the contrast material.

Specimen C: 3 and 4: This specimen is first seen in a P.A., then in a nonattitudinal L.P.O. view. Observe: The left main branch is directed inferiorly in the frontal plane and anteriorly in the horizontal plane. A knife-like incisura is present in both the anterior and inferior parts of the orifice. The presence of an incisura at the orifice produces increased turbulence in the left main branch. Note that the anterior division as in many specimens, continues the course of the left main branch—the posterior division is perpendicular to both. The angle of bifurcation of the left main branch is studied on page 148; in this specimen the posterior division forms a virtual right angle with each of the other two arteries.

The Characteristics of the Orifice

Specimen D: 5: The R.A.O. view: The sharp inferior incisura results from the inferior orientation of the left main branch. The transection lies in the L.A.O.-R.P.O. plane, separating the left and right aortic sinuses and the halves of the posterior aortic sinus.

Specimen E: 6: P.A. view following a frontal transection which has passed through the left main branch: Note the sharp incisura at the lower margin of the orifice. The angle in the aortic wall, seen above the orifice, is produced by the left sinus rim.

Note: The left main branch is also called the main left coronary artery or the left main trunk.

III. The Mode of Attachment of the Proximal Segment of the Right Coronary Artery to the Aorta

Specimen F: 1: A nonattitudinal right lateral view of the aorta, mitral valve, and left ventricle: The septal leaflet of the tricuspid valve has been divided and displaced anteriorly. The drawing of this photograph is seen in **48—1**. The emergence at a right angle to the aortic sinus wall is much more commonly exhibited by the right than by the left coronary artery. A smooth, round orifice results. Apart from our topic, observe: (a) The posterior and anterior leaflets of the mitral valve are approximately equal in width. (b) Without interior lighting, the subvalvular segment of the A.V. membrane (X) can be recognized. (c) The large, long A.V. node artery ascends from the right coronary artery to the right fibrous trigone.

2: A nonattitudinal left lateral view: The line of transection passes through the orifice. The posterior and right aortic leaflets have been removed. The characteristics (of the orifice) just described can be seen.

Specimen G: 3 and **4**: In **3**, a nonattitudinal right lateral view, the great vessels except for their sinuses and much of the right atrium have been removed. Observe: (a) The characteristic proximal segment of the right coronary artery extends from the right aortic sinus, meeting the continuing segment at the junction of the anterior and posterolateral wall of the right ventricle.

4: The atria and the large part of the three free walls of the right ventricle have been removed. Below the right coronary orifice, the posterolateral wall of the right ventricle is closely related to the right half of the right aortic sinus. The left half of the right sinus is in contact with the wall. The aortic sinus-ventricular wall relationship ordinarily precludes the possibility of a right coronary artery paralleling the sinus wall as is seen, not infrequently, in the left main branch.

Specimen H: 5 and **6**: First, the atria and great vessels above their sinuses were removed. A transection then passed through the axis of the left ventricle and the middle of both the left and posterior aortic sinuses. The posterior aortic sinus wall has been excised. **5** is a nonattitudinal right superior examination. **6** is a nonattitudinal R.P.O. view. Observe: (a) The right coronary artery arises from the right aortic sinus (**5**) close to the commissure between the right and posterior leaflets. (b) In both planes, the **proximal segment of the right coronary artery (X)** meets the portion of the sinus from which it arises at a near right angle. It extends anteriorly 1.5 cm, where an obtuse angle marks its junction with **the continuing segment (Y)**. (c) The posterolateral wall of the right ventricle extends almost to the right fibrous trigone, located below the midpoint of the posterior aortic sinus. (d) **The proximal segment is also a part of the right superior segment of the right coronary artery.** It is set apart from the remainder (the continuing portion) of the artery to attract attention to its direction.

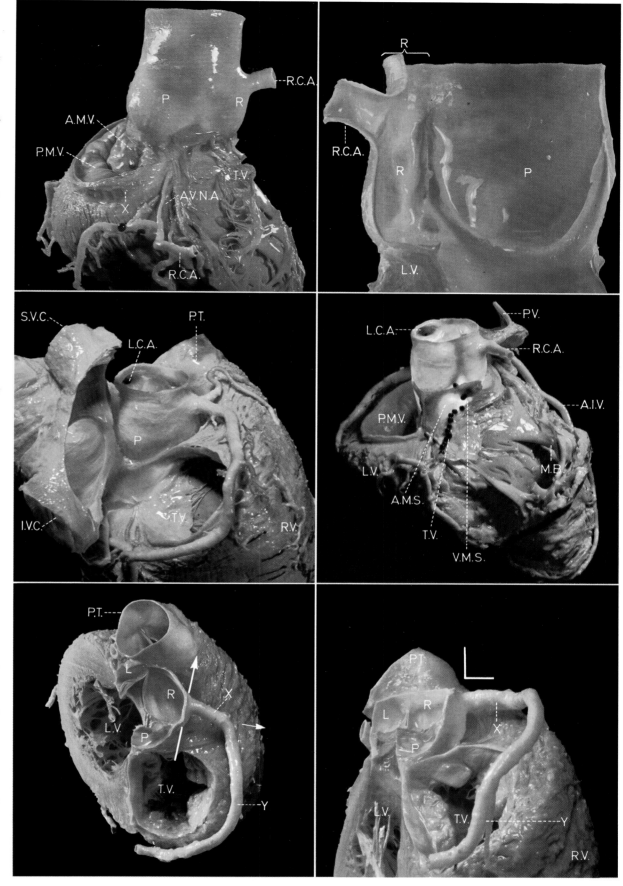

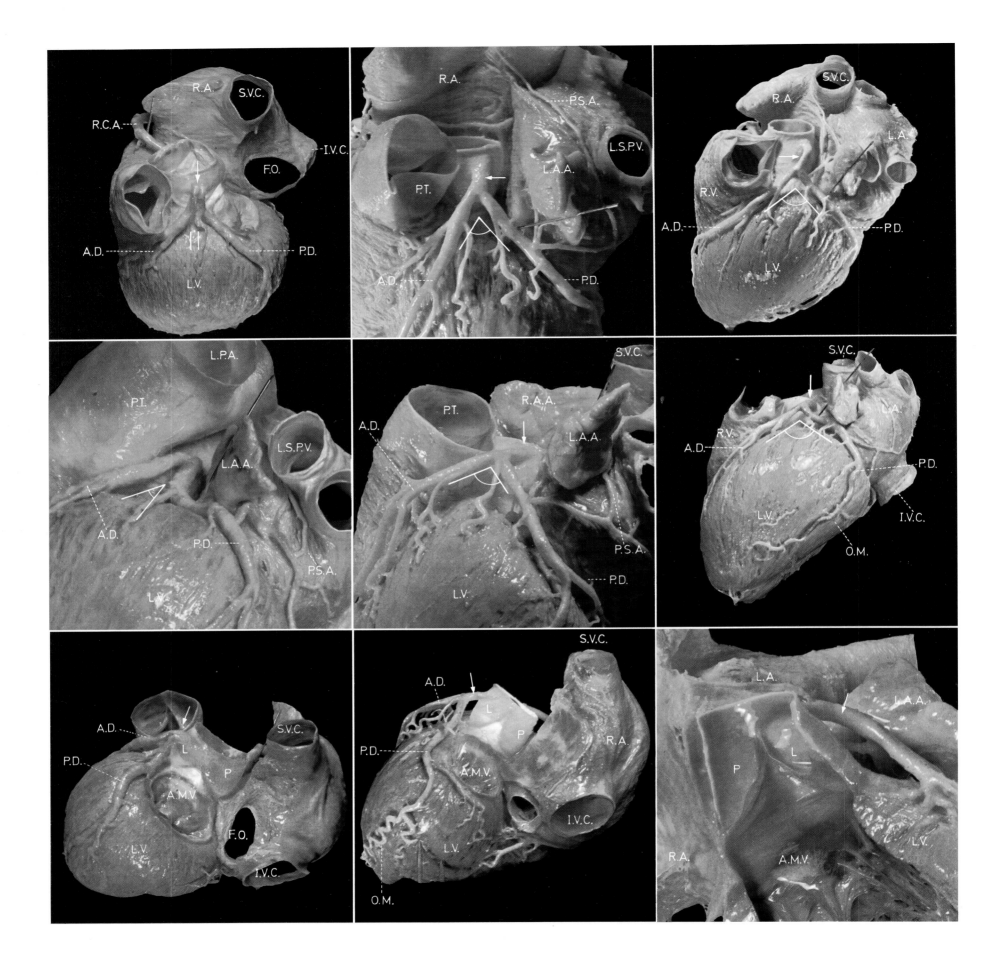

IV. The Mode of Bifurcation and the Axes of the Divisions of the Left Coronary Artery

On page 148, three specimens, A, B, and C, are arranged in three vertical rows. In the three horizontal rows, the views are: upper — left lateral with 45° elevation; middle — left lateral; lower — **7** and **8**, P.A., and **9**, A.P. The great vessels have been removed above the sinuses. In specimen A, the left atrium has been removed in **1** and **7**; black cloth marks the site of the membranous atrial septum (F.O.). Except for its septal wall, the left atrium has been removed in **8**. The entire left aortic sinus and the adjoining half of the posterior are seen in **9**. Observe: (a) As we move across the top row, the lengths of the left main branch (indicated by the arrows) are 2.0, 11.0, and 14.0 mm, and the angles of its bifurcation are 0°, 70°, and 90°. The proximal part of the divisions are optimally seen in these right-angle views. (b) As we move across the middle row, the angles of bifurcation are now 30°, 100°, and 110°. The view is now oblique to the products of bifurcation. (c) In the bottom row the angles formed by the anterior and posterior divisions are quite unlike those seen in the lateral view; they are almost equal in A and B; the divisions are superimposed in C: This difference results from the variation in the contour and axis of the left ventricle and the course of the arteries. In A, the two divisions course tightly applied to the surface of the left ventricle— the epicardial course. In B and C, the artery is separated and superficial to the myocardial surface (see page 179) —this is an aerial course, which is marked in B and moderate in C.

149—1: P.A. view: This specimen is featured on pages 192–196. Observe: (a) The pulmonary ostium is, as it usually is, above the left lateral part of the mitral portion of the ostium of the left ventricle. (b) The posterior division runs on the surface of the left ventricle (the arrow marks the meeting of the two)—this epicardial course is common. (c) Even in this relatively globular heart, **the retropulmonary segment of the anterior division is well above the posterior division**. (d) Note the prominent summit of L.V.

2: Specimen A of page 148 is seen from a P.A. (180°) view, demonstrating the direct vertical descent of the posterior division to reach and course over the surface of the ventricle. Again in this horizontal heart, the posterior division is below the retropulmonary segment of the anterior division. However, despite the angle of bifurcation the divisions are superimposed at their origin.

3: The same specimen is rotated 30° and examined from 210°: The degree of superimposition of the proximal portions of the division has increased; at R.P.O. (225°) it would be complete.

4: The L.A.O. view of specimen C of page 148: The two divisions were superimposed in the A.P. plane (in **148— 9**); however, rotation of 45° results in a decrease in the superimposition in this vertical heart with an aerial pos-

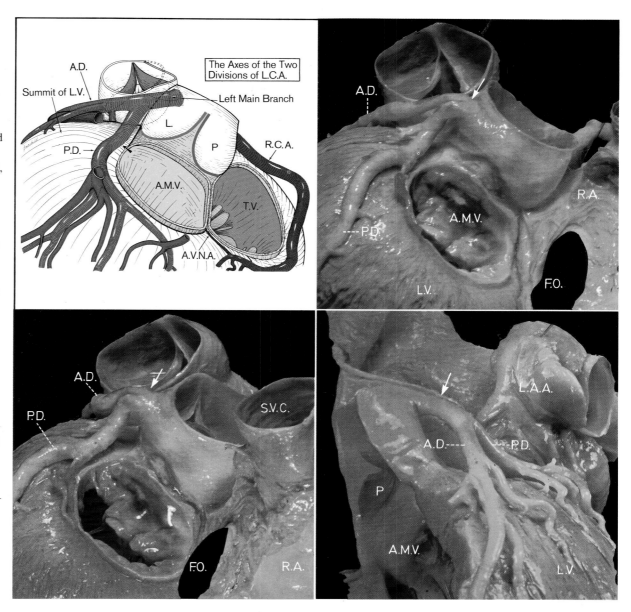

terior division — this is reverse to the findings in specimen A, a horizontal heart whose posterior division pursues an epicardial course. The divisions are still seen obliquely and superimposed at the site of bifurcation.

Conclusions

I. The axes of the retropulmonary segment of the anterior division and the lateral segment of the posterior division, and the relation of the vessels to each other are determined by the following: (1) the relative location of the related pulmonary ostium and the left lateral part of the mitral portion of the ostium of the left ventricle; (2) the shape and disposition of the left ventricle; (3) the course of the arteries in relation to the myocardium— epicardial or aerial; (4) the length, axis, and angle of bifurcation of the left main branch. In each of the horizontal radiographic views, these features must be recognized. Only in this manner will the degree of foreshortening of each branch be recognized — this foreshortening is a resultant of the spatial directions of the branch.

II. A cardinal principle in radiology invokes the necessity of the right-angle examination of structures. **Most often, the proximal portions of the two divisions may be examined optimally not in any of the traditional horizontal plane views, but only when the x-ray tube is placed 45° above its usual left lateral view position** (even the angle formed by the proximal portion of the anterior and posterior divisions of the left coronary artery cannot be accurately measured in the traditional left lateral view [as we have seen on page 148]). Superimposition of the most proximal parts of the products of bifurcation occurs in the three other views.

Comment: The good that results from coronary arteriography—truly an epochal development—perhaps stills the question: Is the information derived from conventional horizontal plane studies definitive? Does a negative study exclude symptom-producing or life-threatening disease? Anatomic studies suggest that the affirmative answer to both questions awaits the application of long-standing radiographic principles.

D. Closing Comments

I. The Size of the Orifices of the Coronary Arteries

The clinician is interested in this measurement, wanting, as he may, to cannulate the vessels for coronary artery perfusion at aortic valve replacement, or to catheterize them for selective coronary arteriography, or to study the effect of coronary artery diameter in the etiology of coronary atherosclerosis.

This following table is not taken from specimens prepared by the perfusion fixation technique described in Chapter 1, which would be highly preferable, but from 100 specimens which were secured after postmortem incision and examination. The data, therefore, probably understate the dimensions seen in the living heart.

Dimension of orifices—100 specimens

	Mean	S.D.	Range
Right coronary artery			
Width	3.7	1.1	0.5–7.0
Height	2.4	0.9	0.5–5.0
Left coronary artery			
Width	4.7	1.2	1.8–8.5
Height	3.2	1.1	1.0–8.5

The data, however, does indicate that the orifices are not round, but elliptical, and the orifice of the left coronary artery is usually larger.

II. The Length of the Left Main Branch

Variations in the number of orifices for the right coronary artery are common; multiple orifices for the left are rare. A short main stem has most of the potential clinical hazards of a double orifice. In a specific study, 100 fresh postmortem specimens were studied and no example was found of multiple orifices in the left aortic sinus. In a much larger number of perfusion-fixed specimens, no example of this variation has been seen. James found one example in a series of 105 hearts. However, a short left main branch is common and is of great clinical significance, posing a problem in coronary arteriography and in coronary artery perfusion during valve replacement. In both instances, a catheter may easily be placed in one or other of the divisions, with resulting lack of opacification or perfusion of the non-cannulated division. In my material, in 100 perfusion-fixed specimens, the left main branch was measured. The results were:

Length of the main coronary artery in 100 specimens

Length (mm)	Number
2– 5	12
6–10	32
11–15	42
16–20	14

Of the last group listed, only 3 were over 17 mm. In a study of 50 hearts, Green, Bernstein and Reppert found the bifurcation of the main trunk 5 mm or less beyond the orifice in 24% of instances. In the specimen shown on page 148, the bifurcation is 2 mm from the coronary orifice.

In a study of 200 hearts, Helwing found the following lengths in mm: 5 or less — 20%; between 6 and 9 — 35%; between 10 and 15 — 33.5%; between 16 and 20 — 11.5%. Spencer and Mallette (1968) stress the importance of recognition of early bifurcation at operation. "Bifurcation within a few millimeters of its ostium was recognized in 6 of the 82 patients".*

III. The Design of the Orifice

From a hemodynamic viewpoint, the design of the attachment of the right coronary artery to the aorta would, in the majority of instances, seem preferable to that of the left. Anatomic considerations may be relevant in the pathogenesis of disease of the right and left coronary arteries. Certainly, in the performance of a bypass from the aorta to a coronary artery, the surgeon attempts to simulate the anatomy usually observed in the right coronary orifice, fashioning the vein graft so that its "proximal segment" is disposed at a right angle to the aorta. Occlusive disease is frequently seen at the junction of the proximal and continuing segment of the right coronary artery, and studies of the configuration and angulation at this site might prove valuable.

In an information-filled article on "Myocardial Infarction Without Atheroclerosis", Cheitlin, McAllister and Castro state "When angina pectoris or myocardial infarction is seen in a young person, congenital abnormalities involving the coronary arteries should immediately be considered. The younger the patient, the more likely the presence of congenital coronary artery anomalies. The most common of these is anomalous origin of the left coronary artery from the pulmonary artery ... resulting in myocardial ischemia and usually myocardial infarction in the first year of life. Occasionally a patient will live to adulthood before either myocardial infarction or death suddenly occurs. ... Similarly, myocardial ischemia and infarction can occur with coronary arterio-cameral fistulae, with low-resistance run-off usually into the right atrium or right ventricle and coronary steal syndrome. Less well recognized is the case of the occasional young man who dies suddenly, usually after exercise, and who at postmortem examination exhibits as the only abnormality the left coronary artery arising from the anterior sinus of Valsalva. In reviewing these cases, some of the patients had previously experienced exertional syncope, chest pain, or myocardial infarction. Recently, we have reviewed the AFIP experience of 51 patients with single or double coronary arteries arising from the same sinus of Valsalva. Sudden, unexpected death occurred in nine of 33 patients (27.3%) with both vessels arising from the anterior sinus of Valsalva and in none of the 18 patients with both vessels from the left sinus of Valsalva. The patients were all males ranging in age from 13 to 36 years. Eight of nine were 22 years of age or younger, and all but one died suddenly and unexpectedly during or immediately following exercise. There was no other explanation for death in these patients. The cause of death is purely speculative. It is possible that the acute posterior leftward passage of the left coronary artery along the wall of the aorta results in a slit-like opening of the left coronary artery. After exercise and increased expansion of the aorta and traction on the left coronary artery with increased ventricular activity, a flap-like closure of the left coronary ostium could occur."

I would add to the interesting speculation referred to by authors: "Flap-like closure of the left coronary ostium" may occur when the artery arises from the left aortic sinus. In many specimens (**145—6, 146—3** and **4, 156—6, 170—2, 209—4**), an acute angle exists between the aorta and the left main branch. When does the acuteness of this angle become critical? In **91—5** and **6,** a sharp incisura exists although the axis of the left main branch is only 15° below the horizontal. The right coronary artery characteristically demonstrates a perpendicular take-off; however, this occurs in the left coronary artery as exemplified in specimens apart from those in chapter 10 (**184—3, 189—1** and **198—3**). Clinicopathologic correlation, regarding the relevance of orifice characteristics, is dependent on what is termed herein as perfusion fixation of hearts. Lev and his associates have drawn attention to "controlled pressure fixation" of hearts (Glagov et al., 1963; Eckner et al., 1969) and its importance.

---

* Spencer, F.C., Mallette, W.: Technical considerations of coronary perfusion during aortic valve replacement. *J. cardiovasc. Surg.* 9, 562, 1968.

Chapter 11: The Arteries to the Atria and to the A.V. Node

Introduction

In 1924, Spalteholz divided the atrial arteries into three groups—the anterior, intermediate (marginal), and posterior. In almost all hearts there is a **main atrial branch** which indeed is the term that Baroldi (1967) prefers for such a vessel. This vessel supplies branches to both atria and the atrial septum, but its most important branch passes through and supplies the S.A. node. The artery passes (either clockwise or counterclockwise) around the superior cavo-atrial junction, and in recognition of this course, Gross in 1921 used the term **"ramus ostiae cavae superiorus"**. Contrariwise in the following year, Crainicianu termed the vessel **"the Keith and Flack artery"**; eschewing eponyms, James in 1961 used the term **"sinus node artery"**. The artery does give a large branch to the terminal muscle bundle; however, Spalteholz in 1924 described the branch supplying the S.A. node as the **"ramus crista terminalis"**. These facts have been stated because these terms appear in medical writing.

I prefer the term **"sinus node artery"**. A student of anatomy should be armed with the knowledge of the origin, course, termination, relations, and mode of branching of an artery. The location of the S.A. node at the superior cavo-atrial junction, a dominating landmark in cardiac anatomy, well defines the termination. The artery can be designated additionally with terms that indicate the origin and predict, to some extent, the course of the

arteries. The **right sinus node artery** is defined as one arising from the right coronary artery. The **left sinus node artery** arises from the proximal 10 mm of the posterior division of the left coronary artery (the circumflex). It ascends on the anterior wall of the left atrium to reach the interatrial muscle bundle, through which it usually courses, en route to the S.A. node. The **posterior sinus node artery** arises from the proximal 50 mm of the posterior division of the left coronary artery, frequently posterior to the lateral wall of the left atrium. Like the left sinus node artery, it usually proceeds intramurally through the main trunk of the interatrial muscle bundle to the superior cavo-atrial junction. Before reaching this muscle bundle, **it is characterized by its course** over the lateral wall of the left atrium between the attachments of the atrial appendage and the left superior pulmonary vein. The clinical significance of this classification will be discussed in the appropriate sections. Although most authors cite a predominance of origin from the right coronary artery, in my dissections, right, left, and posterior sinus node arteries were found in 48, 30, and 22%, respectively.

The atrial arteries serve an important role in the establishment of collateral circulation in occlusive disease of the right or left coronary arteries. This collateral may develop between branches (a) on the anterior walls of the atria, (b) in the atrial septum, and (c) on the posterior surface of the heart. In 50 specimens, Kugel (1927) found a large branch passing as a **low left anterior atrial branch** to reach the interatrial septum, where it "(a) passed posteriorly in the septum to effect an anastomosis at the crux, or (b) effected an anastomosis with a low right anterior atrial artery, or (c) passed posteriorly together with a branch from the latter". Kugel also stated that the artery was important in the blood supply to the adjacent portions of the aortic and mitral valves. He applied the term "arteria anastomotica auricularis magna" to this vessels. However, it is usually referred to as Kugel's artery. The aptness of either term can be questioned. Gross dissection can be carried out satisfactorily to the 1 mm level. However, the demonstration of smaller branches and their anastomosis can only be accomplished by techniques such as the injection and corrosion method. The value of this technique in the definitive portrayal of this particular anatomy can be adduced by the study of page 142 of the monograph of James (1961). Kugel stated that the artery always arose from the proximal left cirumflex or the left sinus node artery, when the latter was present. However, James used the term "Kugel artery" to describe either a low right or a low left anterior atrial branch. These he includes, along with the right intermediate atrial artery and "the left atrial circumflex coronary artery",

as the three atrial arteries which are found in addition to the sinus node artery in most human hearts. In the specimens dissected in my study, virtually all specimens have demonstrated either a right or a left low anterior atrial artery. However, a vessel arising from the proximal left coronary artery, of constant occurrence, and of a size worthy of the term **arteria anastomotica auricularis magna**, has not been seen. It may be concluded that the terms low anterior atrial artery left or right, are preferable.

Four major sites are seen for collateral development: (1) apex of L.V.; (2) the septal wall of L.V.; (3) the anterior wall of the right ventricle; (4) the atria (v.s.). Vessels in the first two sites are involved, not only in "effecting collateral", but in maintaining the vital pumping action of the left ventricle. The collateral in the last two sites are important because they are not involved in the maintenance of the vital function of the left ventricle and both run in low pressure walls, hence during systole a large flow occurs. The atrial vessels are often larger than commonly appreciated.

Throughout this work I use the term minor atrial circumflex for the common, small artery that arises from the lateral part of the posterior division and runs around the left A.V. sulcus, often reaching the crux and supplying the adjacent surfaces of the left atrium and ventricle. (When the posterior division itself courses over the left atrial wall, this course will merit the subdesignation—major atrial circumflex.) A posterior left atrial branch is defined most easily as one which arises on the posterior aspect of the heart and supplies the posterior wall of the left atrium. However, a branch is seen in **204—4** which arises on the lateral surface of the heart and supplies the posterior wall of the left atrium; it runs well above the A.V. sulcus and cannot be termed a minor atrial circumflex—it is termed a posterior left atrial branch. Such a term denotes the supply of the posterior wall of the left atrium with an origin on the lateral or posterior wall. These arteries reach the interatrial septum and may send small branches inferiorly to the posterior wall of the left ventricle. Like the minor atrial circumflex, it may contribute to collateral between both the atrial and ventricular branches of the right and left coronary arteries.

Note: No inconsistency exists in the use of the term minor atrial circumflex and the disavowal of the traditional term, circumflex branch (page 122). The former, by definition, bends around the left atrium and related A.V. sulcus; usually it reaches the posterior interatrial sulcus. The latter reaches the postero-inferior aspect of the heart in only 35% of hearts. The term atrial circumflex is usually used in medical writing.

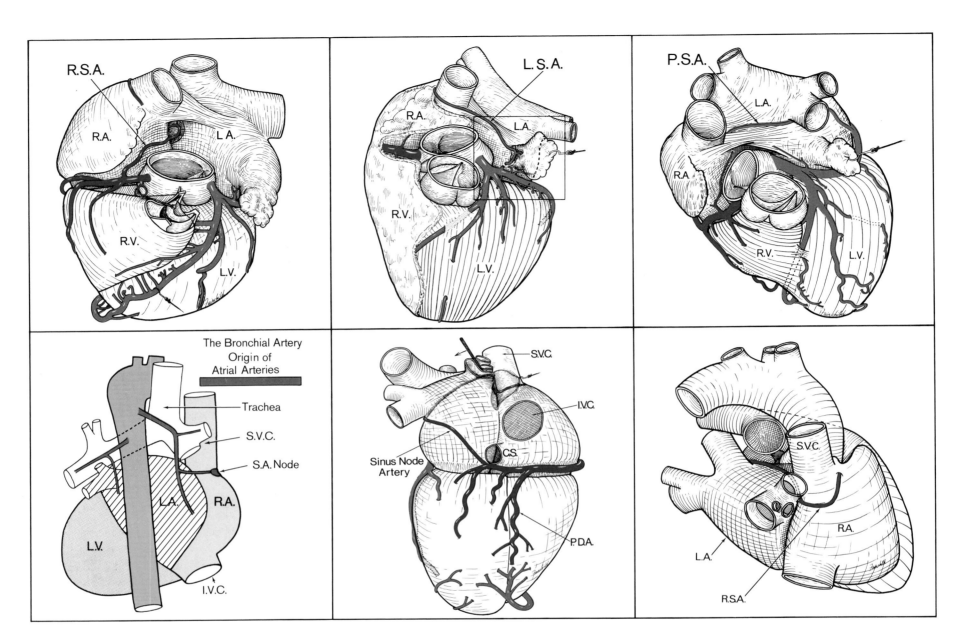

A. The Atrial Arteries

The Origin of the Three Sinus Node Arteries

Drawings of three specimens A, B, and C, **1–3**, demonstrate the mode of origin and course of the sinus node arteries as they are defined herein—note their abbreviations.

1: The Right Sinus Node Artery: Nonattitudinal superior anterior view: The artery originates from the proximal right coronary, passes across the anteromedial wall of the right atrium and, as is usual, when it passes in a counterclockwise manner (in relation to the superior vena cava), it penetrates the atrial septum below the interatrial bundle. See other views of this specimen—**175—5, 6.**

2: The Left Sinus Node Artery: Nonattitudinal left superior view: The artery arises from the proximal portion of the left coronary artery. Characteristically, it courses through the left anterior ramus of the interatrial

muscle bundle and then through the bundle itself; here the artery presents a deviant but important course through the wall of the left atrial appendage—note the clockwise course.

3: The Posterior Sinus Node Artery: Although the site of the origin from the posterior division varies, its initial course over the lateral wall of the left atrium between the atrial appendage and the left superior pulmonary vein is characteristic.

The Unusual Origin of a Sinus Node Artery:

4: 106 specimens were dissected in order to find 100 sinus node arteries. This simple drawing is shown to attract attention to the possibility of their **extracoronary origin**. The artery may arise from a bronchial artery or conceivably directly from the descending thoracic aorta. This drawing has been inspired by the important work of Moberg, which will be discussed on page 162*.

5 and 6: As seen in the inferior view in **5**, the sinus node artery in this specimen arises from the right coronary

artery just beyond the crux. Its termination is seen from a nonattitudinal R.P.O. view in **6**. The unusual origin of the sinus node artery and its course, entirely intramurally from its origin to its termination, represent two additional explanations for failure to identify the sinus node artery. The photographs of the termination of this vessel will be seen on page 154. In **5** a feature is seen which is quite unusual. The posterior A.V. sulci almost form a straight line which is continuous through the crux (see page 68). (This is specimen D.)

---

* An article on the right bronchial artery anatomy by Nathan *et al.* containing photographs and useful drawings merits study. They state, "The course of the bronchial artery always originated at the superior border of the first or second right aortic intercostal artery at a variable distance (0.5 to 5.0 cm) from the aorta."

The Atrial Arteries and Collateral Circulation

Specimen E: 1 and **2**: A superior L.A.O. view: With the exception of the inferior, the walls of the right ventricle have been excised. The papillary muscles of this specimen are seen in **83—6**. Note the location of the **anterior atrial arteries** and their proximity to both the aortic and mitral valves and their potential for intercoronary collateral development.

Specimen F: 3 and **4**: The superior L.A.O. view of the specimen seen on page 206. Observe: (a) The posterior sinus node artery arises inferior to the left inferior pulmonary vein. (b) The left atrial appendage is usually supplied by two small branches which appear susceptible to injury. Traction on these during operation might effect rupture at their origin, with the possible development of dissection in the posterior division of the left coronary artery. (c) The right anterior atrial branch passes across and gives a branch to the anteromedial wall of the right atrium. As it enters the interatrial septum, it contributes a branch to the anterior wall of the left atrium, and a third branch which passes up to anastomose with the posterior sinus node artery at the superior cavo-atrial junction. This is the only specimen I have encountered with collateral at this level, ascertainable by gross dissection. This infrequency suggests that division of the sinus node artery at operation may be a factor in the development of postoperative arrhythmias.

Specimen G: 5: The superior view of a specimen seen in this perspective on page 6 and from a P.A. view on page 15: The right sinus node artery arises 4 mm beyond the origin of the right coronary artery. It passes onto the anteromedial wall of the right atrium, giving a branch to it and the branch to the S.A. node which passes in front of the superior vena cava. It then continues on as a large branch to the atrial septum. The right coronary artery terminates at the crux inferiorly, giving branches to the septum and the A.V. node artery. A posterior atrial branch also reaches the septum from the left coronary artery. **The atrial septum is an important site for the development of intra- and inter-coronary collateral circulation.**

Specimen H: 6: An inferior view: In contrast to the commonly seen minor atrial circumflex branch described on 151, posterior left atrial branches are uncommon. Here a large branch is present; it supplies the entire posterior and part of the superior walls of the atrium in addition to small branches to L.V. **The postero-inferior aspect of the heart is an important area for collateral development.** In addition to the above two arteries, a posterior sinus node artery may often be seen, in arteriograms, playing a vital role maintaining perfusion of the left ventricle in the presence of occlusive disease of the right coronary artery: The potential for this role is seen in **158—4**. This specimen appears in other views in **152—3** and **182—1-4**.

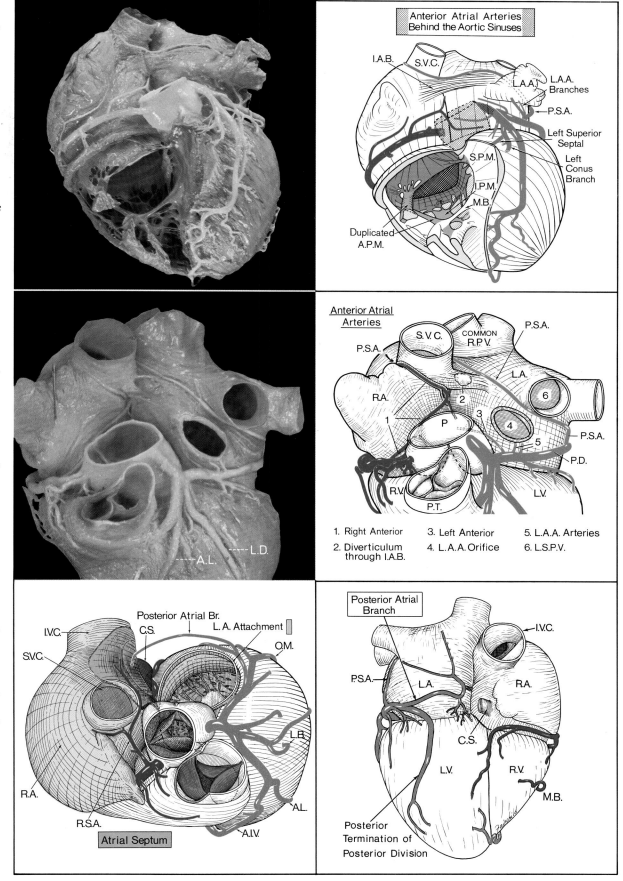

153

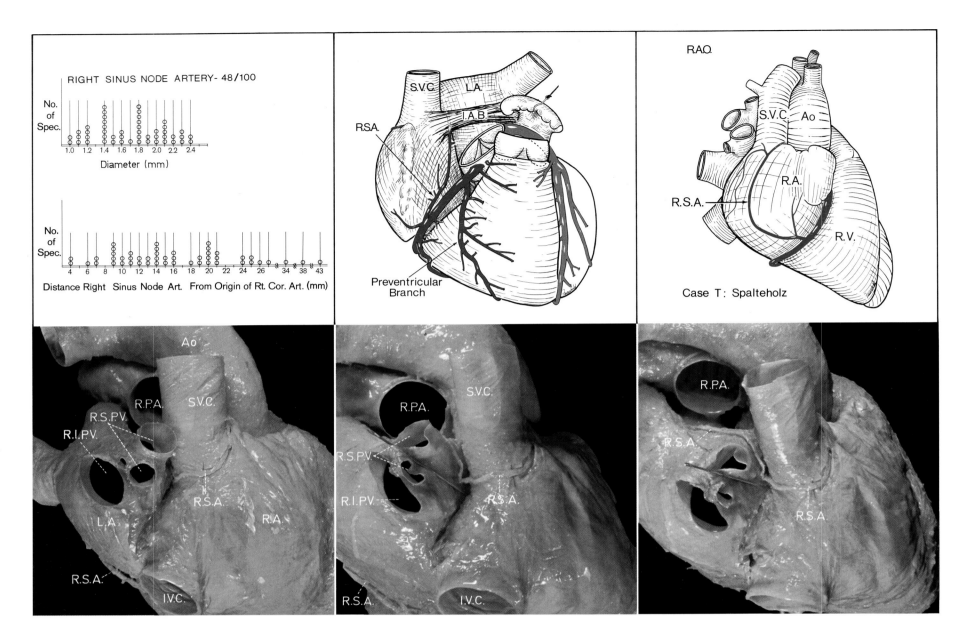

B. The Right Sinus Node Artery

1: These data should refute the statement that sinus node arteries are only 1.0 mm in diameter and should emphasize, first, their potential for the development of collateral circulation and second, the desirability of avoiding their injury at operation. The distance in millimeters between their origin and the orifice of the parent right coronary artery is shown. Three examples of unusual sites of origin of the artery will now be examined.

Specimen A: 2: The artery arises 43 mm from the origin of the right coronary artery—**the most distal origin** in the 100 specimens studied in 1967. A large preventricular branch supplies a large part of the anterior wall of the right ventricle.

3: In the dog, the sinus node artery arises as **an intermediate branch of the right coronary artery**. This is rare in humans. In our dissection, no example of this variant occurred. This drawing depicts the occurrence in a human heart, Case T, described in the monograph of Spalteholz (1924). In the dog, the left coronary artery is dominant: The sinus node artery is often the mode of termination of the right coronary artery. A relationship may exist between sinus node artery injury and postoperative arrhythmia: An oblique right atriotomy incision (directed postero-inferiorly across the lateral wall of the right atrium) will virtually always divide the artery in a dog but almost never in a human. This is an example of the fact that deductions derived from observations made in experiments on animals are not necessarily applicable to man.

Specimen B: 4, **5**, and **6**: Nonattitudinal R.P.O. views of the specimen just examined (**152**—**5** and **6**) in which the sinus node artery arose from the right coronary artery to the left of the crux. In **4** and **5**, the artery may be seen just above its origin and in **6**, the vessel is seen running over the superior aspect of the left atrium. The sinus node artery loops inferiorly into the interatrial septum prior to its passage superiorly to reach the S.A.

node. This course is frequently seen when a sinus node artery, regardless of its site of origin, passes in a counterclockwise manner in relation to the superior vena cava. The artery may be injured by an incision in the left atrial wall for operations on the mitral valve. These photographs demonstrate how the atria may be separated in the posterior interatrial sulcus in this procedure. When the left atrium is large and exposure is satisfactory without this mobilization (in order to avoid the artery), dissection in this area should be avoided.
It has long been my attempt at operation to subject the right atrium and its blood supply to minimal trauma. I have avoided clamping and incising the right atrial appendage, hoping to avoid trauma to the S.A. node by the clamp or a superior extension of the incision; this also may be of importance in reducing the possibility of trauma and occlusion of the right sinus node artery, the potential for which will be examined in four specimens.

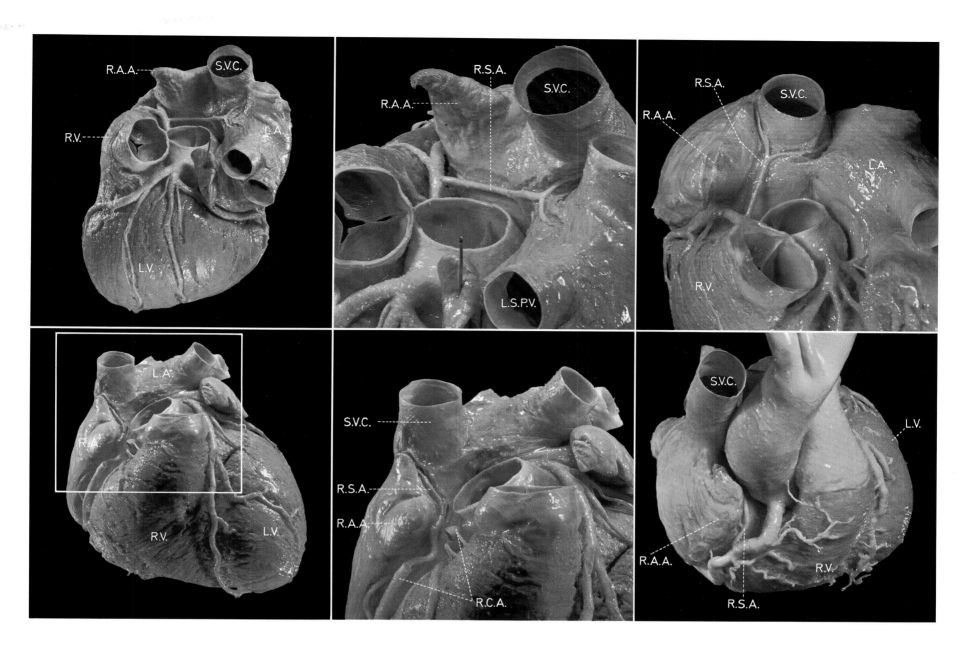

Its Relations to the Right Atrial Appendage— A Surgical Hazard?

Specimen C: 1 and **2**: The superior left lateral view: Observe: (a) The right sinus node artery measures 2.2 mm in diameter. Not infrequently, its caliber exceeds that of the anterior interventricular artery. (b) It arises from the right coronary artery 15 mm beyond its origin; **this places it in contact with the right atrium***. (c) Arteries with a counterclockwise course perforate the septum; they do not ascend anteriorly to the superior cavo-atrial angle; this may also explain their course over the atrial wall at a low level. (d) The size and degree of angularity of the right atrial appendage are variables; here we see their positive occurrence. The combination of anatomic dispositions, (c) and (d), places the artery out of harm's way should the atrial appendage ever be clamped.

Specimen D: 3: A superior L.A.O. view: This specimen has been seen in **153—5**. (a) From its origin only 4 mm beyond the right coronary artery orifice, it (R.S.A.) passes directly through the right coronary fossa, well separated from the right atrial wall, to the superior cavo-atrial junction, where the branch to the sinus node passes in a clockwise manner in relation to the superior vena cava. The appendage is large (it may be seen in **153—5**) but its angularity is less than that of Specimen C. The artery could be injured if a clamp encroached on the superior cavo-atrial angle.

Specimen E: 4 and **5**: An elevated anterior view of the third specimen, from which one inch of the right coronary artery has been removed to display the origin and course of the sinus node artery as it passes close to the summit of the poorly developed right atrial appendage. The artery pursues an intramural course enroute to the S.A. node and can be seen in **88—5** and **6** within the muscle. In passing note the large size of the anterior interventricular (A.I.V.) branch and anterolateral branches of the left coronary artery. **Comment**: (a) The origin of the artery is 25 mm beyond the orifice of its parent vessel. (b) The atrial appendage is small and blunt. (c) The artery passes in a clockwise course around the superior

vena cava. Each of these factors increases the risk of injury to the risk of injury to the artery their combination would probably make sinus node artery injury a certainty if the atrial appendage were to be clamped and excised.

Specimen F: 6: An elevated right superior view: Arising from the continuing segment of the right coronary artery, the sinus node artery passes posteriorly, in contact with and at a high level on the atrial appendage—the potential for its injury is evident.

---

* In the presence of a proximal origin, the artery usually traverses the fat in the right coronary fossa, as shown in **3**.

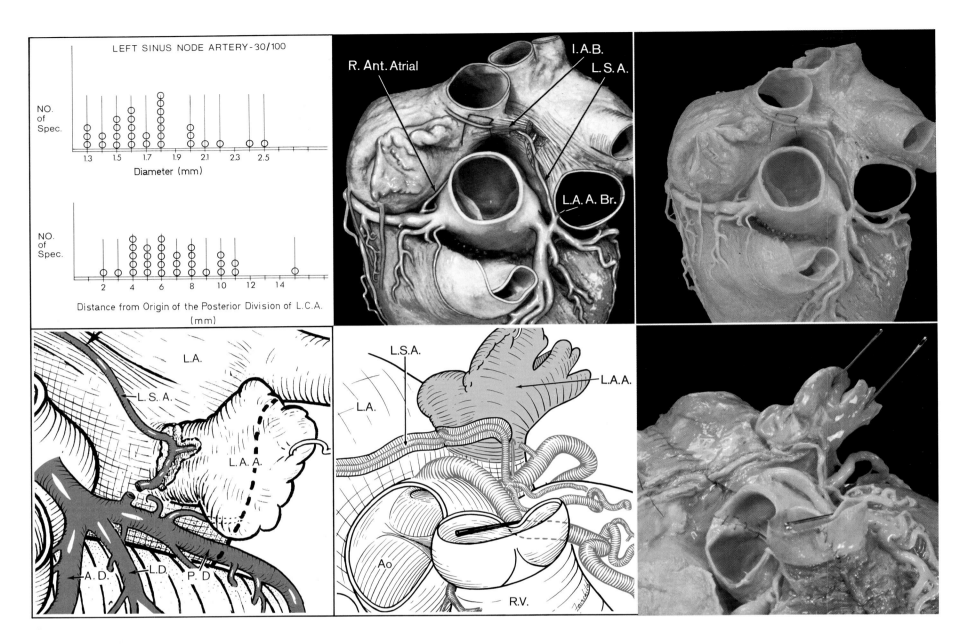

C. The Left Sinus Node Artery and Its Relation to the Left Atrial Appendage

1: This mode of origin was present in 30 of the 100 specimens in which a sinus node artery was identified. The size of sinus node arteries appears unrelated to their site of origin. The artery arises from the first few millimeters of the posterior division of the left coronary artery*. It arises alone or in connection with an artery to the left atrial appendage. It passes to the right, and in most specimens, after a short course, commences an intramural course in the interatrial muscle bundle as shown in the specimens on this page.

Specimen A: 2–3: **2** is a retouched photograph of **3**. The left atrial appendage has been removed at the site of its attachment to the atrium. The sinus node artery arises along with the artery to the former. The two "draw" the posterior division of the left coronary artery towards the atrio-appendageal junction. In three instances, two

of which are shown next, the artery passed through the wall of the left atrial appendage.

Specimen B: 4: This area has been excerpted from the specimen in 152—2, which provides orientation for this specimen.

Specimen C: 5 and **6** are nonattitudinal anterosuperior views.

In order to avoid a cul de sac in which a thrombus may develop, ligation or amputation is effected at the orifice of the appendage—this would certainly divide the sinus node arteries shown here. Ligation or amputation of the appendage is carried out when this structure is used as an avenue for closed operations on the mitral valve or used as a site of introduction of a decompression catheter (see page 28). When the mitral valve is exposed through other incisions, the appendage has been removed in order to reduce the hazard of thromboembolism. Both a left and a posterior sinus node artery may course in the wall of the left atrium at the antero-inferior or superior margins of the orifice of the append-

age, and both may be damaged when the latter is ligated or amputated; this hazard exists in 52% of hearts in this study.

The S.A. node, lying postero-inferior to the superior cavo-atrial angle, and its arterial blood supply may be injured by the incisions in the right atrium which are used for caval cannulation as well as for exposure of the right atrium. As seen on the next page, in my practice, the two small incisions for the cannulation are made in the oblique vascular watershed in the lateral wall of the atrium (not in the appendage). This method of caval cannulation is used in all cardiac operations with the exception of the creation of a baffle in transposition of the great vessels. If these incisions are joined, good exposure of the right atrial cavity results; also transatrial closure of ventricular septal defects may be accomplished.

---

* In our dissections, a careful search for nonterminal branches of the left main branch has been fruitless—such an origin for the sinus node artery has been reported, and are seen in arteriograms.

D. The Avoidance of Trauma to the S.A. Node and Its Blood Supply

I. The Optimal Location for a Superior Vena Cava Tape

In **1–4** four specimens are seen. **5** is the drawing of **3** and **4**. The views are **1**—255°; **2**—240°; **3** and **4**—270°.
Anatomic Features: (a) In **1** and **2** the superior cavo-atrial angle is at the level of the inferior wall of the right pulmonary artery as it passes posterior to the superior vena cava—**the usual relationship.** In **3** and **4** the angle is deviated above and below its usual level. (b) The superior vena cava: In **1**, the azygos vein demarcates its short upper and long lower segments. In **3** and **4**, the atrial muscle ascends its wall—the increased hazard to an accompanying S.A. node is evident.

The Surgical Inference: As stated on page 131, if the superior vena cava is to be encircled with a tape for a snare, the dissection should not be carried into the retrocaval recess—the easy way—instead it should be carried out at a much higher level. This is possible because the inferior segment of the superior vena cava is long. Hence, regardless of variations in the height of the superior cavo-atrial angle, the related S.A. node will not be injured.

II. The Optimal Location for Right Atrial Incisions

6: R.A.O. view: The red beads indicate the site of the S.A. node posteroinferior to the superior cavo-atrial angle. The **right atrial appendage** is unusually large and anteriorly located in this specimen; note the variation in its size in the five specimens on this page. However, as stated on page 154, this structure is not used for caval cannulation; the method I prefer is shown in this photograph. The purse-string sutures are placed obliquely in the less-vascular zone of the lateral wall of the right atrium. Their ends face each other; they are used for snares. The blue beads indicate the site of incisions for the insertion of the catheters. If the right atrium is to be opened, tapes around the cuffed vena cava-catheters are tightened; the snares are removed from the atrial purse-string sutures; the upper and lower components of which are grasped and drawn apart; the bridge of right atrial wall between the cannulation incisions is divided. An adequate atriotomy results. At the conclusion of the intracardiac procedure, the purse-string sutures are brought obliquely through the apposed walls, used as snares, then tied down after the catheters are removed. This procedure results in minimal trauma to the atrium and its blood supply and is easily performed. This technique obviates the need for an additional incision (to expose the interior of the atrium) which further impairs the blood supply of the atrium and may injure the S.A. node artery (which may loop inferiorly) or the S.A. node itself. Following operations for the closure of atrial septal defects, a significant incidence of permanent arrhythmia has been reported; working through this oblique vascular watershed of the right atrium, freedom from this complication has resulted.

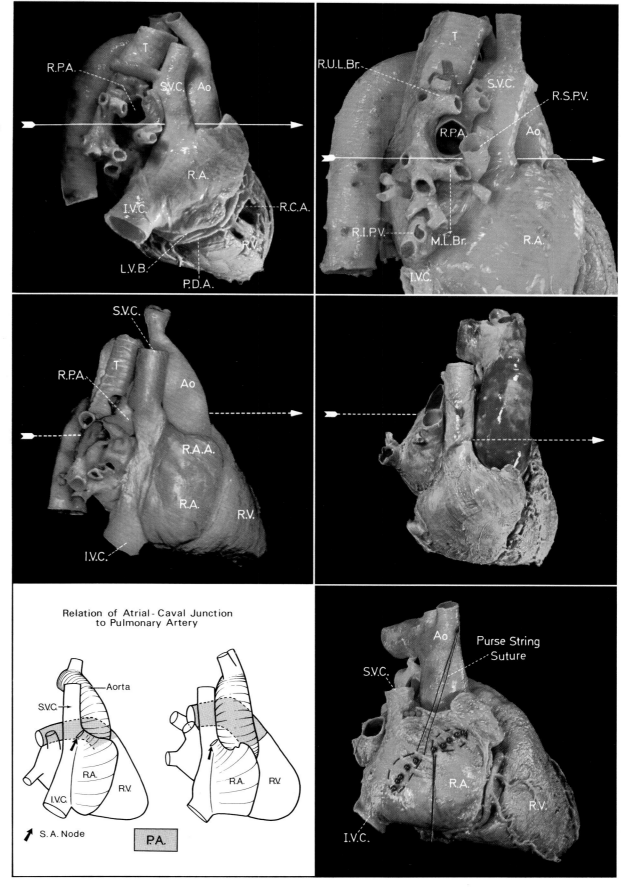

Relation of Atrial-Caval Junction to Pulmonary Artery

S.A. Node

P.A.

157

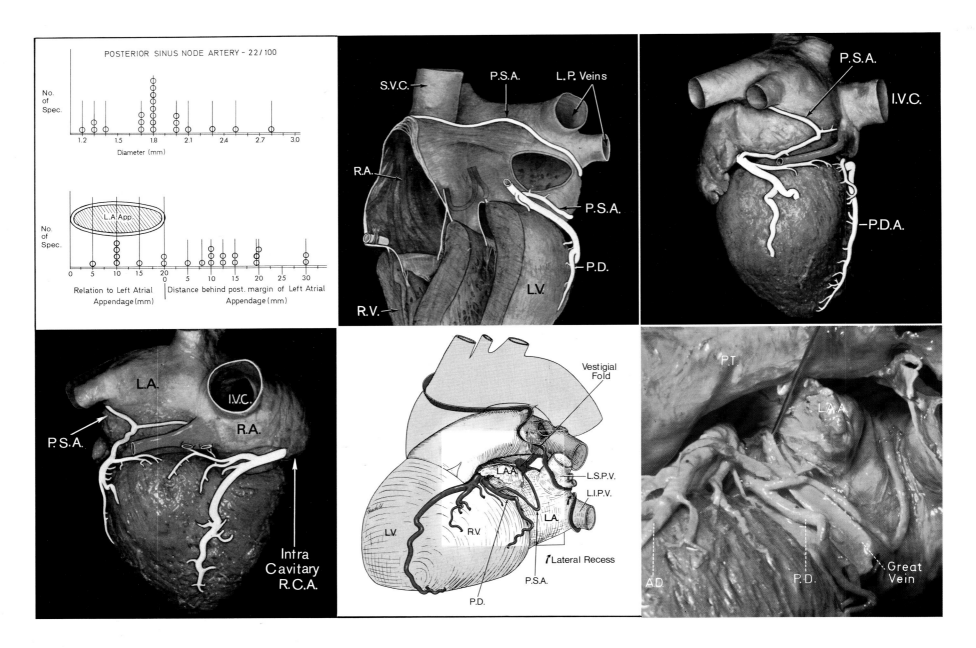

E. The Posterior Sinus Node Artery

1: (a) Four of the 22 specimens had a diameter larger than 2 mm. (b) In 8 specimens, the artery arose inferior to the left appendage attachment. In the remainder, the distance in millimeters behind the posterior margin of the appendage is shown.

Specimen A: 2–4: The mode of transection of this specimen should be seen on page 186. The posterior segment is seen in **2**, a left lateral nonattitudinal view and in **3** and **4** the obtuse margin and inferior views. Observe: (a) The posterior sinus node artery (P.S.A.) arises under the midpoint of the attachment of the left atrial appendage. The vessel then runs almost to the midpoint of the posterior wall of the left atrium before it recurs, passing close to the origin of the left inferior pulmonary vein en route to the sinus node. It gives off a posterior branch which runs to the atrial septum. The artery, hence, provides blood supply to a large area of the left atrium, the interatrial septum, and a portion of the right atrial wall—truly a main atrial artery.

Specimen B: 5 and **6:** This specimen is seen on page **127**—**3–6** showing the pericardial reflections on the right. The highlighted area in the drawing shows the area examined in **6**. The 2.2-mm posterior sinus node artery arises below the appendageal attachment from the 3.2-mm posterior division. It passes posteriorly on the atrial wall, then recurs at an acute angle, passing superiorly between the atrial appendage and the left superior pulmonary vein, continuing upward through the inferior attachment of the vestigial fold of the left superior vena cava. It is interesting to note that the artery on the lateral wall of the left atrium, in this specimen and in many others, follows the course of the left superior cardinal vein of the fetus and the oblique left atrial vein of adults.

As seen in **5** and **127**—**6**, the layer of pericardium between the proximal parts of the pulmonary arteries and the left atrium has been removed. In this specimen the upper attachment of the vestigial fold is to the right pulmonary artery.

Mode of Origin

In 22 specimens the origin of the posterior sinus node artery was as follows: (a) 7 specimens—**minor atrial circumflex**—**159**—**2** is an example thereof; in **159**—**3–6** the posterior wall branch may be considered an offshoot of the sinus node artery; (b) 10 specimens—the **lateral segment of the posterior division** which terminates as the posterior branch (6) or the obtuse marginal branch (4); (c) 5 specimens—the **posterior segment of the posterior division** which terminates as the posterior branch (3) and the posterior descending (2).

It has not been customary to separately classify the posterior sinus node artery—five examples are seen on these two pages—five other examples are present in this work: **141**—**1** and **2; 152**—**3** and **6; 188**—**3; 189**—**1–6; 206**—**1–6.**

Specimen C: 1: Nonattitudinal left lateral view: Observe: The posterior sinus node artery arises posterior to the attachment of the left atrial appendage from the posterior division which terminates at the crux, demonstrating a balanced pattern of supply, as shown on page 177—**5** and **6**. The sinus node artery abuts on the left superior pulmonary vein.

Specimen D: 2: A left lateral view: Observe: The artery is a branch of a minor atrial circumflex (M.A.C.). It impinges on the common left pulmonary vein.

Specimen E: 3–6: This specimen is seen in **3** and **4** from a left superior view, in **5** from an L.P.O. view, and in **6** from the superior view. Observe: (a) The posterior sinus node artery arises, together with the two appendageal branches, below the left atrial appendage and passes posteriorly, contributing a posterior branch which reaches the interatrial septum, as seen in **5**. (b) The artery crosses the attachment of the left superior pulmonary vein, as seen in **3**, **4**, and **6**. (c) Regardless of the exact site of origin of the posterior sinus node artery (from the posterior division), the artery must pass from the left, anteriorly across the superior aspect of the left atrium to reach the sinus node, as seen in **6**. (d) The artery passes in a clockwise manner around the superior vena cava, as shown in **3**. (e) A relatively large right anterior atrial branch (X) is seen in **3** and **4**. (f) In **4**, a needle deflecting the atrial appendage penetrates the unusually large left fibrous trigone, which results from the unusual posterior site of the attachment of the left atrium to the aorto-ventricular membrane. This anatomical variation is seen in 15—**5** and **6**.

In the performance of radical intrapericardial left pneumonectomy, resection of a considerable part of the left atrium in relation to the pulmonary veins is frequently necessary. Such procedures will divide the artery examined on this page. The artery may be injured where it is related to the orifice of the left atrial appendage when excision of the latter is performed. It will be divided when a left lateral atriotomy is used for open operations on the mitral valve.

The Three Sinus Node Arteries—Summary

1. **Size**—no difference is seen in the diameter of the three sinus node arteries
2. **Course in relation to the superior vena cava:** When counterclockwise, the artery may be injured by the conventional incision for mitral valve operations. When clockwise, it may be injured when the right atrial appendage is clamped. The findings in this group of 100 specimens are:

    Right sinus node artery (48 specimens): clockwise—15; counterclockwise—25; twin encircling branches—8

    Left sinus node artery (30 specimens): all passed clockwise

    Posterior sinus node arteries (22 specimens): clockwise—10; counterclockwise—12

Note the striking disparity in the course (in relation to the superior vena cava) of the sinus node arteries which originate from the left coronary artery.

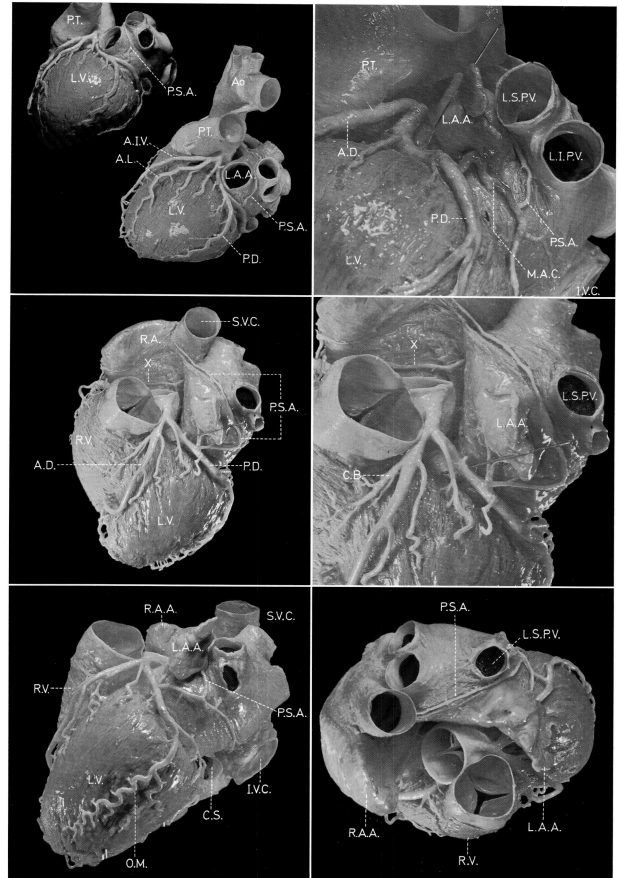

← A.V. Node Artery in Relation to L.V. Ostium

A.V. Node Artery

Inferior Wall of R.A.

F. The A.V. Node Artery

I. Its Relation to the Ostium of the Left Ventricle and the Mitral Valve

The relation of the integrity of this artery to the maintenance of normal conduction has not been established. Anatomic studies utilizing injection corrosion and microradiographic techniques suggest the presence of important collateral from the anterior atrial arteries. In patients with obliterative disease of the trunk (right or left coronary artery) supplying the A.V. node branch, complete heart block is seen accompanying acute myocardial infarction. The total incidence is roughly 3%; however, with right coronary artery disease the incidence is approximately 10%. With disease of the anterior or division the block results from ischemia of the bundle branches. The conduction disturbances seen in patients after open heart surgery are often attributed to metabolic derangement: The possibility exists of a simpler anatomic explanation—one based on the acute interruption of the artery to the A.V. node. The collateral circulation into the arterial bed beyond the site of a chronic occlusion of the parent trunk proximally, provides flow through the A.V. node artery, hence the virtual absence of associated conduction disturbances cannot be adduced to summarily reject this consideration.

Specimen A: 1: A 255° view is seen after removal of the right atrium: The beads identify the following: blue and red = anterior and posterior margins of atrial apposition; adjacent lower red and blue = the right fibrous trigone; the same red = the location of the A.V. node. Note the features of the A.V. node artery (A.V.N.A.) seen between the two red beads: (a) **It arises from a dominant left coronary artery.** (b) It is 30 mm long; the length is inversely related to the degree of anterosuperior extension of the parent trunk into the crux—as seen on page 71 it may, as a result, be very short. (c) It is tightly applied to the confluence of the chambers and the mitral valve attachment.

Specimen B: 2: A superior P.A. view of a specimen with a **dominant left coronary artery**. In its distal 5 mm, the A.V. node artery is in contact with the mitral valve attachment. This specimen is seen after removal of the left atrium, and these two photographs demonstrate the location of the A.V. node artery and its artery of origin in relation to the atrial septum, an important site for the development of collateral circulation.

Specimen C: 3 and 4: Superior R.P.O. view: Although **it arises from a dominant right coronary artery**, the A.V. node artery is closely related to the mitral portion of the ostium of L.V. I have never seen the A.V. node branch arise from the trunk of a right coronary artery proximal to the origin of the posterior descending branch.

Specimen D: 5 and 6: Nonattitudinal R.P.O. view: A **balanced type of arterial distribution** is present. The right atrial wall has been elevated from the posterior superior process of the left ventricle. The A.V. node artery is exposed, hugging the left atrial attachment to the A.V. membrane. In conclusion, regardless of its origin, the A.V. node artery may be in contact with the attachment of the mitral valve. It is incorrect to equate the origin of the A.V. node artery with dominance (right or left)—it arises from the left, not only in left dominance (12%), but in the balanced pattern (17% in this study).

II. Its Relation to the Posterior Superior Process of the Left Ventricle and the Tricuspid Valve

Specimen E: 1 and **2:** Right lateral view: The right coronary artery ascends onto the posterior superior process of the left ventricle. The shorter A.V. node artery resulting, crosses the latter, coming into contact with the mitral valve attachment in its terminal few millimeters only. Note the superior direction of the artery and the superior orientation of the ostium of the left ventricle, along which courses the His bundle and, more anteriorly, the first division of the right bundle. Frequently, it is stated that these latter structures are oriented in an antero-inferior direction because of the failure to examine them in an attitudinal manner. A portion of the right atrial wall remains in contact with the process, and between the two structures runs the "superior" septal artery. (The preferred term is posterior septal artery. See page 173.)

Specimen F: 3 and **4:** A superior P.A. view: This specimen appears in other views on page 198. Here, note the A.V. node artery running through the midzone of the posterior superior process of the left ventricle, well separated from both A.V. valves.

Specimen G: 5: An inferior view: Two needles elevate the inferior wall of the right atrium. The A.V. node artery again courses through the midzone of the crux, well away from the attachments of both A.V. valves.

Specimen H: 6: A left inferior view: The A.V. node artery runs in contact with the inferior wall of the right atrium. The fat-filled area between the inferior wall and the posterior superior process of L.V. is seen in transected specimens, **102—3** and **4** and **104—3** and **4**. The A.V. node artery may be located intramurally in the right atrial wall. In passing, note that the posterior descending branch is accompanied by two veins.

Note: The A.V. node artery supplies the A.V. node and the His bundle. Since the latter is found in the attachment of the membranous septum to the ostium of the left ventricle, the artery has been called the **ramus septi fibrosi.**

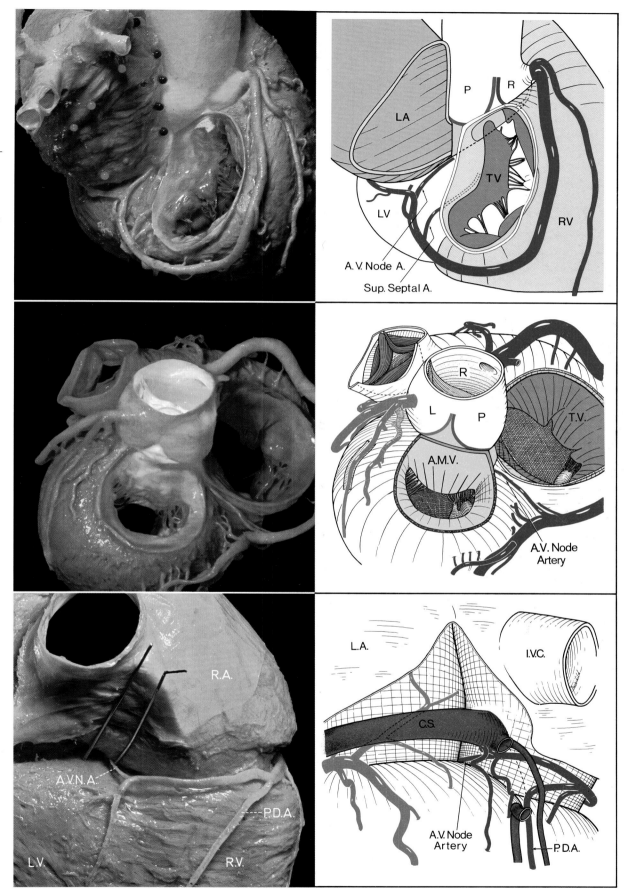

G. Clinical Comments

The bronchial arteries pass from the aorta to the posterior aspect of the right and left main bronchi. They are not far from the left atrium: this relationship can be studied on page 126. In an examination of 40 postmortem specimens, Moberg found anastomosis between the bronchial arteries and the heart at the ventricular level in every instance. He also found and demonstrated extracardial anastomosis between the internal mammary and the heart at the ventricular level in 4 out of 49 specimens, and at the atrial level in 15 specimens. Johnsson carried out selective bronchial artery opacification in two patients, one with complete obstruction of the anterior descending branch, and one with obstruction of the right main coronary artery. In both patients opacification of the artery beyond the obstruction resulted. The studies of these workers, apart from the evident clinical implications, are interesting anatomically in that they may explain the failure of identification of a sinus node artery during the dissection of a specimen. In one of the patients of Johnsson, the collateral route was through the sinus node artery. Moberg states that the site of anastomosis usually is at the atrial level. The sinus node artery, hence, may arise from the bronchial artery, and it is not inconceivable that a separate origin for the atrial arteries from the aorta may be identified in the future.

The following is found in Moberg's article (1968): "The first description of extracardial anastomoses dates back to v. Haller 1803. He found communications between the coronary arteries and the mediastinal vessels. The first more comprehensive study was made by Hudson, Moritz & Wearn 1932. Working with human postmortem material they ... stated that anastomoses were found between the coronary arteries and the pericardiophrenic branches of the internal mammary arteries, the anterior mediastinal, pericardial, bronchial, superior and inferior phrenic, intercostal and oesophageal branches of the aorta. ... In conclusion the authors stated that "this rich potential extracardiac coronary collateral circulation is probably of significance in compensating for sclerosis of the large trunks of the coronary arteries". Recently Petelenz (1963, 1965) studied anastomoses between the bronchial and the coronary arteries in 100 adult subjects. The results of postmortem contrast injection into the bronchial arteries were that in 37 specimens contrast medium "reached the heart but did not spread in it" and in 40 specimens contrast medium 'covered (to different degrees) the auricular surface'. The right coronary artery was filled in 10 hearts and the left in 4 more. In 26 specimens contrast medium was visible in the region of the sinus node".

Moberg also noted that subsequent to the presentation of his own studies in 1963, "Bjork (1966) reviewed 200 coronary angiographies on living subjects. An anastomotic flow from the bronchial to the coronary arteries was identified in 73. ... In 14 subjects with coronary atheromatosis the anastomoses had a diameter of at least 2 mm as measured from the angiograms".

Ferrer has used the metaphor the sick sinus syndrome, in which are grouped a variety of conditions attributable to a failing sinus node, which may result from anatomical lesions, inherited or acquired. The latter are much more common and are seen in coronary, rheumatic, myopathic, or collagenous heart diseases. Characteristic of this syndrome are: (1) persistent severe sinus bradycardia; (2) sinus arrest and replacement by atrial or junctional rhythms; (3) sinus arrest, without rescue by other rhythms and consequent standstill, and (4) atrial fibrillation which may be refractory to cardioversion.* Arrhythmias following cardiac operations are frequently attributed to metabolic factors. The atrial fibrillation accompanying mitral valve dysfunction may not be abolished by cardioversion following virtual normalization of cardiac function by valve replacement. It is possible that injury to the sinus node or to its blood supply may be the proximate cause of the complicating or persisting arrhythmia. Attention has been directed here to the anatomic dispositions of the sinus node arteries which would be conducive to their interruption. It is axiomatic that the surgeon should accomplish his goal with minimal disturbance to anatomic structures.

The various incisions which are made in the left atrium for mitral valve operations may now be reviewed in relation to the sinus node arteries. (1) The most common incision used today enters the right lateral or septal wall of the left atrium; if the posterior interatrial groove is dissected, a sinus node artery (regardless of its origin) with a counterclockwise course will often loop down into the groove and be divided. (2) A transseptal incision, (see page 64) incising the right atrial and septal walls transversely would seem disadvantageous when mitral valve replacement is used in patients with associated occlusive coronary artery disease: The arterial collaterals in the atrial septum will be divided. (3) A superior approach, passing through the interatrial bundle will probably interrupt the continuity of sinus node arteries arising from the left coronary artery. (4) A left approach is used by most surgeons for closed procedures on the mitral valve. Either a left or a posterior sinus node artery may be damaged or occluded when the appendage is closed. In the open technique, an incision is made in the appendage and extended posteriorly, and a posterior sinus node artery will, in most instances, be divided. (5) A posterior incision may be made between the pulmonary veins, and here, no sinus node artery will be divided unless a posterior artery (P.S.A.) loops far posteriorly, as is seen in **158—2–4**. When the right lateral or the superior walls are used for the insertion of a catheter for decompression of the left heart, injury to a sinus node artery may occur.

The location of the A.V. node artery was examined in 60 specimens. In 28, the artery ran in contact with the ostium of L.V.; hence, in jeopardy during mitral valve replacement. In 20, the artery ran through the middle of the fat-filled space between the inferior wall of the right atrium and the posterior superior process of the left ventricle. In 12, the artery ran along the inferior wall of the right atrium, adjacent to, but not in contact with the attachment of the tricuspid valve. Therefore, conduction abnormalities would seem unlikely from encirclement of the artery in tricuspid valve replacement. When (the septal leaflet of) the tricuspid valve is attached to the A.V. membrane far posteriorly, the placement of sutures for its replacement could result in injury to the A.V. node and the His bundle. The placement of deep sutures during replacement of either the mitral or tricuspid valve must be avoided: Recall also that major coronary trunks may follow the margins of the posterior superior process of the left ventricle as demonstrated on page 71. Occlusion of such branches could result in infarction of large areas of the left ventricle.

---

* The above material is largely derived from a valuable editorial in the J.A.M.A.—see the reference.

Chapter 12 : The Branches of the Coronary Arteries

Introduction

The designation of a branch should include its origin and the border or sector of the wall of the ventricle on which it courses. For example, the **anterior interventricular** branch of the anterior division and **obtuse marginal** branch of the posterior division course over the borders of the lateral wall. A **lateral** branch of either the anterior or posterior division descends in the 90° sector of this wall; similarly **anterolateral** branches of the anterior division and **posterolateral** branches of both divisions cross the sectors implied.

If we are hoping to effect precision in our assessment of the effects of disease or its treatment, we cannot be satisfied with enumeration of the number of the trunks or branches involved: Their role in perfusion of the left ventricle requires quantitation. **In this exercise, the following five observations are important.** *

A: The Respective Roles of the Right and Left Coronary Arteries

To this determination, the term **dominant** has been applied; it has been much maligned, but, nevertheless, is commonly used. The anatomy of the crux is critical in its consideration. When the posterior descending is a branch of the left coronary artery, the latter supplies the entire left ventricle and is, not inappropriately, termed a **dominant left.** When the right supplies the posterior descending, but no branches to the left ventricle, the term **balanced** is used—this term is derived by convention and is not descriptive. The term **dominant right,** however, is misleading; this term is applied to a right coronary artery which supplies the posterior descending branch and any portion of the posterior wall of L.V.; when it supplies even 5% of this wall, the designation still applies. When it is recalled that more than 75% of the septal wall is usually supplied by the left coronary artery, it is apparent that a dominant right coronary artery may supply only 5 to 10% of the entire left ventricle! In our 100 specimens, the incidence of right, balanced, and left was 71%, 17%, and 12%. Attempts have been made to subdivide the dominant right group; however, the varying geometric patterns found result in much imprecision in this exercise. In 71 specimens, the percentage of the posterior wall supplied by the right coronary artery was estimated after exclusion of the area extending 2.0 cm above the apex. Type I—less than 20%=21; Type II—between 20–80%=43; Type III—in excess of 80%=7. The right may occasionally supply an area of the lateral wall.

B: The Dominance of the Divisions of the Left Coronary

Artery was estimated by measuring the external diameter at their origin. The anterior was larger in 48%, the posterior was larger in 22% and the two were equal in 30%. The limitation of this measurement as an indicator of perfusion fractions should, however, be realized.

C: The Relative Size of Major Branches of the Right Coronary Artery and Each Division of the Left Coronary Artery

As an example, wide variations occur in the relative size of the L.V. branch and posterior descending branch of the right coronary artery.

D: The Pattern of Branches to the Three Walls of the Ventricle

1. The posterior wall: (a) A dominant branch may be seen: It may be located on either border (i.e., a large obtuse marginal or a large posterior descending branch) or be found between the borders. (b) A large branch may be found on each border. (c) Multiple large branches, or multiple small branches may occur. **II. The**

lateral wall: (a) A large posterior border artery (obtuse marginal) may dominate—the anterior I.V. branch and the anterolateral branch are small. (b) A large lateral branch or a large lateral division may be the dominant artery to the wall: Obtuse marginal and anterolateral are not present. (c) Two large border branches: The anterior interventricular and obtuse marginal are large; small branches intervene. (d) Between an anterior interventricular and posterior (wall) branch—both unremarkable in size—only a multitude of small branches about 1.0 mm in size) extend onto the wall. (e) Multiple large branches are present. **III. The Septal Wall:** In the absence of a dominant left coronary artery, an additional expression of the relative role of the right and left coronary is afforded by comparison of the size of the arteries in the interventricular sulci.

E: Relative Size of Adjacent Branches

A large anterolateral branch may usurp the supply area and be associated with diminution in the size of the anterior interventricular branch. The reverse may occur. On page 170, quickly scan the arteries between the interventricular grooves. (1) On the anterior half of the lateral wall, large antero-lateral arteries are present—their large size may be associated with a reduction in caliber of the anterior I.V. branch; this has not occurred. (2) No arteries run in the posterior I.V. groove; however, the products of bifurcation of the right coronary are large and supply the posterior aspect of the ventricles. (3) The diameter of the obtuse marginal is less than that usually seen; it fails to reach its usual termination—the apex. The diminution in its dimensions seems appropriate to the large size of the arteries seen in (1) and (2). These reciprocal dimensions should always be noted but they must not delude us into expecting a constant predictable pattern.

The **septal branches** are of great clinical importance. (1) They perfuse the septal wall, approximately 30% of the mass of the left ventricle. (2) They provide a vital area for the development of collateral circulation between the right and left coronary arteries, since in approximately 90% of hearts, the posterior descending branch arises from the right. (3) They supply the A.V. portion of the conduction system. (4) They run 3 to 4 mm under the surface of the right ventricle and are vulnerable to injury in operations requiring division of infundibular muscle—e.g., the tetralogy of Fallot. (5) In a coronary arteriogram, the motion of the septal arteries may be used to study septal wall function.

---

* All patterns described will be encountered in specimens in the following chapters, and the pages on which they appear are listed in the index.

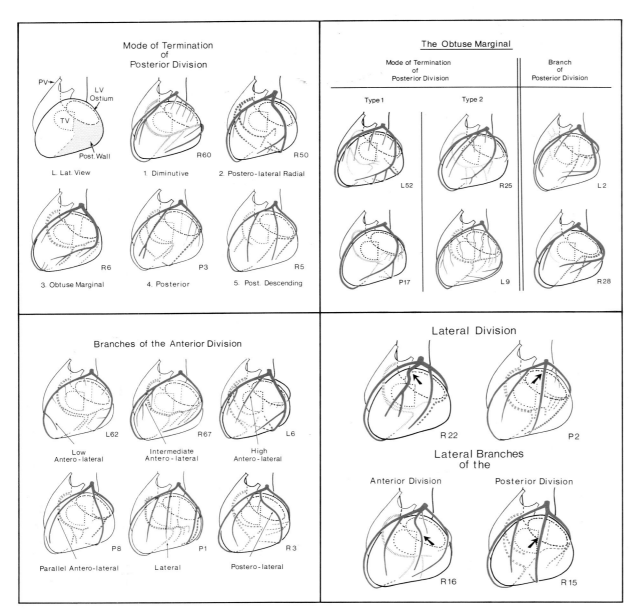

Mode of Termination of Posterior Division

L. Lat. View — PV, LV Ostium, TV, Post. Wall

R60 — 1. Diminutive
R50 — 2. Postero-lateral Radial
R6 — 3. Obtuse Marginal
P3 — 4. Posterior
R5 — 5. Post. Descending

The Obtuse Marginal

Mode of Termination of Posterior Division | Branch of Posterior Division

Type 1 — L52, P17
Type 2 — R25, L9
L2, R28

Branches of the Anterior Division

L62 — Low Antero-lateral
R67 — Intermediate Antero-lateral
L6 — High Antero-lateral
P8 — Parallel Antero-lateral
P1 — Lateral
R3 — Postero-lateral

Lateral Division

R22, P2

Lateral Branches of the

Anterior Division — R16
Posterior Division — R15

A. Terminology and General Plan

I. The Terminology and Mode of Branching of the Left Coronary Artery

1: Mode of termination of the posterior division: The orientation diagram: **Simulation of the left lateral view** of a coronary arteriogram is intended. Each diagram contains the tricuspid, left ventricular, and pulmonary ostia, the anatomic landmarks for the right coronary artery, the posterior division, and the anterior division, respectively. The stippled area shows the location of the posterior wall of L.V. The right coronary artery is blue; the left coronary artery is red. We see diagramatically the arterial plan of specimens, which are all seen later in photographs.

The posterior division displays five basic modes of termination: (1) The **diminutive posterior division** supplies a small area of the posterosuperior portion of the lateral wall of L.V. (2) The **posterolateral radial** artery passes radially or obliquely around the long axis of the left

ventricle enroute to the middle of the posterior I.V. sulcus. Passing directly posterolaterally from its origin, it bears little relation to the A.V. sulcus. It usually is associated with what I term a minor atrial circumflex branch, approximately 1.0 mm in size, which roughly follows the ostium of L.V. to the crux; is it not inappropriate to call this the circumflex artery and the 4.5-mm vessel, which supplies large areas of the lateral and posterior walls of L.V., the branch? (3) The **obtuse marginal** follows this margin and often reaches the apex. (4) The posterior division reaches the posterior aspect of the heart and terminates as a **posterior branch** to the left ventricle. The "balanced type" of supply usually falls into this group (see pages 69 and 177). (5) The posterior division reaches the posterior I.V. groove and terminates as the **posterior descending branch.**

2: The obtuse marginal artery may be the mode of termination of the posterior division or be a branch of a division which terminates as a "posterior branch" or more commonly as the posterior descending branch as

seen here. Running along the boundary (the obtuse margin) between the lateral and posterior wall, variations occur in the extent of the supply to these walls. In type 1 large, and in type 2 insignificant areas of the posterior wall are supplied.

3: When a branch of the anterior division proceeds to the anterolateral portion of the lateral wall, it should be termed an **anterolateral branch.** These are subdivided into (1) high, (2) intermediate, and (3) low—when they arise from (1) the retropulmonary segment, (2) the upper or (3) the lower half of the anterior interventricular segment (of the anterior division). A branch running parallel and close to the anterior interventricular branch is termed a parallel anterolateral. Anterolateral branches are frequently termed "diagonal". In geometry, a diagonal line joins the nonadjacent vertices of a rectilinear figure, hence a diagonal artery could be directed antero-inferiorly or postero-inferiorly; the abandonment of this designation is suggested. When branches descend in the lateral or the posterolateral sectors of the lateral wall, they are termed the **lateral** or **posterolateral branches** of the anterior division. They usually arise from the retropulmonary segment. "Left anterior descending" seems a poor term to describe the artery seen in specimen R3.

4: When the left main branch trifurcates, I term the intermediate artery **the lateral division.** It has been termed the diagonal branch. This creates confusion with (what are described here as) anterolateral branches; also, the vessel usually descends vertically, not diagonally, across the lateral wall of L.V. The term "median" also has been used. Median may be synonymous with intermediate; however, its association in anatomy with the median plane may create confusion. The lateral division should be differentiated from, and are less common than, lateral branches of the anterior and posterior divisions.

The lateral branches of the anterior division have been termed the first diagonal branch—the anterolateral branch being the second diagonal branch. Lateral branches of the posterior division are large and were found in 16 of 100 hearts.*

Note: On the next 45 pages, specimens exemplify the various branches defined here. The specimens from which these four figures were made are as follows: The specimen number (normal type e.g. R60) precedes the figure number (bold type) and page number (normal type) where the specimen appears.

1. R60 = **166—4, 36—1, 59—3** and **4, 199—4–6**; R50 = **167—5C**, 200, 201; R6 = 187; P3 = **166—4, 152—3, 153—6**; R5 = **175—5** and 6.

2. L52 = **166—5**, 204; R25 = 170; L2 = 208; P17 = **166—5**, 184, 185; L9 = **188—2**; R28 = 209.

3. L62 = 176, 177; R67 = **174—1–4**; L6 = **167—5A**, 202, 203; P8 = **166—4, 69—6**; **188—3**; P1 = **166—3**, 192—196; R3 = **167—4B**, 177.

4. R22 = 180, 181; P2 = 206; R16 = 168; R15 = **167—5B**, 169.

* See the comments on terminology in the addendum on page 178.

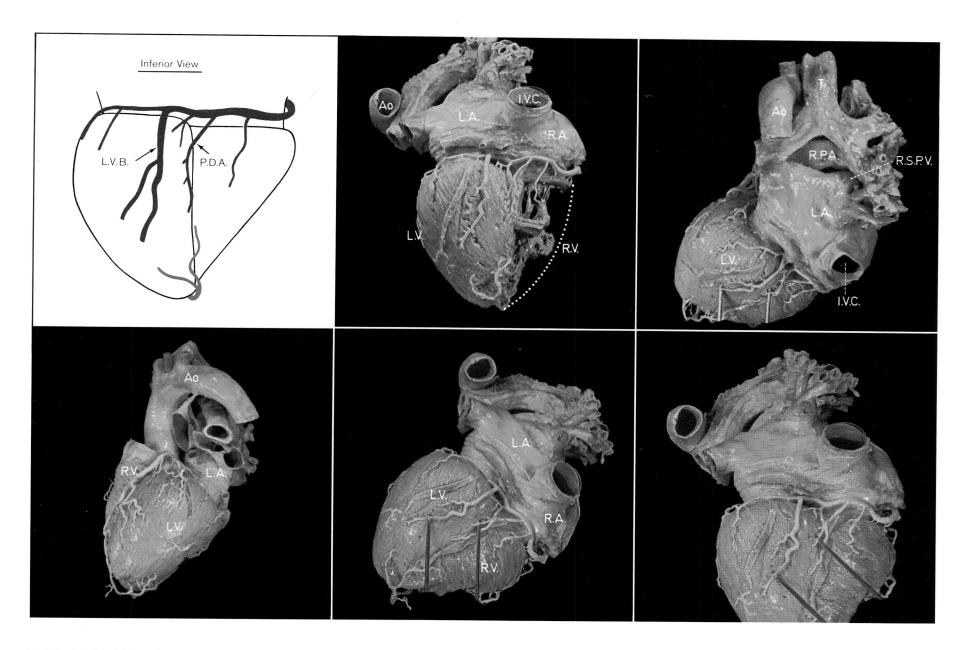

Inferior View

L.V.B.   P.D.A.

Ao   L.A.   I.V.C.   R.A.

L.V.   R.V.

Ao   R.P.A.   R.S.P.V.   L.A.   L.V.   I.V.C.

Ao   R.V.   L.A.   L.V.

L.A.   L.V.   R.A.   R.V.

II. The Optimal Examination of a Wall of the Left Ventricle and Its Related Vessels

This matter is discussed in relation to the lateral wall (pages 29 and 149) and the septal wall (page 173). We will now simulate the effect of tilting the x-ray tube, or the patient, in the study of the posterior wall of L.V.

1 and **2**: Inferior view: The axes of the vessels and the axis of posterior wall of L.V. are parallel. The vessel axis (see **166—5**) determines the optimal view in a horizontal plane examination; in this perpendicular plane examination—the optimal laboratory view—the axis is immaterial. In **2**, the inferior wall has been largely removed to establish the relation of the "posterior descending artery" to the septal wall—the sulcus is usually not recognizable.

3: P.A. view: Here, in contrast to **2**, the branches on the posterior wall are seen obliquely and end-on. In passing, note that the tracheal bifurcation is 2.8 cm above the left atrium.

4: Left lateral view: The plane of the posterior wall of L.V. is elevated 45° above the horizontal. This angle determines the angle of elevation.

5: The P.A. view is seen after **the specimen has been rotated 45° anteriorly** on its transverse axis. The plane of the posterior wall is now at a right angle to the line of examination. The interventricular and A.V. sulci are oblique.

6: The photograph shown in 5 has been rotated 45°: The disposition of structures in this view and the optimal laboratory view in **2** is identical.

Summary:
I. **The planes of the three walls of the left ventricle**
(1) **The posterior wall** is essentially uniplanar; in contradistinction, two areas require identification in each of the other two walls. These areas will be designated A, which requires an elevated view, and B, which is well seen in a horizontal plane view.

(2) **The lateral wall**
A—**the area adjoining the summit** is seen on page 29; the related, highly important proximal parts of the divisions of the left coronary artery are seen in **148—1–6** and **155—1**.
B—**the area of steep descent** is seen in **107—5** and in many photographs.
(3) **The septal wall**: An arbitrary demarcation—a horizontal line intersecting the superior papillary muscle—can be visualized in **115—4**.
A—**the prepulmonic area** is distinguished by the crossing of the large (not uncommonly 2.0 mm in diameter) left superior septal artery.
B—**the inferior septal area**, optimally seen in an R.A.O. horizontal plane view—see page 173.
II. **The angle of elevation** of the plane of examination
(a) varies inversely with the axis of L.V. in a frontal plane.
(b) The angle will not be as large for the prepulmonic as that needed for the area of the summit.
Note: This specimen is diagrammed—R 18 (**167—1**) and shown in **199—1–3**.

165

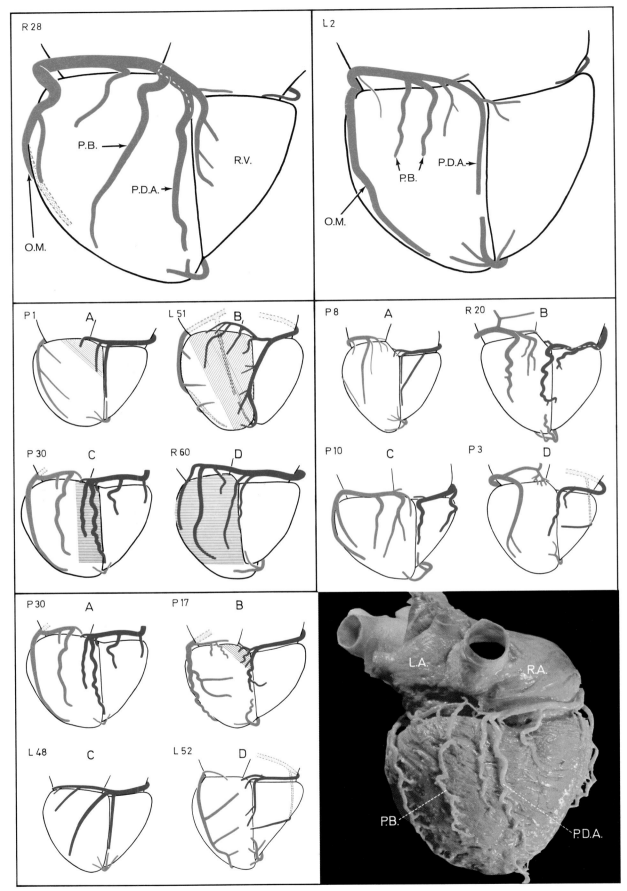

III. The Arterial Branches to the Posterior Wall of the Left Ventricle

The anatomy of the crux (seen on page 68) is a prerequisite to the study and understanding of this matter. These drawings are derived from specimens shown in photographs in the atlas except for P3 (in **4**) which appears in a drawing (**153—6**).

1 and **2**: Inferior view of two specimens seen on pages 208 and 209: The left coronary artery supplies the posterior descending branch, branches to the inferior wall of the right ventricle, and the entire left ventricle, and to it is applied the term, **dominant left coronary artery**. Such arteries show variations in their branches—two examples are: (a) In **1**, the posterior descending is larger than the anterior interventricular branch, suggesting its larger than usual role in the supply of the septum. In **2**, the reverse occurs. (b) As seen in both specimens, an obtuse marginal branch is commonly present; this branch may be large—in **2** it is larger than either the posterior part of the posterior division or the posterior descending branch.

3: The dominant right pattern: Note the variations in both the size and shape of the area supplied. In the presence of a diminutive posterior division of the left, the right coronary artery may contribute to the supply of the lateral wall of L.V.—see D.

4: The balanced pattern of supply: In these four specimens, the right coronary artery provides the posterior descending branch which supplies only a small area of L.V. adjoining the posterior I.V. groove. The left supplies the remainder of the left ventricle and the A.V. node—the node does not always (as is often stated) receive its supply from the vessel which supplies the posterior descending branch. This misconception may be attributable to an incomplete knowledge of the anatomy of the crux.

5: The arteries on the posterior wall of L.V. may be parallel as in A, at right angles as in B or oblique to the axis of the wall, as in C and D.

6: This is a photograph from which the drawings **5A** and **3C** depicting the parallel axis was made. Branches passing from the right coronary artery in the posterior right A.V. sulcus to the inferior wall of the right ventricle are uncommon. Such a branch is seen here. The posterior I.V. sulcus or junction (page 85) is not recognizable and its ends are ill-defined. The artery labelled P.D.A. (posterior descending artery) may lie to the left of this junction.

On the next page, **the variations in the origin and course and occurrence of the posterior descending branch** will be divided into four groups: (1) **orthotopic**, (2) **retroventricular**, (3) **circum-marginal**, and (4) **absence**. In the orthotopic, the branch is located in the atrioventricular and interventricular sulci. In the retroventricular, the branch crosses the inferior wall of the right ventricle. In the circum-marginal, the branch arises anteriorly, crossing the anterior wall, the acute margin, and the inferior wall of the right ventricle en route to the posterior interventricular groove.

IV. The Posterior Descending Coronary Branch of the Right Coronary Artery—Its Variations

6 consists of theoretical possibilities. **3 B** is reported but not encountered in my dissections. All other specimens, from which the tracings were derived are found in photographs except for R 1 in **4**, which is shown in the drawing **181—6**.

1: The relative size of the posterior descending and left ventricular branches: With proximal obstruction, the surgeon commonly brings the graft to the main artery to the right of the crux. Cases will be seen, however, where it may be preferable to graft into the posterior descending or a left ventricular branch below the A.V. sulcus. Four variations may be seen which affect the possibilities for a distal anastomosis. In **1 A**, multiple, small, nongraftable, distal branches are present. In **1 B**, the posterior descending is the large graftable branch. In **1 C**, the left ventricular branch is dominant. In **1 D**, both the posterior descending and the left ventricular branches are large and suitable for anastomosis. When the left coronary artery is dominant, this determination may still be made. R 18 occupies page 165.

2: This is a photograph of the specimen seen in **1 A**.

3: Orthotopic variations: 3A, the "classical" posterior descending coronary artery, occupying the upper two thirds of the posterior interventricular groove—the anterior interventricular branch occupies the lower third; **3B,** the anterior interventricular branch, recurring high on the posterior surface; **3C,** dominance of the posterior descending artery; and **3D,** the origin of the vessel at the acute margin, whence it runs parallel with the parent trunk to the crux. Variation **4D** is common; variations **3B** and **3C** are uncommon.

4: The retroventricular variations: The artery may arise at the midpoint of the posterior right A.V. sulcus, or, as shown in the remaining three specimens, at the acute margin. From the acute margin, the artery may pass directly and obliquely to the I.V. groove, or first run along the acute margin and then medially to the groove. The specimen in **2** above in an example of the latter. These patterns are all very common. In **4B** and **C**, two arteries run in the groove sequentially.

5: The circum-marginal P.D.A.: This vessel may constitute, or contribute to, the supply of the area of the posterior I.V. groove and septum. In L 6, both the left and right coronary arteries first give off a smaller branch which runs in relation to the left ventricular and tricuspid ostia; the arteries then pass obliquely or radially around the obtuse and acute margins to reach the posterior I.V. groove.

6: 6A, very rarely, a large branch of the right coronary artery supplies the septum, and branches from this could replace the posterior descending. **6B,** the anterior division of the left coronary artery supplies the entire ventricular septum, and no posterior branch is present. **6C,** is another theoretic possibility.

Note: This artery fails to run in the posterior I.V. groove so frequently that the less descriptive term "posterior descending" is preferable to "posterior interventricular branch".

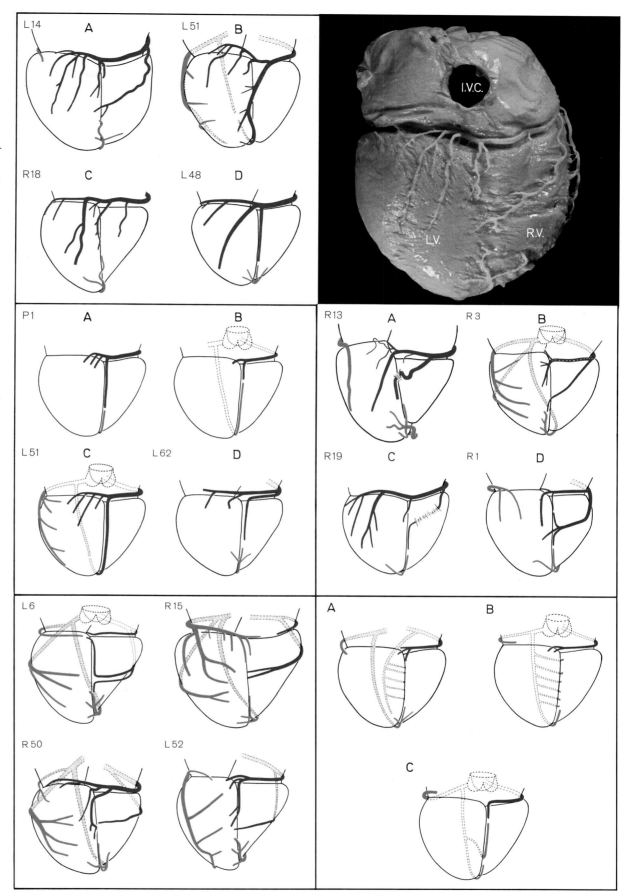

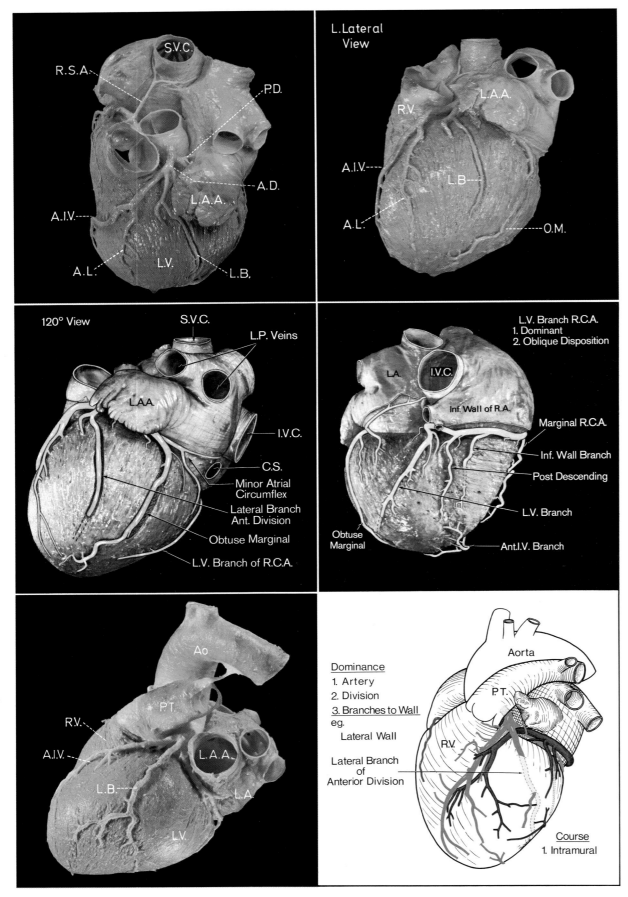

B. The Branches of the Anterior Division of the Left Coronary Artery

I. The Lateral Branch of the Anterior Division

On the four pages, 168–170, three specimens will be featured to exemplify the three types of branches from the anterior division to the free wall of the ventricle. These are (a) the anterolateral, (b) the posterolateral, and (c) the lateral. A fourth specimen demonstrates that a lateral branch may arise from the posterior division. In these specimens, we will coincidentally observe (a) the relative size of the posterior descending and L.V. branches of the right coronary artery, (b) the relation of the axis of the posterior wall of L.V. to that of its arterial branches, and (c) four variations of the posterior descending branch.

Specimen A: This specimen (shown in **1–4**) is also seen on pages **6—1–6, 15—1–4, 153—5** and R16 in **164—4**.

1: Superior left lateral view: The 5-mm-long left main branch is directed almost in the plane of the aorta. From the anterior division, a 3-mm lateral branch passes across the lateral wall of L.V. The posterior division courses directly to the ostium of the left ventricle, running with the latter to the obtuse margin, where it terminates as the obtuse marginal artery.

2: The lateral branch descends almost vertically across the lateral wall of L.V. in an intramural location. The obtuse marginal courses over the postero-inferior aspect of the obtuse margin, reaching the apex.

3: 120° view: The lateral branch extends only to the obtuse margin. The obtuse marginal branch courses intramurally. Note the large size of the left atrial appendage, its disposition in a frontal plane, and its attachment posteriorly on the lateral wall of the left atrium.

4: Inferior view: Observe: (a) The inferior right vertricular branch is unusual. Usually, only fine, intramural branches extend from the acute margin and the A.V. sulcus to supply the inferior wall. These are not seen in gross dissections. (b) The left ventricular branch: (1) it is larger than the posterior descending; (2) its oblique course is common—the triangular area of the posterior wall of L.V. between it and the obtuse marginal artery is devoid of significant branches. This is a common finding—an occluded trunk should not be suspected.

Specimen B, 5 and **Specimen C, 6** are nonattitudinal views. Observe: (a) When a wall of the left ventricle, in this instance the lateral, is examined, a branch will frequently tower above all others in size and apparent importance. A lateral branch commonly fills such a role. In specimen C, the size in external diameter of the three arteries in the coronary fossa are: the lateral branch = 3.5 mm; the continuing anterior division = 4.0 mm; the posterior division = 3.0 mm. In specimen B, the lateral branch is 4 mm in size. Comment: Lateral branches of the anterior division are: (1) **common**—see page 178; (2) **large**—these specimens are typical; (3) seen in an **intramural, vertical** course as they descend the lateral wall of L.V. (4) They must be differentiated from a lateral branch of the posterior division.

The Lateral Branch of the Posterior Division

Specimen D—1–6 is seen, R 15 in **164—4** and **167—5**.

1: A nonattitudinal superior left lateral view: The left main branch is 8 mm in both diameter and length. High in the interventricular groove, the anterior division gives off an intermediate anterolateral branch (A.L.). The posterior division essentially bifurcates into a larger lateral (L.B.) and a large branch seen running in the lateral left A.V. sulcus. This is one of the few specimens where the posterior division is found in the depth of the A.V. sulcus—when the posterior left A.V. sulcus is reached (see **6**) it ascends onto the wall of the left atrium, however.

2: The left main branch emerges from the middle of the sinus, extending slightly anteriorly but at right angles to the wall of the sinus. The red bead marks the site of the commissure between the left and posterior aortic annuli. This specimen is seen in **25—2** as an example of clockwise annular rotation.

3: A left lateral view: Observe: (a) The large intermediate anterolateral branch courses intramurally in the 75° sector. The lateral branch of the posterior division passes vertically across the left ventricle, ending, not at the obtuse margin as did the lateral branch in the specimen in **168—1–4**, but continuing (see **169—6**) around the margin to reach the posterior I.V. groove.

4: Superior R.A.O. view: A rod retracts the right atrial appendage to disclose the large right sinus node artery. The conus branch (C.B.) passes intramurally like branches to the anterior wall of R.V. often do; hence, it is not seen in the next view.

5: R.A.O. view: After giving off a small branch which continues in the right A.V. sulcus, **the right coronary terminates as the large circum-marginal branch (M.B.)** which passes around the acute margin on its way to the posterior I.V. groove.

6: The lateral branch of the posterior division, a product of bifurcation, courses around the obtuse margin of L.V. to reach the posterior I.V. groove. After giving off an L.V. branch which passes intramurally and obliquely towards the apex, the second product of this bifurcation continues above the A.V. sulcus to supply a small intramural posterior descending branch—a dominant left pattern. With complete proximal obstruction, filling by collateral of the distal branches may not be seen. Imagine the consternation of the surgeon should he, anticipating a large posterior descending branch, attempt to bring a graft to it. Note that four arteries reach the posterior I.V. groove!

The axes of the arteries on the posterior wall of L.V. are disposed parallel, at a right angle, and oblique to its axis—an example of the need for the right-angle examination of this surface of the left ventricle and its arterial branches. In each and all of the conventional views which are made in a horizontal plane (of the patient and his heart), some vessel will be seen foreshortened.

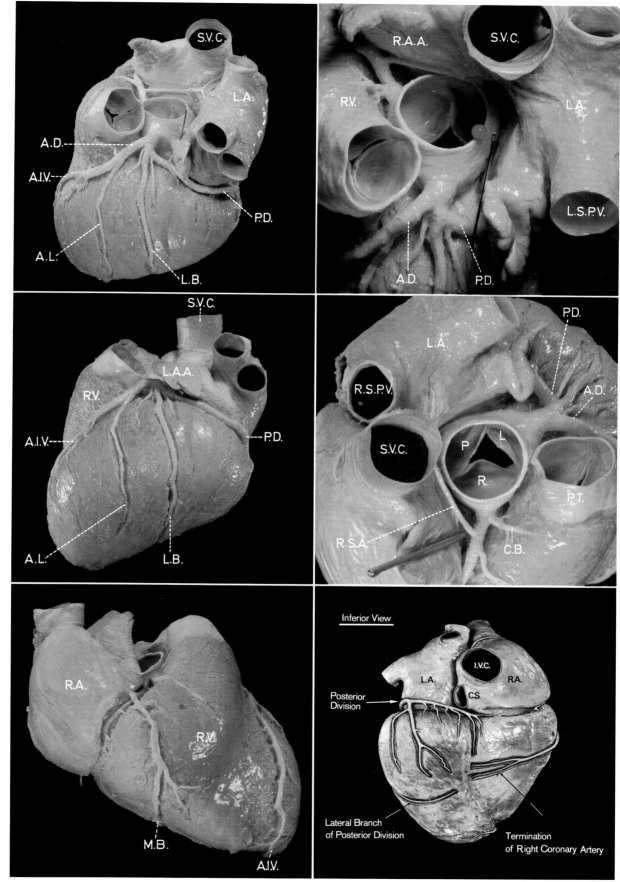

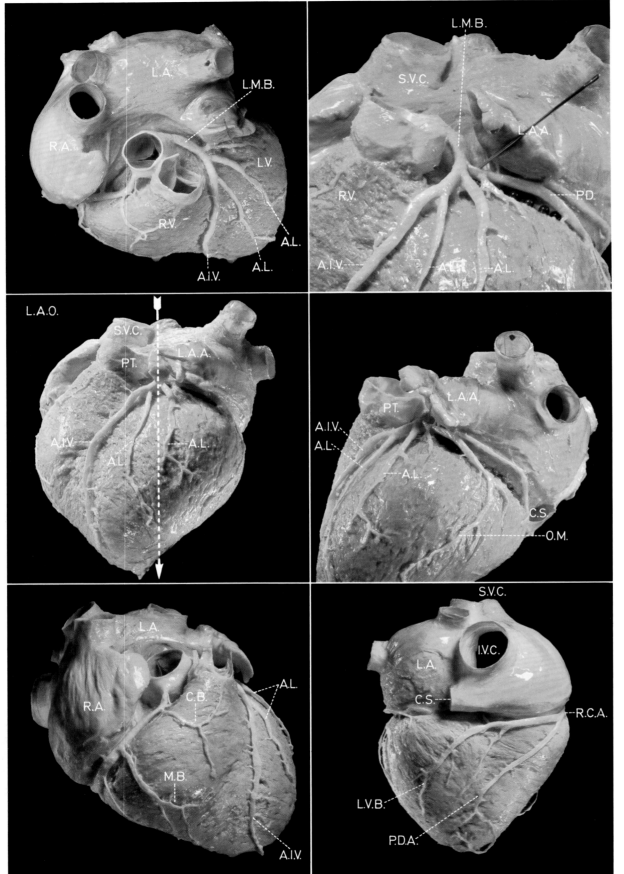

II. The Anterolateral Branches
of the Anterior Division

Specimen A: 1–6

1: In this superior view, the disposition of the vessels in the horizontal plane is seen. Observe: (a) The left main branch (L.M.B.) arises posterior to the midpoint of the left aortic sinus and is angled 30° anteriorly. (b) Two high anterolateral branches are given off (behind the pulmonary valve). The upper is directed towards 60°, continuing the course of the left main branch; the lower is directed towards 30°. (c) The right sinus node artery arises 36 mm beyond the origin of the right coronary artery—it runs counterclockwise around the superior vena cava—these two circumstances place it low on the anteromedial wall of the right atrium. Clamping the prominent appendage would not injure the artery. (e) In passing, note that the pulmonary annuli are rotated 30° clockwise from their usual location.

2: L.A.O. view with 10° elevation: (a) The left main branch is well seen because of its inferior axis. (b) The anterolateral branches are large. (c) The posterior division impinges on the retracted left atrial appendage.

3: L.A.O. view: The two anterolateral branches run on either side of the vertical line bisecting the field of examination: the anterior I.V. branch is well to the right—proximally it is not intramural! The appendage lies in place.

4: Left lateral view: The posterior division, after giving off a minor atrial circumflex branch, terminates as an obtuse marginal artery. The large atrial appendage is in a sagittal plane and covers the left coronary fossa. The reduction in size and proximal termination (it fails to reach the apex) of the obtuse marginal are concordant with the well-developed branches of the anterior division to the lateral wall of L.V.

5: A superior R.A.O. view: Although there are wide variations in the number and the location of origin of the branches to the anterior wall of R.V., frequently, as seen here, two branches dominate, an infundibular and a marginal. Here the former branch arises 2 cm below the orifice. The term, marginal branch, is imprecise; it may imply either the origin at, or the supply of the wall at and above, the acute margin.

6: The inferior view: At the acute margin, the right coronary artery bifurcates; the lower branch runs obliquely to the posterior I.V. sulcus (see 167—4). The larger upper branch continues in the posterior right A.V. sulcus to the crux, whence it crosses the left ventricular wall obliquely, anteroinferior to the posterior left A.V. sulcus, and reaches the obtuse margin.
The left ventricle may be divided (see page 33) into lateral, posterior, and septal walls which comprise approximately 40%, 30%, and 30% of its mass. In the next specimen, the contribution of the various arterial components to its total perfusion will be estimated. The computations are not exact but can be offered as evidence that the separation of coronary disease into three groups with "one-", "two-", or "three-vessel disease" is so imprecise as to be of little value.

170

III. The Posterolateral Branch of the Anterior Division

Specimen B—1–6, is R3 in **164–3** and **167–4**

1: The left lateral arteriographic simulation: The lateral wall of L.V. receives two large branches from the anterior division—the anterolateral and the posterolateral. The posterior division terminates as a posterolateral radial branch which wraps around the ventricle devolving into three branches which provide the major supply to its posterior wall.

2: Inferior view: The 2.5 mm posterolateral branch, in addition to supplying a major portion of the lateral wall, supplies about 15% of the posterior wall of L.V. as shown by the stippled area.

3: A superior lateral view: Just beyond its origin, the posterolateral branch (P.L.B.) gives off a 1.5 mm branch. It then passes intramurally where it remains for the remainder of its course. A large intermediate anterolateral branch is present.

4: An inferior view of the obtuse margin, showing the radial or circummarginal course of the posterior division above and the posterolateral branch below.

5: The right coronary artery supplies two large lower branches to the anterior wall of R.V.—one originates at the midpoint of the anterior right A.V. sulcus and the second at the acute margin. Contrast the large anterior interventricular artery and the small branches of the right coronary artery in the posterior I.V. sulcus.

6: An inferior view (its drawing is seen in **2**): Observe: (a) The right coronary artery bifurcates at the acute margin. (b) The branches from the left coronary artery to the posterior wall of the left ventricle exhibit a transverse disposition, in contrast to the oblique course of the L.V. branches from the right coronary artery in the specimen in **170—6**.

The Perfusion Partition of the Left Ventricle

The Right and Left Coronary Arteries: The "dominant right" supplies the A.V. node and about 5% of the posterior wall of L.V. Examination of the arteries in the I.V. grooves suggests that approximately 90% of the septal wall is supplied by the anterior division; hence, only 4.5% (1.5% and 3%) of L.V. is supplied by the right.

The Divisions of the Left Coronary Artery: (1) The posterior division supplies approximately 80% of the posterior and 10% of the lateral walls—i.e., 24% and 4%=28% of L.V. (2) The anterior division, therefore, supplies 67.5% of L.V. The potentially large role of the anterior division requires emphasis. Is not the (presumed descriptive) term, left anterior descending, less appropriate than the more general term, anterior division, in the designation of this artery?
In a conventional horizontal plane arteriogram this posterolateral branch might be misinterpreted as a branch of the posterior division.

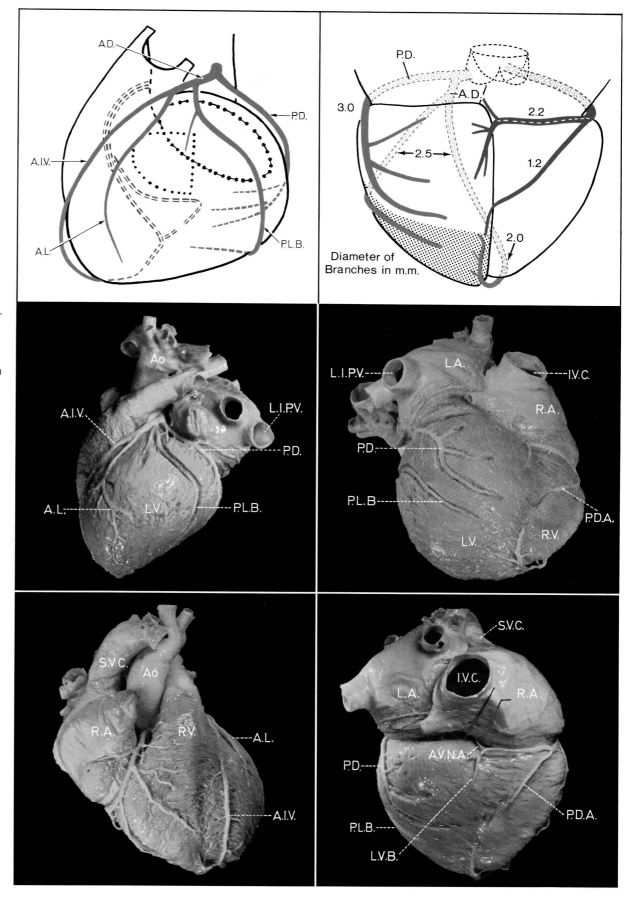

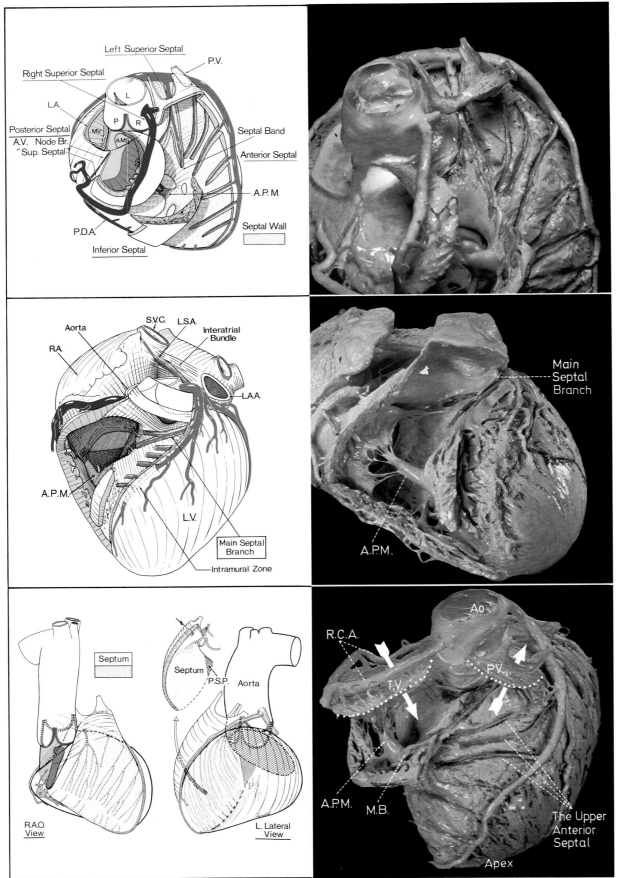

C. The Septal Branches

Except for **3, 4,** and **5,** all photographs and drawings on these two pages are from a single specimen from which the right ventricular walls have been removed, leaving a rim in relation to both the tricuspid and pulmonary ostia and a strut projecting from the inferior attachment from which the inferior and anterior papillary muscles arise. In **173—2,** the tricuspid rim has been removed.

1 and **2:** A superior R.A.O. view: The septal branches at the five attachments of the right ventricle to the A.V. unit are underlined in the drawing. In **2,** observe: (a) The 2.0-mm **left superior septal branch** arises at a right angle from the anterior division. In dogs, this branch is constant and supplies 75% of the septal wall. In the human hearts dissected in this study, a main septal branch of 1.5 mm or larger was found in 64 of 100 specimens. In 38, it entered the septum behind the pulmonary valve. It supplies the second and third divisions of the right bundle branch and may also provide branches to the first division and even the His bundle. It bifurcates into upper and lower branches. The former is directed towards the left ventricular ostium; the latter passes through the septal muscle band; it and the upper four anterior septal branches are directed towards and supply the anterior papillary muscle. Examine the left superior septal artery in **173—1, 2.**

3 and **4:** Superior L.A.O. and A.P. views: In 26 of the above 64 specimens, **the main septal branch** arose in the proximal 2 cm of the anterior interventricular groove, where the anterior interventricular branch usually courses intramurally. If the latter artery is dissected in this area, injury to the septal branch must be avoided. Occlusive disease of the anterior division most commonly occurs in its proximal 4 cm. The presence of a main septal branch and its relation to (a) the site of occlusion and (b) to the origin of the branches to the lateral wall is of obvious clinical importance. Geens and co-workers, in a study of 47 specimens, found a main septal artery in all—30% arose posterior to the pulmonary attachment and 70% in the upper anterior interventricular groove.

Note: This specimen occupies all of page 85.

5: In this drawing of an arteriogram, the six anterior septal branches are approximately 60 mm in length—the inferior septal branches barely penetrate the thickness of the left ventricular wall. Note the disposition of the septum in these views—particularly its upper portion.

6: A superior L.A.O. view: The septal wall and its branches continue the contour of the left ventricle. The predominant course of the upper anterior branches is towards the moderator band: They supply the anterior and often the inferior papillary muscle: Farrer-Brown emphasized their importance in the supply of the anterior wall of the right ventricle in occlusive disease of the right coronary artery.

Note: The terms septal arteries and septal branches are used here synonymously.

I. The Relation of Septal Arteries to the Operative Correction of the Tetralogy of Fallot

(1) In a normal heart (**80**—3 and 4), a **short posterior wall of the infundibulum** may be seen; this is a characteristic of the tetralogy of Fallot. When the main septal artery is a "left superior septal" (see **172**—2 and 6), it may be divided coincident to the resection of the muscle of this wall. The division of this 2.0-mm artery may effect myocardial infarction and represent the cause of cardiac failure in the postoperative period; pulmonary valvular insufficiency or the effects of ventriculotomy may not be the causative factors! (2) In a normal heart (**80**—1), **large high trabeculae** are present. In the above malformation, the septal band is often fragmented into multiple constraining trabeculae which require resection—an anterior main septal artery (see **172**—3 and 4), coursing through the base of one of these trabeculae, may be divided. (c) The three highest anterior septal branches, in relation to the septal band, are also in jeopardy.

Note: Many surgeons avoid resection of the muscle of the posterior infundibular wall; however, as suggested here, septal artery injury may occur when the trabeculae are divided at too deep a level.

II. The Attitudinal Examination of the Septal Arteries

1 and 2: R.A.O. view: In **2**, of the walls of the right ventricle, only the strut, to which the papillary muscles are attached, remains. Observe: The upper division of the left superior septal supplies the first division of the right bundle branch and extends posteriorly to the area of the His bundle. The arrow is shown to suggest that the popular terminology used to describe septal arteries results from the nonattitudinal examination of the heart with the apex below and the arrow disposed vertically. The terms in common use, anterior, posterior, and superior, should preferably be anterior, inferior, and posterior.

3 and 4: The specimen is shown from 30° to emphasize the distance between the **right margin of the septum** and the anterior interventricular groove in the L.A.O. examination. In cineangiograms, the motion of the septal arteries affords some information regarding the function of the septal wall.

5 and 6: A.P. view: The **right superior septal artery** is shown in the drawing to indicate its course and the proximity of the right coronary artery to the ventricular septum. (It was not seen in the specimen, which is not surprising in the presence of the large left superior septal branch.) In the bovine heart, this artery may supply 50% of the septal wall. In humans, the vessel is usually small in size and infrequent in occurrence (incidences are 12 and 20%—see Rodriguez *et al.*). **The inferior septal arteries** in the equine heart are large and predominate in the supply of the septum. In human hearts, the posterior descending branch may be larger than the anterior interventricular—a more equine type of pattern may occur. In the pig, the anterior and inferior septal branches share equally in the supply of the septum (Fehn *et al.*).

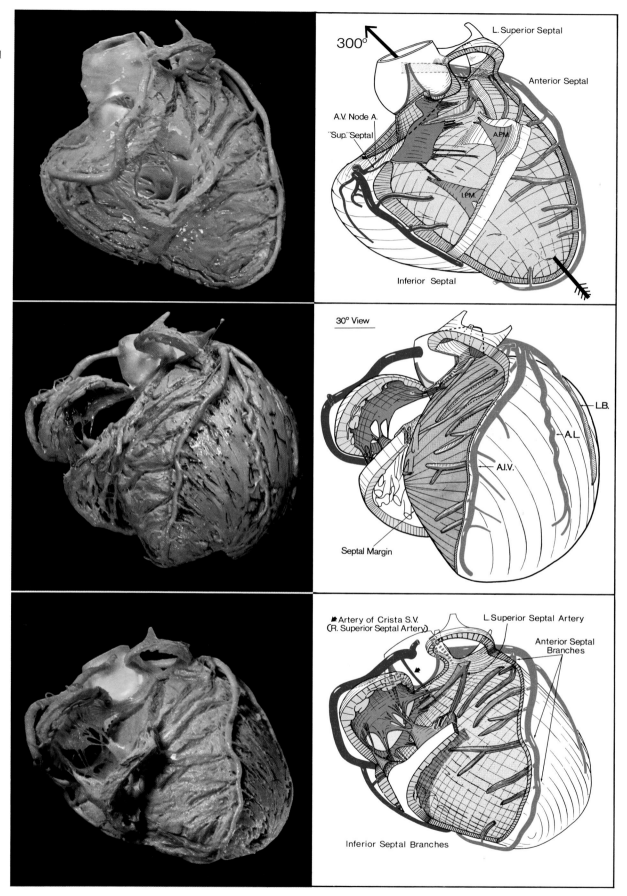

173

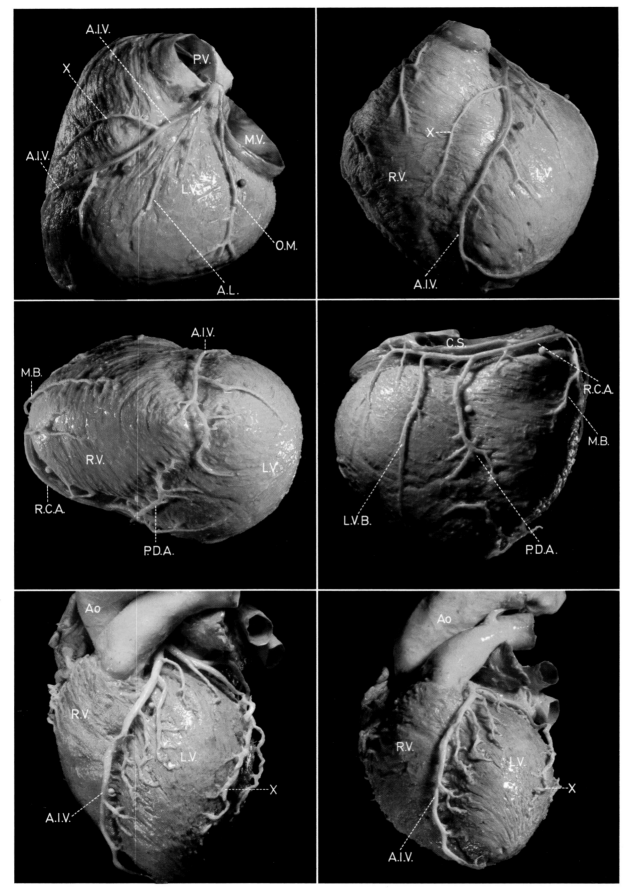

D. Variations in the Size and the Number of Branches

I. Variations in the Size of Branches— The Small Artery Heart

The size of an artery is of interest to the surgeon in the selection of patients for a bypass graft; it affects the area of supply (hence the need for surgery) and often determines whether a vein or the internal mammary artery will be used for the bypass. In coronary arteriograms, great discrepancy in size is seen within groups of the same weight, sex, and activity level. In some hearts, all the arterial branches are small in caliber—as demonstrated in specimen A. The second specimen, B, of almost identical weight, is presented for comparison. 3-mm beads are placed in relation to the branches to obviate the numerical description of their diameter. Note the contrast in the size of their arteries.

Specimen A: Views: **1:** Superior left lateral, **2:** L.A.O., **3:** Apex, and **4:** Inferior. The heart, without the atria and great vessels, weighs 260 grams. All the arteries are small. In **1** and **2:** The anterior interventricular supplies a relatively large branch (X), the left preventricular (see page **201—3**), to the right ventricle, the right 4/5 of which is usually supplied by the right coronary artery. Small arteries supply the right ventricle; these are much better studied when the injection and corrosion technique is used. In **4**, note the linear disposition of the right coronary artery as it passes superficially in relation to the crux; a U-shaped bend is not present. Such a bend has been emphasized and demonstrated in photographs by James—my repeated reference to its absence is not an attempt to deny its existence but to suggest that the relation of coronary arteries to the ostia of the ventricles is the fundamental consideration in this, as in all areas.

Specimen B: In **5** and **6**, the views selected are similar to **1** and **2**. At the time of the photography, this specimen was the best available to use for comparison with specimen A; however, more striking examples appear in this work: On page 205 (**1–4**), a specimen appears with unusually large normal branches. On that same page (**205—5**), a lateral view of this specimen (**174—5–6**) is used in portraying a **lateral axial branch** whose course divides the lateral wall of L.V. into anterosuperior and postero-inferior halves—it is seen here and is marked X.

As seen on the next page, it is helpful to compare **the size of the anterior interventricular and posterior descending branches**. A graft may be contemplated into either, usually the former. In the presence of proximal occlusive disease, the distal artery may be poorly, or not visualized in arteriograms; hence, it would be valuable if its size could be predicted. The following anatomic features are compatible with, although not determinative of, a small anterior interventricular branch—(1) a large posterior descending branch, (2) a large anterolateral branch located adjacent to the anterior interventricular groove, and (3) a large left superior septal branch. These observations are also of interest in assessing the pattern of blood supply of the ventricular septum.

174

II. Variations in the Size of the Anterior Interventricular Artery

Specimen C: 1 and **2:** A.P. and inferior views: The size of anterior I.V. branch is small. The posterior descending branch is dominant, supplying the lower 3 cm of the anterior I.V. groove—this is exceptional—it usually terminates at or just above the junction of the intermediate and lower thirds of the posterior I.V. groove. The variations in its origin and course, however (described on page 167), are numerous in their variety and occurrence.

Note: The anterior division is better shown in **61—6**.

Specimen D: 3: Superior A.P. view: A parallel anterolateral branch runs near and almost parallel to the smaller anterior I.V. branch. These two branches may be superimposed in the R.A.O. and lateral views but are separated in the L.A.O. view. A "parallel branch" may not only be confused with the interventricular branch in diagnostic studies and at operation, but also may be associated with diminution in size of the latter, as is seen here.

Specimen E: 4: An A.P. view of the aorta and ventricles: The large anterior interventricular branch is accompanied by a small parallel anterolateral branch. This is an example of heat injury to the aorta. The right coronary artery demonstrates the common pattern of branching, with large infundibular and marginal vessels.

Specimen F: 5 and **6**
5: The left lateral and inferior views: A dominant left pattern is seen. Of immediate interest is the presence of the multiple small branches which arise from the myocardial aspect of the large anterior interventricular branch. When the latter is disposed in an aerial or a superficial course, these branches may be dissected out. When it winds tightly around the I.V. groove, the vessels passing to the septum and to the adjoining right and left ventricular walls are short and may easily be injured if the artery is elevated above the surface of the ventricle. Examine the superior view of this specimen—**152—1**.

6: The lateral view: The above vessels and the left superior septal can be noted. Anterolateral and lateral branches additionally arise from this division. These are associated with a less well-developed obtuse marginal branch from the posterior division. The anterior interventricular is larger than the posterior descending branch. Since the branches of the anterior division are large and numerous, the diameter of the anterior division exceeds that of the posterior. This relationship is discussed on page 208. Note: In specimen C, one might assume from the examination of the arteries in the interventricular grooves that the origin of septal supply is predominately from below; however, a large left superior septal branch may be present to negate such an assumption.

Note: The specimens on these two pages are shown elsewhere: A = R 67 (**164—3**); B = **205—5**; C = L 51 (**166—3**) and **167—1** and **3**; D = **7—1-6, 31—4-7**; E = **108—5** and **6, 119—5** and **6, 168—5**; F = R 5 (**164—1**).

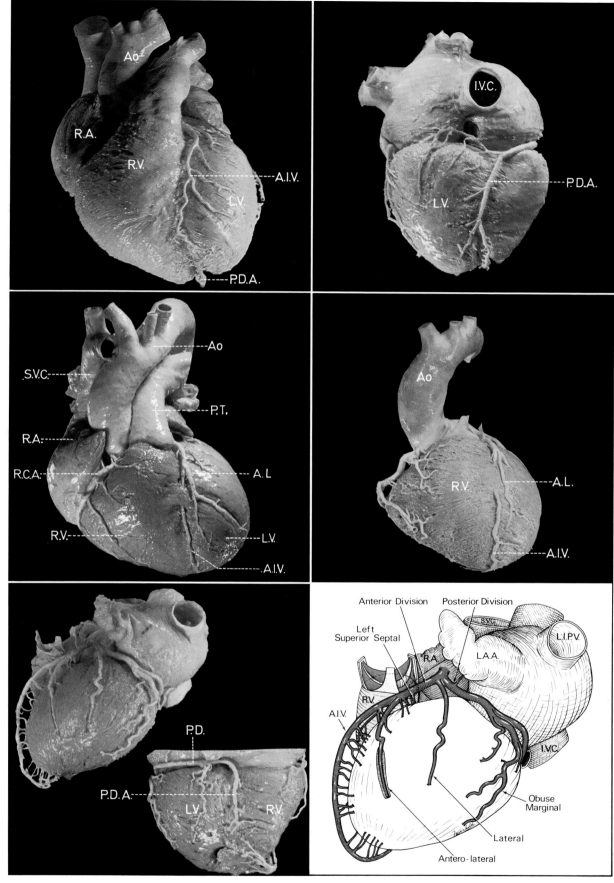

175

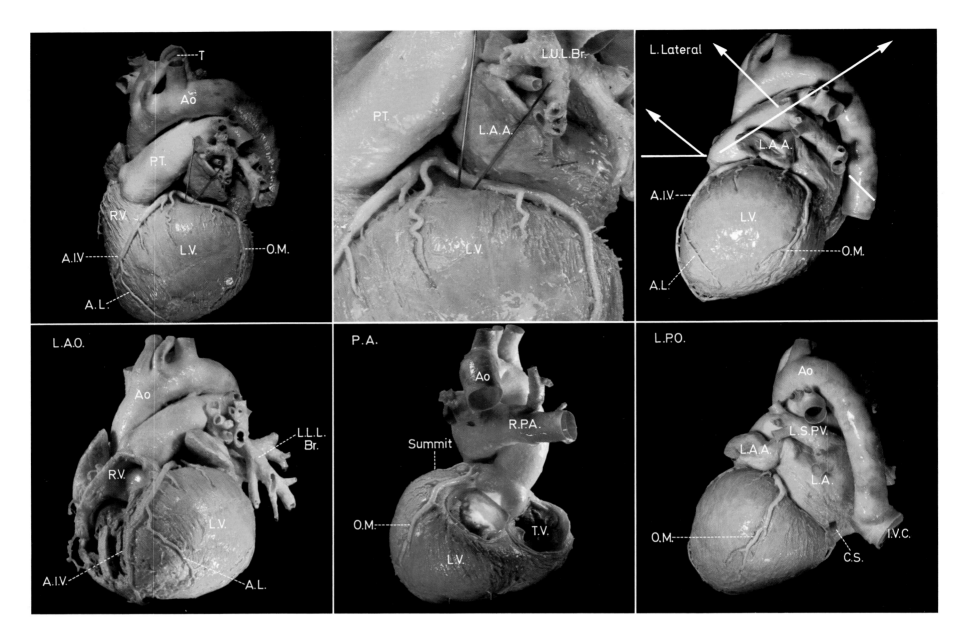

III. Variation in the Number of Branches—
The Sparsely Branched Heart

Specimen A, 1–6 and **177—1–4**, is the stoutly muscled, 360-gram heart of a 220-pound, muscular, previously healthy, male accident victim; in this large heart, the arteries are sparse and relatively small—in specimen B the opposite occurs. Specimen A is also a good example of a horizontal heart; it is shown in greater detail to demonstrate (a) the shape of the left ventricle and (b) the characteristic reduction in the vertical dimension of the right atrium, right ventricle, and left ventricle and the reciprocal elongation of the superior vena cava, the pulmonary trunk, and the ascending aorta. See page 79.
1: A superior left lateral view shows only four small (1.5 mm) branches between the low anterolateral and the obtuse marginal branch. A 2.1-mm left sinus node artery was present.

2: From the same perspective, closer inspection is afforded of these small branches and the 5.5-mm anterior and the 4.0-mm posterior divisions. The scale is 1:1.

3: An attitudinal left lateral view: The anterior wall of the right ventricle has been removed. Just above the apex, a 2-mm, low anterolateral branch (A.L.) is present. The only other significant branch is the obtuse marginal (O.M.). Apart from our primary topic, the arrows indicate (1) the obliquity of the pulmonary veins, and (2) the axes of the pulmonary ostium and trunk.

4: L.A.O. view: Observe: (a) The low anterolateral branch winds around the apex. (b) The left lower lobe bronchi (L.L.L. Br.) extend posteroinferiorly in the thorax. (c) Note the shape of the massive, globular left ventricle in this view.

5: P.A. view after removal of the atria and the postero-lateral wall of the right ventricle: Observe: (a) the well-developed left ventricle with its prominent summit; (b) the axes of the conjoined atrial attachment and the antero-superior segment of the left atrial attachment to the A.V. membrane form an angle of 110° (see page 47). The latter is seen between the transilluminated intervalvular trigone above and the anterior leaflet of the mitral valve below;

(c) the contour and spiral disposition of the great vessels. The isolated atria are seen in **59—1**. (d) The anterosuperior attachment of the left atrium, which overlies the intervalvular attachment of the anterior leaflet of the mitral valve, is perpendicular to the axes of both the base-apex length of the leaflet and the aortic bulb and the remainder of the lower half of the ascending aorta.

6: L.P.O. view: The obtuse marginal branch is 3.5 mm in diameter as it commences its intramural course. The obtuse margin is midway between the upper and lower borders of L.V. in this, the mirror image of which is seen in the R.A.O. view of an arteriogram. In its upper course the artery follows the margin. The posterior division gives no additional epicardial branches in the region of the A.V. sulcus such as a minor atrial circumflex branch.

Specimen A on this page is seen in L62 (**167—4**) and Specimen B is seen in P10 (**166—4**).

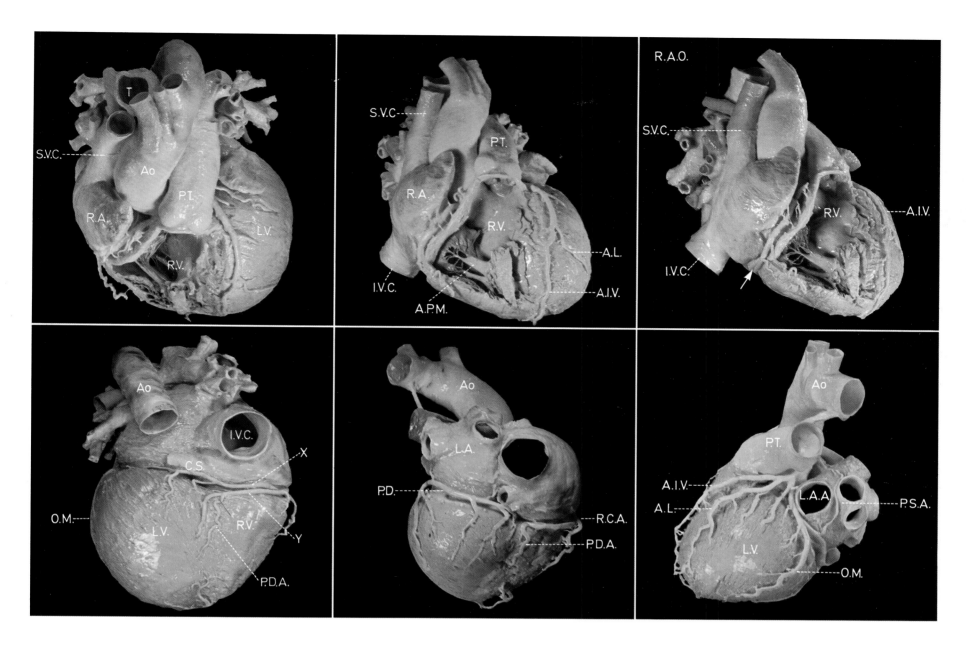

1: Superior view: The origin of the right coronary artery is seen. Note the great vessels in this view and in **176—1, 3,** and **4.** They are elongated.

2: 345° view: Observe: (a) The anterior interventricular branch (A.I.V.) is relatively large; it is 2.5 mm in diameter as it recurs to the posterior I.V. groove; it is larger than the posterior descending. (b) Note the inferior location of the anterior papillary muscle (A.P.M.).

3: An R.A.O. view: The 3.5-mm right coronary artery divides at the acute margin into the two branches (see arrow). In this horizontal heart, note the following: (1) The infundibulum of the right ventricle is shortened. (2) The pulmonary trunk is elongated; the angle of elevation of its axis is large (see **176—3**). (3) The right atrium is shortened—it extends slightly above the infundibulum (c.f. **77—5** and **6**). (4) The superior vena cava, like the pulmonary trunk, is elongated.

4: Inferior view: At the acute margin, the right coronary bifurcates; two branches, each 3.2 mm in diameter, run together in the posterior right A.V. sulcus to the crux. The upper branch (X) proceeds to the junction of the

lateral and middle thirds of the posterior left A.V. sulcus. The lower branch (Y) runs to the crux, where it provides the posterior descending and a parallel left ventricular branch. The branches to the posterior surface of the heart are unimpressive in size and number. Bifurcation of the right coronary artery at the acute margin is common; this is an example of one of the four patterns of the orthotopic type of the posterior descending artery described on page 167. The importance of recognizing this variation is apparent if confusion in the study of arteriograms and at operation is to be avoided.
This specimen shows (1) a large artery in the anterior interventricular groove, (2) a 3.5 mm obtuse marginal branch, and (3) an unimpressive 1.8-mm posterior descending branch and two similar-sized branches passing to the posterior wall of L.V. These few branches provided flow for this large well-muscled heart of a physically active, healthy man. When this paucity of large branches is encountered at arteriography, it does not, therefore, indicate occlusion at the take-off of a nonvisualized branch.

A Small Heart with Copious, Large Branches—A Contrast

Specimen B: 5 and **6:** The inferior view and the left lateral nonattitudinal view: A 220-gram heart of an inactive female patient who evidenced no signs of heart disease. Observe: (a) Six branches, each 3-mm or larger in diameter, are present between the anterior interventricular branch and the posterior descending branch of the right coronary artery. (b) Here, as in **160—5** and **6,** we see **one of the two types of the balanced pattern of circulation**—the posterior division terminates as a posterior branch which proximates and parallels the posterior descending branch. In **the second type** the posterior branch is well separated from the posterior descending. As defined (**166—4**), in both types the posterior descending branch originates from the right coronary artery and the A.V. node and the entire left ventricle, with the exception of tiny branches from the posterior descending, are supplied by the left coronary artery (page 69).

E. A Review of Branches

I. The Incidence of the Branches of the Left Coronary Artery in 100 Specimens

The branches 2.0 mm or larger in external diameter were recorded. In 9 instances a lateral division was present; no vessel was so classified unless it was comparable in size to the anterior or the posterior division. From the anterior division no branches of this size were found in 16 hearts; in 84 hearts, the following 127 branches were found. In 4 hearts the posterior division measured less than 2.0 mm in diameter. In the remaining 96 hearts the following 136 branches were found.

Anterior Division		Posterior Division	
Anterolateral		Lateral branch	16
Low	3	Posterolateral radial	5
Intermediate	59	Obtuse marginal	73
High	43	Posterior branch	30
Lateral	20	Posterior descending	12
Posterolateral	2		

Comment: The inclusion of hearts of different size creates difficulties when a size criterion is used for the branches. However, the following points seem important: (1) Anterolateral branches are common. (2) Lateral branches, though less common, are large and require emphasis. (3) The obtuse marginal branch is the commonest branch of the posterior division. (4) **The lateral view:** Many years ago, attention was directed to its importance in the x-ray examination of the chest; perhaps its value in the cineradiographic examination of the coronary arteries requires emphasis. It is useful in the separation of the branches on the lateral wall of the left ventricle and in the recognition of their division of origin.

II. The Anterior Interventricular Artery

The anterior interventricular sulcus has been reviewed on page 86. Now we will review the relationship of the artery to the sulcus. The aptness of the term, anterior interventricular branch (or artery) may be assayed by the examination of ten specimens. In the first five, the anterior wall of the right ventricle is in place; in the second five, it has been removed in one or more of the photographs. **In the first group**, the reverse-S course of the anterior division is seen on pages 202 and 209. The artery is seen in relation to the incisura in **174—1–4**. The large size the artery may attain is seen in **174—5** and **6** and **205—5**. **The second group** is made up of the following specimens: (a) pages 114, 115, and **76—5** and **6**; (b) pages 184 and 185; (c) pages 176 and 177; (d) **2—1–3**; **111—5**, and **6** and **208—6**; (e) **78—1** and **3**. It may be concluded, following this survey, that the term anterior interventricular artery is descriptive.

III. The Posterior Descending Branch

Lacking a suitable alternative, the traditional term, posterior descending branch, or artery, is used to denote either an artery running in the sulcus or an artery contributing to the supply of the sulcal area. The variations in (a) the origin, (b) the course, and (c) the number are great and in some instances none of the implications of the term posterior descending branch apply: (a) The artery may **arise anteriorly** and exhibit an important part of its course related to the anterior wall of the right ventricle. (b) The acute margin is inferior to the posterior I.V. sulcus (**31—1–3**); therefore, in many specimens (see page **167—5**) **the artery ascends.** (c) Often the term **denotes multiple branches.** The term posterior interventricular branch, evoking precise and often inappropriate inferences, seems more undesirable.

In coronary arteriography, multiple branches may descend in the axis of L.V. (see **166—5**) and the identification of the posterior descending branch may be difficult. What anatomic guides are of value in the identification of the posterior interventricular sulcus. (a) **The coronary sinus orifice** (seen on page 190) is (1) a variable distance above the ostium of L.V.—10 mm in the first specimen and 4 mm in the second. (2) It is located above the inferior commissure—both structures are 10 mm postero-inferior to the right fibrous trigone and the A.V. node. The orifice is probably the best available clinical guide (in arteriography) for the upper end of the posterior interventricular sulcus or junction. (b) **The posterior interventricular vein** has been termed the middle vein. (This term is certainly not descriptive, evoking the question: Middle of what? Even when the heart is viewed with the apex dependent, the vein bisects no surface or structure.) (1) In approximately 2/3 of hearts, it arises on the anterior surface of L.V. and in 1/3 at the apex. (2) It usually lies on the left side of the posterior descending artery. (3) It is always (James) superficial to the arteries in the crux. Its course between the terminus of the coronary sinus and the apical incisura roughly delineates the posterior interventricular "sulcus". Studies are needed to determine if, in fact, the coronary sinus orifice and the vein provide reliable arteriographic guides to the "sulcus".

IV. The Relation of Major Arterial Trunks to the Right Lateral Division of the Ostium of L.V.

During mitral valve replacement, we have noted the danger of arterial injury (a) in relation to the superior commissure (page **61, 62**) where a large vessel is often 2–3 mm from the ostium of L.V. and (b) at the right lateral border of the ostium where the A.V. node artery may be encircled by a suture (page 160). The arterial-ostial relationship may now be examined in each of the three arterial patterns.

A Dominant Left Coronary Artery

As a rule, it courses above the posterior division of L.V. When it reaches the crux, the A.V. node artery extends to the right fibrous trigone and the main trunk skirts the posterior margin of the posterosuperior process of L.V. and terminates as the posterior descending branch (**169—6, 175—5, 207—4**, pages 208, 209).

A Balanced Pattern

In **160—5** and **6**, the trunk runs in contact with the inferior commissure of the mitral valve. The relationship is less close in **177—5** and **6** and in **207—2**; essentially only the A.V. node artery is in jeopardy.

A Dominant Right Coronary Artery

Type III: Examine **174—4, 190—1**, and **199—4**: The superficial relationship would probably make arterial injury unlikely. Only in **205—4** is a centrally directed U-shaped bend present. Such a bend is often referred to. It is not often found in specimens; however, when present it is important—placing the trunk in jeopardy during valve replacement—see extreme examples on page 71.

Type II arteries are seen in **167—2, 181—5**, and **190—4** only in the first is the centrally directed U-shaped bend present. In contrast to the ostial course in the above specimens—a substial course is seen in **170—6, 198—3** (both Type III) and in **187—6** (Type II).

Addendum: The terminology used in this atlas was sent to the publisher in 1972; it was derived from observations made on gross specimens during the preceding 10 years and is consistent with observations made in coronary arteriograms. In the comprehensive reporting system prepared by a committee of the American Heart Association (April, 1975), the terms (in addition to those described on page 163) which are at variance with those used by me, will be noted. Those of the committee will be stated first: (1) posterolateral branch of circumflex = posterior branch (P.B.) of the posterior division; (2) atrial circumflex = minor atrial circumflex; (3) main left coronary artery = left main branch. As mentioned before, branch and artery are used synonymously. When is a vessel a branch or an artery? Perhaps the term, left main trunk, may be preferable to either. (4) The committee has divided the right coronary artery and the two divisions of the left into segments which are similar in plan to the spatial divisions used in this work; however, the details of their method requires examination of their report.

Chapter 13: The Course and Relations of the Branches of the Coronary Arteries

Introduction

A. The course of the coronary arteries in relation to the myocardium may be:

1. **The epicardial**—running essentially in contact with the surface of the myocardium.
2. **Intramural**—included here is the intraseptal course.
3. **Aerial**—running above the myocardial surface.
4. **Intracavitary.**

The intramural course was first described by Geiringer, who used the term "mural coronary". He noted that Tandler dismissed the phenomenon with the following remark "... only sometimes can one see a few myocardial fibres cross over them (the main coronary branches)

bridge fashion". Geiringer also quotes Crainicianu, "Sometimes however, I was able to observe how for example the Ramus descendens of the left coronary artery viz., after a variable course, digs itself more or less deeply into the cardiac muscle along the course of the interventricular groove to reappear on the surface after a few centimetres. In such a case I have asked myself what influence muscular contractions may have on the circulation in a big artery which finds itself in such an anatomical position." Geiringer answered, following his own study, that atheroma occurred only rarely in the intramural segment where the intima was thinner than in corresponding epicardial branches. Polacek has emphasized the frequency of the course and its effect on the histology of the artery—he used the term myocardial **bridges** and loops in reference to long ventricular and short atrial muscle segments covering an artery. In 1956, Edwards, *et al.*, in a study of 15 examples, found a lack of freedom from atheroma in the intramural segment. In 1958, Amplatz and Anderson reported the "angiographic appearance of myocardial **bridging**". I have long been impressed by the frequency of the intramural artery in specimens. However, I have never recognized an "intramural artery" in the arteriograms of patients in whom I encountered one later at operation. The aerial coronary, however, located peripheral to the myocardial blush, can be easily seen in arteriograms.

B. The relation of the veins to the coronary arteries is of apparent importance at operation. Also of interest is their relation to major anatomic landmarks, and the degree to which they provide radiographic identification of the latter. The cardiac veins consist of three systems: (1) The Thebesian: These small vessels drain a variable portion of the right atrium and ventricle and empty directly and usually individually into these chambers. The internal openings, foramina venarum minimarum, are best seen on the septal wall of the right atrium. (2) Anterior cardiac veins receive blood from the right two-thirds of the anterior wall of the right ventricle. (3) The vastly larger coronary system drains the remainder of the heart.

C. The major landmarks for consideration in the course and relation to arteries are:

1. **Anatomic**
   (a) The aortic sinuses
   (b) The three ostia
     (1) left ventricular
     (2) right ventricular—tricuspid and pulmonary
   (c) The three walls of the left ventricle
   (d) The three walls of the right ventricle
   (e) The three margins—obtuse, acute, and septal
   (f) Sulci—anterior and posterior interventricular
          —anterior and posterior interatrial
   (g) Others—the superior cavo-atrial angle
           —the summit of the left ventricle

2. **Radiographic borders**
   (a) The borders of the left ventricle
   (b) The borders of the heart

Anatomic terms should be descriptive and refer to the anatomic position. However in radiographic examinations of the heart we can define borders which refer to those parts which form the border in the specific views. Identification of vessels is facilitated if our knowledge embodies their relationship to these different borders. This fact strengthens the judgment that preliminary examination is needed in fixed views—I favor the classic radiographic ones.

Optimal examination of a vessel is carried out at a right angle to it. Hence, it is essential in the examination of each radiographic view to be constantly aware of the direction of the vessel. The direction is determined by its course, which can be established in relationship to the great anatomic landmarks and to the contour of the left ventricle in particular. As this study proceeds, it will be obvious that as a result of the multidirectional course of the arteries, multiple views in the horizontal plane are essential, and optimal examination of many segments of the vessels can only be afforded when either the x-ray tube or the patient is tilted to afford a right-angle examination (see remarks on pages 149 and 165).

Although aortic root injections are rarely used for the study of the coronary arteries in adults, filling of segments of both the right and left arteries may occur in selective studies as a result of collateral flow resulting from occlusive disease. Hence, their relations to each other are important; these are seen in the final five pages which are comprised of composite drawings made by the superimposition of photographs of the two opposite aspects of each of the four classic radiographic planes of examination.

In the study of a selective left arteriogram the following observations are made (a similiar method is used in the study of the right):

(1) In the first view studied, the number of branches is noted.

(2) Armed with the knowledge of anatomic landmarks and their relationship to the radiographic landmarks in each view the location of each branch may be predicted. After all view are examined the definitive identification of each branch is made.

(3) The role of each branch in the perfusion of one or more wall is quantitated.

(4) As a corollary the pattern of supply of each of the three walls is established.

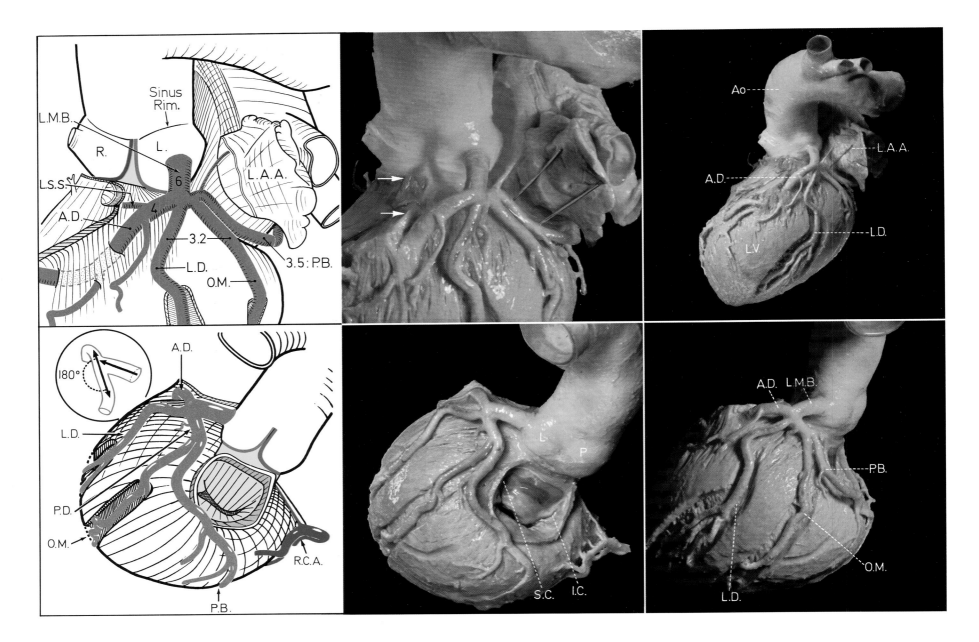

A. The Course of the Coronary Arteries in Relation to the Myocardium

I. The Intramural Course

Specimen A: In **1, 2, 3** the right heart has been removed—the pulmonary attachment extends between the arrows in **2**. In **4, 5, 6** the left atrium has also been removed. In **181—1–4**, the intact specimen appears.

1, 2, and 3: Superior left lateral view: Observe: (a) **The left main branch:** (1) Its origin is in the anterior half of the sinus, halfway between the sinus rim and the nadir of the left annulus (L). This low origin is unusual in humans. (2) It is 6 mm in diameter, 14 mm in length, and lies in a frontal plane. (3) It trifurcates. (b) **The anterior division:** (1) The retropulmonary segment extends anterolaterally behind the pulmonary attachment of the right ventricle. As it reaches the anterior I.V. groove, it promptly passes intramurally. (2) Two anterolateral branches (both 1.5 mm in diameter) are given off during this intramural course. (c) **The lateral division** (L.D.): A characteristic loop is seen just before

it commences its intramural course; this loop leads a surgeon to an intramural artery. (d) The **posterior division** almost immediately bifurcates into an obtuse marginal (O.M.) and a posterior branch (P.B.). (e) The external diameter of these vessels is indicated in mm. In the area of examination, the four main branches have a combined cross section which exceeds that of the main branch by 33%.

4 and 5: Nonattitudinal left posterior views: Observe: (a) The anterior and posterior divisions form an angle of 180°. (b) As the posterior division is directed to the ostium of L.V. above the superior commissure of the mitral valve, it forms an acute angle with the left main branch. (c) Note the large size of the obtuse marginal artery.

6: 120° view: (a) The occurrence of trifurcation has been questioned; this specimen is presented as positive evidence for this event. The intermediate vessel, **the lateral division**, must be differentiated from the more common

lateral branches of an anterior or posterior division. (b) Note the loops in both the lateral division and the obtuse marginal above their entrance into the muscle.

The intramural course of branches is frequently seen and **the following generalizations may be made** from my material: (a) **This course has been invariably seen** in (1) lateral divisions, (2) posterolateral radial branches, and with only a few exceptions in (3) lateral branches of either division. (b) **In a majority of specimens this course is seen** in the proximal 2–3 cm of the anterior interventricular groove. (c) An incidence of approximately 10–15% is seen in the anterior interventricular branch distal to its proximal 2–3 cm and in anterolateral branches. (d) In perhaps 5–10% of specimens the obtuse marginal branch runs within the muscle, as does the posterior descending branch. (e) **It has never been observed** in (1) branches from the right coronary artery to the L.V., or (2) L.V. branches from the posterior division which run in the axis of the ventricle to supply its posterior wall.

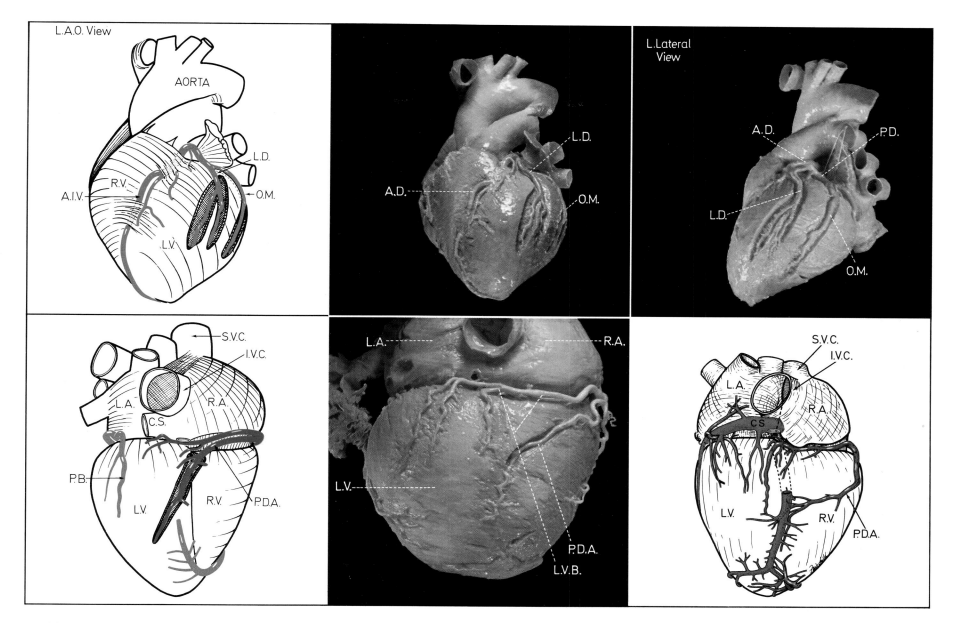

1 and 2: L.A.O. view: (a) Note the location of the lateral division and the obtuse marginal branch in this view. (b) The anterior interventricular branch (A.I.V.) courses intramurally in its proximal 24 mm and again in its midportion. This vessel is still 3 mm in diameter as it recurs to the posterior wall! (c) The two anterolateral branches are small.

3: Left lateral view: **The lateral division**: (1) Below, it runs in the axis of the ventricle; more often, a vertical course is seen. (2) As is usual, it is associated with small anterolateral branches. (3) When a lateral division is present, the posterior division is usually large and terminates either as a posterior branch to the left ventricle, as seen in this specimen, or as a posterior descending branch associated with a posterior branch to L.V. In either case, between the lateral division and the posterior branch to L.V., usually only small branches are seen—in this specimen however a large obtuse marginal branch is found. This specimen is diagrammed in **164—4** (R 22).

4: Inferior view: Observe: (a) In viewing the posterior aspect, the heart is rotated to the left to show the division

of the right coronary artery into posterior descending and left ventricular branches at the acute margin, whence they demonstrate a parallel course to the crux; this is seen in the specimen found on pages 176 and 177. (b) The posterior descending branch follows an intramural course. (c) The posterior division terminates as a posterior left ventricular branch; note its axial course—such branches have not been found in an intramural course.

Comment: (a) The **intramural course** is seen in the posterior descending branch of the right and in all branches of the left coronary artery with the exception of the continuing posterior branch which courses parallel to the axis of L.V. It has been suggested that the intramural course protects an artery from atheroma formation and causes occlusion simulation at arteriography. Beyond debate, however, is the fact that on external examination of the heart at operation, such vessels are hidden and may be divided by incisions in the right or left ventricle (branches to the anterior and inferior walls of the right ventricle often pursue an intramural course). Of importance also is the frequent necessity to expose

an intramural branch during operations for the correction of coronary artery occlusive disease. (b) **The branches of the left coronary artery are numerous and large**, in contrast to two specimens featured on the preceding four pages, where one displayed a general reduction in size—the "small artery heart"—and the other specimen demonstrated the reduction in the number of branches—"the sparsely branched heart". Vessel size certainly affects the ease of implantation of a vein graft at operation, and may be of significance in the time of onset and incidence of symptomatic occlusive disease.

5: **Specimen B** and 6: **Specimen C**: Observe: (a) When bifurcation occurs at the acute margin, the posterior descending may course (1) parallel to the L.V. branch in the A.V. sulcus—see **4**; (2) diagonally across the inferior wall of the right ventricle—see **5**; (3) the products of bifurcation and the posterior I.V. groove may form a rectangular figure—see **6**. (b) In **5**, note the rectilinear course of the left ventricular branch across the posterior A.V. sulci and the presence of three small branches which descend to supply this strongly muscled heart.

181

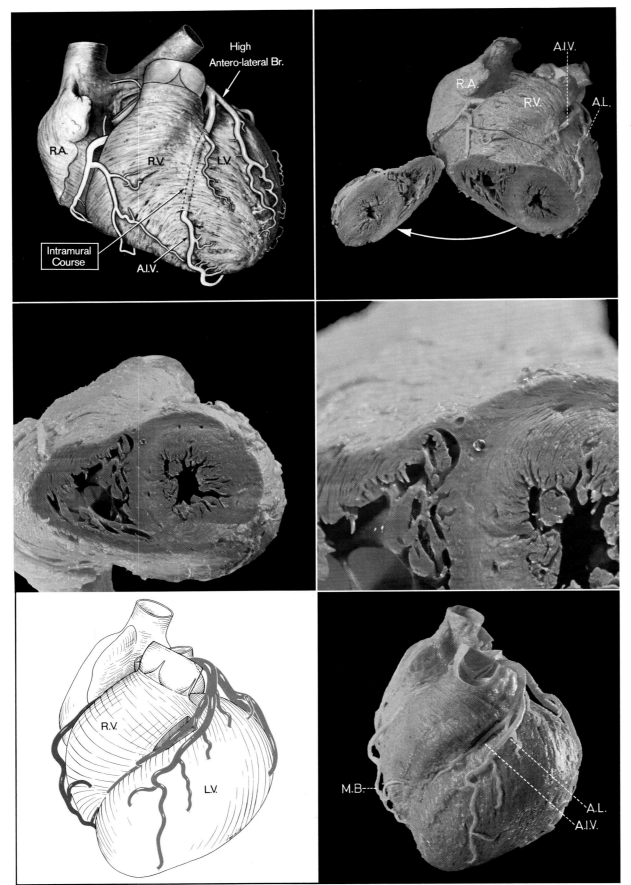

The Intramural Course
of the Anterior Interventricular Branch

Specimen A: 1–4

1: An A.P. view, retouched: The extensive intramural course of the artery is shown. This can also be seen in photograph **2**, which depicts the site of transection of the specimen. In **3** and **4**, observe: The artery is separated from the right ventricular cavity by the width of the head of a household pin. In aorto-coronary bypass operations, during the dissection of an anterior interventricular branch found in an intramural location, instances of penetration of the right ventricular cavity have occurred; repair of the resulting defect, without loss of the artery in the groove, may be difficult. This specimen demonstrates that such a dissection should be carried out with care.

Examine two additional views of this specimen, **152—3** and **153—6** and observe the following: (a) The supply of the lateral wall of L.V. is dominated by a large (3.5 mm) anterolateral branch (see **1** and **2** on this page and **152—3**). (b) On the posterior surface of L.V. (**153—6**), one large branch dominates—the posterior branch. On the borders of this wall, the posterior descending and the obtuse marginal are minuscule. See page 163. D.

Specimen B: 5 and **6**: High L.A.O. views: (a) The **anterior interventricular branch**: In the proximal 3 cm of the anterior I.V. groove, the artery runs intramurally. In the lower $^1/_3$ of the groove, a twig from the marginal branch (of R.C.A.) is present. (b) **The anterolateral branch**: (1) It is large. (2) It supplies and encircles the apex to reach the posterior I.V. groove. (3) In the R.A.O. view, this artery is usually above, but may be mistaken for the anterior interventricular branch. If disease is suspected in the latter, a graft could, by error, be sutured into the former. (4) In the presence of a large anterolateral branch, the anterior interventricular branch may be small.

Comment: In the majority of the specimens dissected, the intramural course was seen in the upper 2–3 mm of the interventricular groove. The artery may run for a short distance intramurally in the groove below this level. It has been suggested that bypass procedures to the anterior interventricular artery can be carried out with a beating heart by elevating the artery from the myocardium. In addition to the presence of the numerous septal branches which arise from the myocardial aspect of the artery, the common occurrence of the intramural location of this vessel should also be recalled when such a procedure is envisioned.

Before examining specimen C on the next page, review pages 138 and 139. The anomalous intraseptal artery to be studied accompanies the retroaortic translocation of the posterior division to the right aortic sinus, the "anomalous circumflex coronary artery". In **136—4**, the transseptal course was included as a possible route for anomalous arteries, and this is an example thereof. The branches with an anomalous origin and course are red and white striped.

The Intraseptal Course
of the Anterior Interventricular Branch

Specimen C, 1–6, is examined attitudinally. The atria, great vessels above their sinuses, and the anterior wall of the right ventricle have been removed.

1 and 2: L.A.O. view: A small branch, arising from an independent right aortic sinus orifice, passes anterior to the infundibulum, reaching the upper interventricular groove. Behind the pulmonary trunk, the 3.2-mm anomalous branch of the anterior division enters the septum. In this view, it would not be differentiated from a normal anterior interventricular branch. The remainder of the anterior division passes over the left ventricle as a lateral branch. The "anomalous circumflex" (P.D.) is above the ostium of L.V.

3 and 4: A.P. view: The anomalous septal artery, which replaces the anterior interventricular branch, enters the ventricular septum behind the posterior pulmonary leaflet. The vessel descends vertically in the septal wall, midway between the left cardiac border and the anterior right A.V. sulcus. Note the distance between the anterior I.V. sulcus and (1) the left cardiac border and (2) the anomalous septal artery.

5 and 6: R.A.O. view: The right aortic sinus is delimited inferiorly by the transilluminated right anterior fibrous trigone (yellow in **5**). Observe: Three orifices are present in the right aortic sinus: (a) the combined orifice for the right coronary and the "anomalous circumflex"; separate orifices for (b) the upper conal branch, and (c) the branch which passes across the conus to the anterior interventricular groove. The anomalous vessel in the septum is set back 1.5 cm from the surface of the anterior I.V. groove. Inferiorly, it emerges to follow the groove to the apex.

The incidence of this rare variation is unknown. However, its presence and misinterpretation as an anterior interventricular artery could effect a real surgical dilemma if a bypass into such a vessel were attempted. **The intramural course, rather than the intraseptal, might be suspected.** The identification of its lower extension onto the interventricular groove would be unlikely and the hazard of prospecting in the interventricular groove has already been indicated. The identification of such an artery is possible if, in the examination of an arteriogram, one observes the discipline of always establishing the location of the great surgical landmarks of the heart. In the A.P. view, the anterior interventricular groove is located to the left of the left ventricular ostium. In this specimen, when the mirror image of the P.A. view and the A.P. view were superimposed, it was evident that the artery descended vertically within the outline of the ostium. In the R.A.O. view, the vessel is displaced to the right of the anterior interventricular groove. It is so distant to the left cardiac border of the heart that suspicion should arise that this vessel is not in the groove.

Note: Hwang described a case of a solitary right coronary artery in which the anterior division traversed the ventricular septum (the posterior division passed behind the ostia of T.V. and L.V.)—these courses are seen in **143—3).**

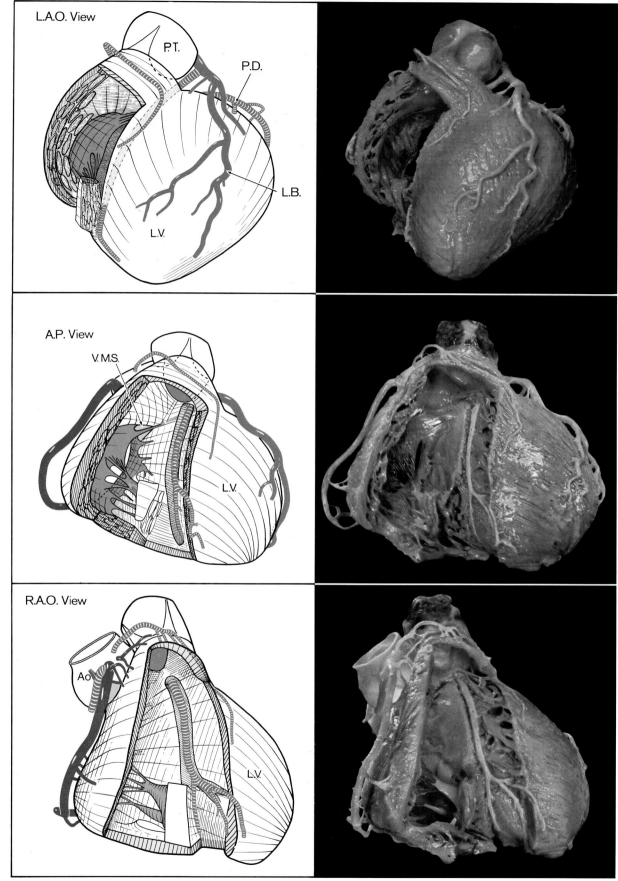

L.A.O. View — P.T., P.D., L.B., L.V.

A.P. View — V.M.S., L.V.

R.A.O. View — Ao, L.V.

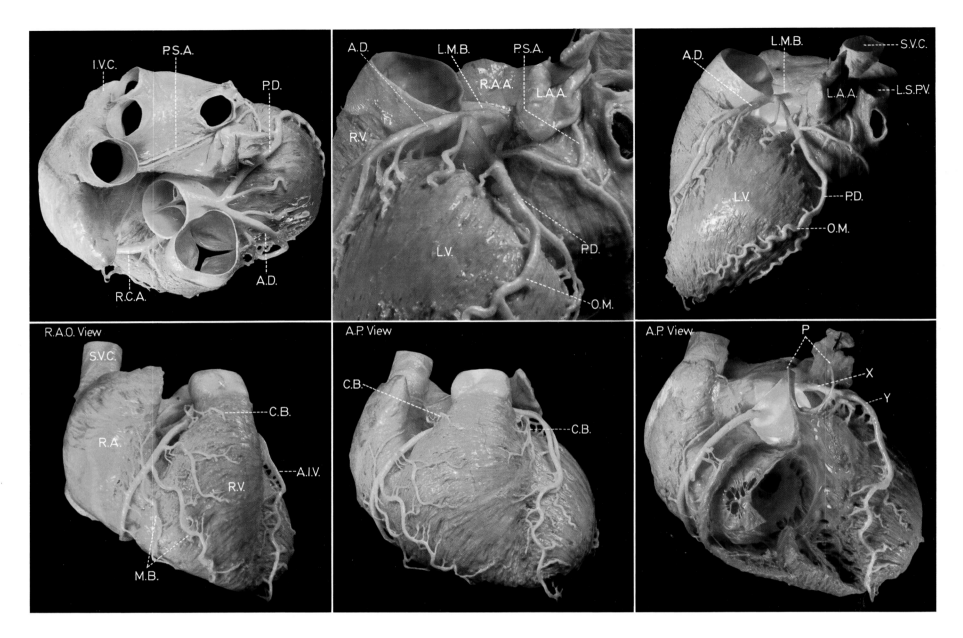

II. The Aerial Coronary Artery

A single specimen is seen on these two pages. The great vessels have been removed above their sinuses. This specimen will be examined in detail because it summates many of the features of the right and left coronary arteries described to this point, in addition to providing an example of the aerial course.

1: Superior view: Observe: (a) The anterior division (A.D.) is separated from the left ventricle by more than 1 cm in much of its course. (b) The posterior sinus node artery (P.S.A.) is directed anteriorly and to the right as it passes over the left atrium. It is located intramurally in the interatrial muscle bundle. (c) The proximal segment of the right coronary artery (R.C.A.), 1.5 cm in length, extends from the surface of the aortic sinus at a right angle. Its junction with the continuing segment is marked by an obtuse angle.

2: Left lateral view: (a) Both the anterior (A.D.) and posterior (P.D.) divisions are high above the ventricular

wall. (b) The posterior division terminates as the obtuse marginal artery. (c) Note the large atrial branch arising below the infolded atrial appendage (L.A.A.). Between the latter and the pulmonary veins, the posterior sinus node artery (P.S.A.) ascends on the atrial wall: its large branch continues to the posterior wall of the left atrium.

3: Left lateral view: The lighting is designed to demonstrate: (a) the height of the posterior division above the surface of the left ventricle; (b) the anterior and horizontal axis of the left main branch (L.M.B.) (which appears as a dark band silhouetted against the transilluminated aortic sinuses).

4: R.A.O. view: The right coronary artery supplies four superficially located branches—an upper infundibular (C.B.), an intermediate, and two marginal (M.B.) to the anterior wall of the right ventricle. The latter two pass obliquely to the acute margin. A small right anterior atrial branch is present.

5 and **6**: A.P. views: In **6**, the anterior and posterolateral walls of the right ventricle and the pulmonary valve, with the exception of the posterior annulus (P), have been removed. Observe: (a) The retropulmonary (X) and (anterior) interventricular (Y) segments of the anterior division are seen in their aerial course high above the surface of the ventricle. (b) All the branches to the right ventricle (from both the right and left coronary arteries) are superficial in location. (c) The left infundibular or conal branches (C.B.) are well seen. Important collateral circulation across the anterior wall of the right ventricle occurs between the following: (1) the right and left conal branches, (2) the marginal branches and the apical complex (see page 208) and the septal arteries in relation to the attachment of the anterior papillary muscle. (d) For the details of the interior of the right ventricle, see **153**—**1–2**.

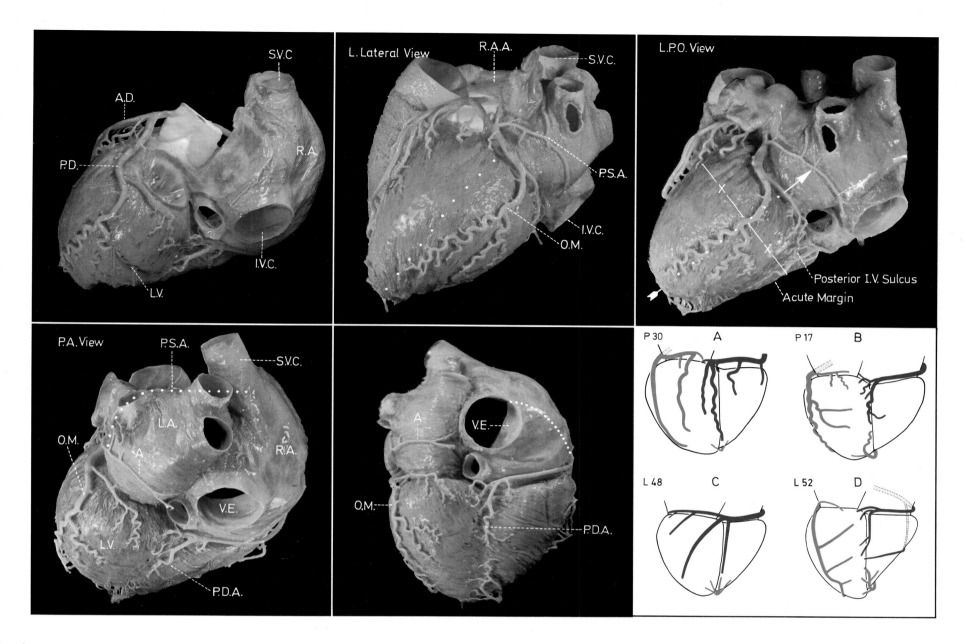

1: Superior P.A. view: The left atrium, with the exception of its septal wall, has been removed, disclosing the aerial course of both divisions of the left coronary artery.

In 2, 3, and 4, we will (a) plot the course of (1) the obtuse marginal artery and (2) the posterior sinus node artery and (b) observe the course of the large high atrial branch.

2: Left lateral view: A dotted line is roughly midway between the anterosuperior and the postero-inferior borders of the left ventricle. Observe: (a) **In this view, the obtuse marginal artery runs along the junction of the upper $^3/_4$ and the lower $^1/_4$ of the lateral wall of L.V.** (b) Plot the course of the posterior sinus node artery from its origin to the superior cavoatrial angle.

3: L.P.O. view: An incomplete arrow marks the axis of the obtuse margin; the arrow is approximately midway between the anterosuperior border of the left ventricle and the acute margin. Note the proximity of the postero-inferior border of the left ventricle to the margin.

4: The P.A. view is seen before removal of the left atrium. Observe: (a) A large atrial branch (A) passes from its origin (from the sinus node artery) to the atrial septum. (b) In this view, the obtuse marginal artery runs along the posterior aspect of the left border of L.V. (c) Visualize the course of the posterior sinus node artery (marked by white dots). Along the lateral wall of the left atrium, it is almost vertical; during its horizontal path across the superior wall it is above the level of the aortic sinuses, hence above the area visualized in a coronary arteriogram.

5: The inferior view: Observe: (a) The posterior wall of the left ventricle is, in large part, supplied by branches which originate from the obtuse marginal artery (Type I) and cross the wall perpendicular to its axis. The specimen (1) attracts attention to the large area of L.V. which may be supplied by this artery and (2) may be used to champion the view that the cause of clarity and precision is served by thinking of the origin, course, termina-

tion and mode of branching of the posterior division rather than attempting to locate a branch which can be termed the circumflex, although it be only 1 mm in diameter, and to term the obtuse marginal a branch thereof, although it be 3,5 mm in diameter. (b) The triangular area of L.V. below its posterior superior process is supplied by the right coronary artery. This is a common pattern of supply. When the area is infarcted, the most common type of posterior ischemic aneurysm may result. (c) Note the valve of the inferior vena cava (V.E.); it extends above the anterior portion of the orifice; its attachment forms the posterior border of the inferior wall of the right atrium; the lateral border of this wall is indicated by the curved dotted line.

6: This drawing depicts the relationship of the axes of the left ventricular branches supplied by the right or left coronary artery to the axis of the posterior wall of the left ventricle. The vessels may be parallel, perpendicular, or oblique to the axis of L.V. B is a tracing of 5.

185

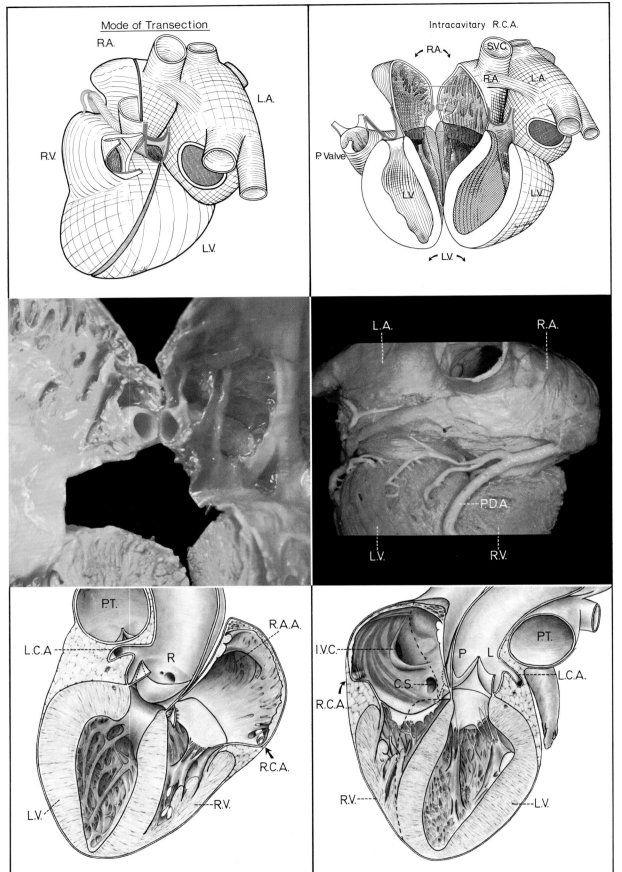

Mode of Transection

R.A.

L.A.

R.V.

L.V.

Intracavitary R.C.A.

P. Valve

SVC

RA

RA

LA

LV

LV

L.A.

R.A.

P.D.A.

L.V.

R.V.

P.T.

L.C.A

R

R.A.A.

R.C.A.

L.V.

R.V.

I.V.C.

C.S.

R.C.A.

R.V.

P

L

P.T.

L.C.A.

L.V.

III. The Intracavitary Course

The Intracavitary Course of the Right Coronary Artery

Specimen A: 1–6: This specimen was used some years ago to study the cross-sectional anatomy of the heart, at a time when my interest in coronary artery anatomy had not received the stimulus of the surgical developments of recent years.

1: Superior left lateral view: The transection passed through the midpoint of the left aortic annulus and the commissure of the posterior and right annuli.

2: The two segments are distracted. The square area outlined in red will be seen in photograph **3**.

3: 1.2:1.0 magnification: Observe: (a) For a distance of 27 mm, the artery runs in the cavity of the right ventricle. (b) The artery is 7.0 mm in diameter.

4: The inferior view: Observe: (a) The right coronary artery emerges on the surface of the posterior right A.V. sulcus to the left of the acute margin. (b) After giving off small L.V. branches, the artery terminates as an unusually large (5.0 mm) posterior descending artery (which is associated with a small anterior interventricular branch). This specimen is an example of a dominant right coronary Type I; this classification and term might obscure the important role of its posterior descending branch in myocardial perfusion and conceivably blunt the necessity of its revascularization. This is another example of the problems which may be incurred by the use of the term, dominance, in reference to the right and left coronary arteries. As stated on page 133 the role of every branch in the perfusion of the left ventricle requires quantitation.

5 and **6**: The halftone drawings were made from the tracings of the photograph; otherwise, the "unappreciated" artery would, perhaps, have been unrecorded in the drawing.

The right coronary artery enters the cavity of the right ventricle at the acute margin and emerges on the posterior aspect of the heart. This area may be selected for the anastomosis in a bypass procedure for coronary artery occlusive disease because the posterior descending branch is frequently given off here or a short distance beyond in the posterior right A.V. sulcus, and the surgeon may wish to make the anastomosis proximal to its origin. The dissection of such a vessel could lead the operating surgeon into the interior of the right atrium. This development could result in air in the venous lines; however, the problem could be coped with much more easily than could entrance into the cavity of the right ventricle resulting from the dissection of an intramural anterior interventricular branch.

This is the only specimen of an intracavitary right coronary artery I have encountered. There have been, however, three examples of this course in the anterior interventricular branch, one of which is seen on the next page.

The Intracavitary Course
of the Anterior Interventricular Branch

Specimen B: 1–6

1 and **2**: Nonattitudinal left superior views: To expose
the artery, the rectangle of the anterior wall of the right
ventricle, seen between the four dots, has been removed.
The anterior interventricular branch very commonly
courses intramurally in the upper 1 to 3 cm of the interventricular groove. However, in this heart it is located
9 mm below the surface, running within the cavity of the
infundibulum for 3.5 cm of its course.

3 and **4**: The heart has been transected. The septal wall,
at the bottom of photograph **4**, is 16 mm in width. This
measurement can be used to visually gauge the depth of
the interventricular branch. When the surgeon considers
exposing the artery in the proximal few centimeters of
the anterior interventricular groove, he recalls three anatomic facts: (1) It may be intramural—and rarely intracavitary. (2) The main septal artery, or (3) a large anterolateral branch may arise here—both may be injured
in the dissection.

Apart from the present topic, this specimen demonstrates important features of **the blood supply of the left
ventricle.**

5: Left lateral view: Observe: (a) The dotted line runs
midway between the anterosuperior and postero-inferior
borders of the left ventricle. In this lateral view, the
obtuse margin is at the junction of the upper three-
quarters and the lower one-quarter of the area between
these borders. (b) The obtuse marginal artery Type II,
gives only two small branches to the posterior wall of
L.V. It is 4.2 mm in diameter.

6: The inferior view: Observe: (a) The right coronary
artery is superficial at the crux. (b) Its two large left
ventricular branches are disposed obliquely on the posterior wall. (c) The triangle of the posterior wall between
points A, B, and C is supplied by small branches of the
right and the posterior division. This is a common arrangement—the absence of substantial arteries need not
evoke concern that an occluded vessel is unrecognized.
On page 176, a strongly muscled heart was seen possessing **a minimum of large branches to the myocardium**—
this same phenomenon is seen in the lateral wall of this
sturdily structured specimen. (1) **The lateral wall**: The
2-mm anterolateral, the minuscule superior branches,
and the 4-mm obtuse marginal branch supply this wall.
The latter branch is dominant in the perfusion of the
wall. It meets an apical branch of the anterior interventricular branch. (2) **The posterior wall**: The major supply
is from the right coronary artery. Only a small branch
arises from the obtuse marginal branch. (3) **The septal wall**: Just below the red pin in **2**, the sudden diminution in size of the anterior interventricular branch is
attributable to the provision of a 2.4-mm, left main septal branch. The anterior and posterior interventricular
branches measure 2 and 2.4cm, respectively, **suggesting**
a greater role than usual for the latter in the supply of
this wall.

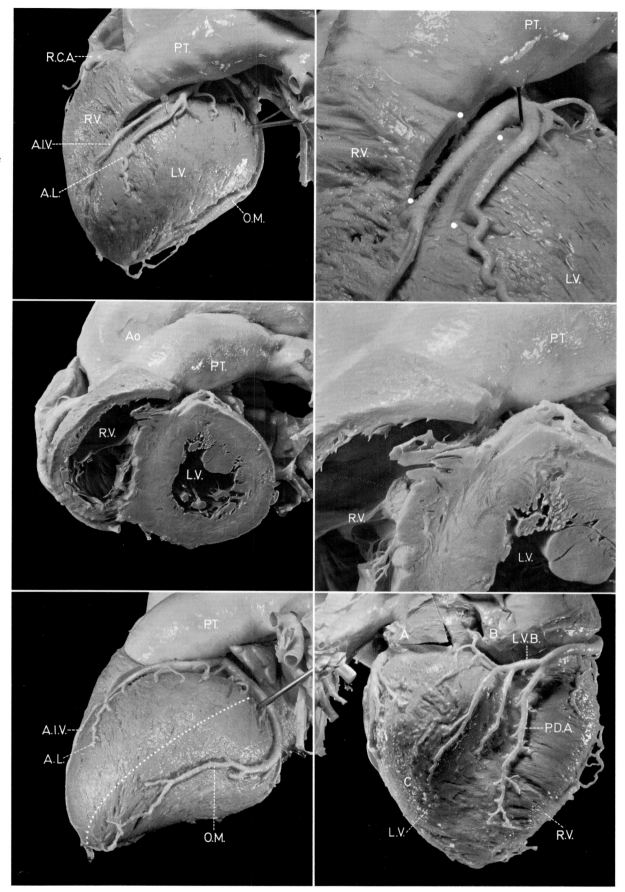

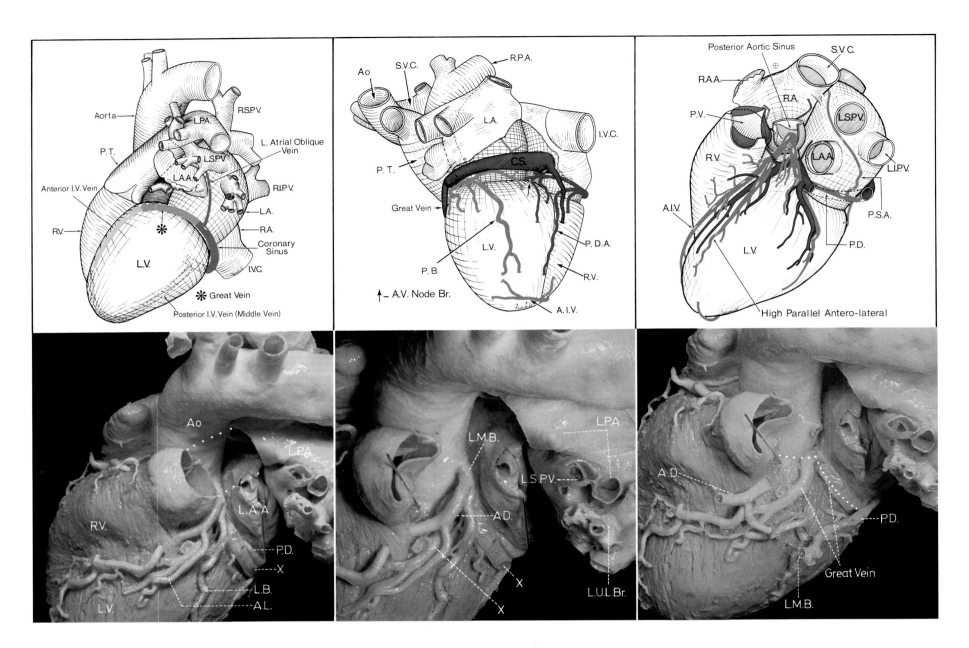

B. The Relation of the Coronary Arteries to the Cardiac Veins

I. Introduction

Specimen A: 1: Left lateral attitudinal view: This is a simulation of the veins seen in the venous phase of a left lateral view of a coronary arteriogram. **The great vein** is supreme, coursing medial to or over the summit of the left ventricle in relation to the proximal portions of the divisions of the left coronary arteries. It extends from the anterior interventricular groove where it merges with the anterior interventricular vein, to just beyond the obtuse margin where it becomes the coronary sinus. **The left atrial oblique vein** marks the junction of the great vein and the coronary sinus; it is usually present (95% of specimens—Baroldi) though only 1.0 mm in size; only a cord may remain. It and the cord in the vestigial fold of the pericardium delineate the course of the left superior cardinal vein in the fetus and a persisting left superior vena cava in the adult heart. The latter is commonly associated with congenital defects whose correc-

tion requires a right cardiotomy. Flow through the vein requires either diversion by cannulation through the coronary sinus or temporary interruption when the vein communicates freely with the right superior vena cava.

Specimen B: 2: Inferior L.P.O. view: At the obtuse margin, **the great vein** passes from the wall of the left ventricle to the wall of the left atrium.

II. The Relation of the Great Vein to the Ostium of the Left Ventricle

Specimen C: 3: Superior L.P.O. view: Parts of the right and left aortic sinus walls (pink) are removed; the left main branch stands, separated from its origin. (a) An obtuse bend, directed into the left coronary fossa, is normally present in the vein. In this specimen, an acute bend extends far into the fossa, deep to the divisions of the left coronary artery. (b) The posterior division is of interest; after supplying a small branch to the obtuse margin, it runs over the atrial wall, high above its attachment. To arteries pursuing this course, the sub-designation, major atrial circumflex, is given. As seen in

69—6, the artery terminates as a posterior branch. This course and this mode of termination are discussed on pages 206 and 207.

Specimen D: 4, 5, and **6**: A superior left lateral nonattitudinal view: An even more marked example of the intrusion of the great vein (X) into the left coronary fossa is seen. Note the two walls, roof, and floor of the fossa.

4: A segment of the pulmonary trunk has been removed. The proximal segment of the anterior interventricular branch and the lateral branch of the posterior division (L.B.) run intramurally.

5: The posterior pulmonary sinus has been inverted. The great vein weaves between the left coronary artery branches. The lateral branch of the posterior division and the anterolateral branch are large.

6: The arteries have been divided and everted. The ostium of L.V. is indicated by dots; lying on it is the diaphanous great vein which effects contact with the aorta.

III. The Relation of the Great Vein and the Left Coronary Artery

Specimen E: 1–6: This specimen is seen in detail in drawings on pages 192–196; it is shown here before and after removal of a major segment of the great vein. The veins and arteries have been filled with blue and red injectate.

1 and **2**: Superior left lateral views: Observe: The great vein is lateral to both the retropulmonary segment of the anterior division and the lateral portion of the posterior division and interdigitates with their branches—**this is the usual relationship.**

3 and **4**: High L.P.O. views: The great vein crosses the lateral margin of the left coronary fossa on the summit of the left ventricle. The posterior sinus node artery is seen in all six drawings and photographs on this page. In **3**, note the distortion of the left main coronary artery resulting from the cannulation incidental to infusion of the colored plastic material (see page 1).

5 and **6**: P.A. attitudinal views: The spatial disposition of the great vein is seen. The muscle-walled coronary sinus, in contrast to the veins, does not appear blue because of the greater thickness of its wall. At the obtuse margin, the great vein crosses from the wall of the left ventricle to the wall of the left atrium. Here the vein is close to the ostium of L.V. In the absence of the left atrial oblique vein the junction of the coronary sinus and great vein is marked by the valve described by Vieussens (1641–1715) and denoted herein by his name. This, one of the few uses of an eponym in this work, stems from lack of a reasonable alternative. The valve described by Thebesius (1686–1732) is better termed the coronary sinus valve. See the bottom of page 87.

Observe: (1) In specimen D, the great vein reaches the ostium of L.V. in relation to the left fibrous trigone; it could be injured during aortic or mitral valve replacement and, as the patient is heparinized, the hematoma could be large. The posterior division is also in a position of danger. (2) In specimens C and D, the vein is deep to the proximal portions of the divisions, not superficial, as seen in specimen E on this page. In addition to this variable relationship, the vein often interdigitates with the lateral wall branches of both divisions and, as James showed in his monograph (1961), the vein may form loops around the arteries. It is apparent that the great vein is an important factor in discouraging the surgeon from anastomosing a vein graft to an artery in the left coronary fossa.

Before leaving this specimen, examine the left coronary artery. The retropulmonary segment of the anterior division runs anterolaterally; from it, a large lateral branch crosses the lateral wall of L.V. An intermediate anterolateral branch extends in the 60° sector; the posterior division terminates on the posterior wall of L.V. as a posterior branch—a smaller branch proceeds to the apex below the obtuse margin.

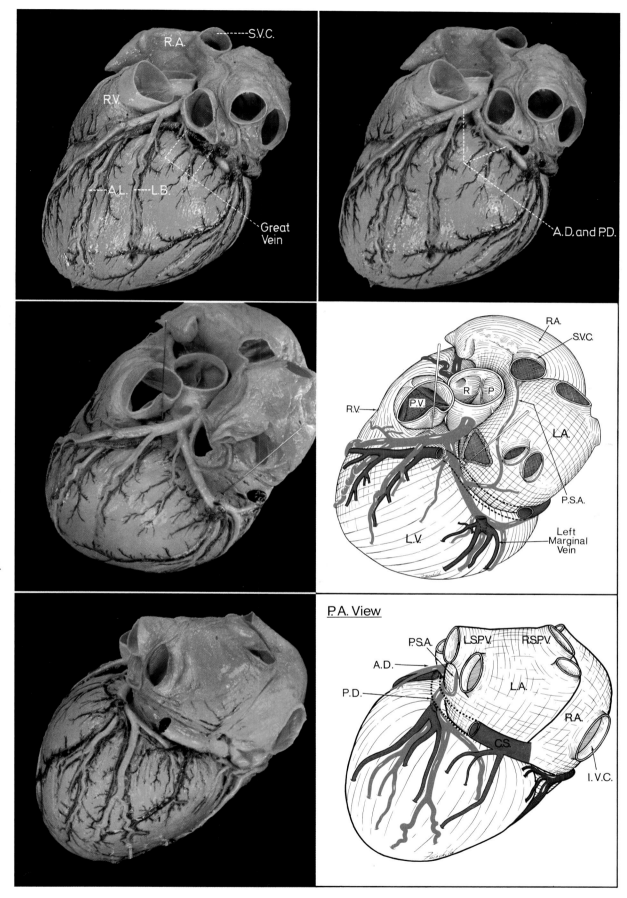

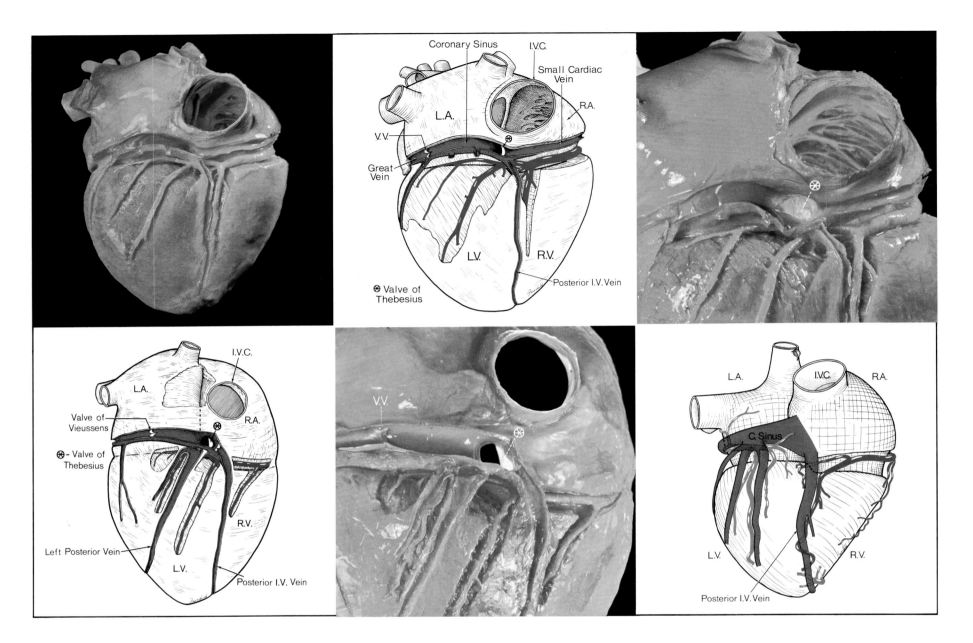

Coronary Sinus I.V.C.

Small Cardiac Vein

L.A.

R.A.

V.V.

Great Vein

L.V. R.V.

⊗ Valve of Thebesius

Posterior I.V. Vein

I.V.C.

L.A.

Valve of Vieussens

R.A.

⊗ - Valve of Thebesius

R.V.

Left Posterior Vein

L.V.

Posterior I.V. Vein

V.V.

⊗

L.A. I.V.C. R.A.

C. Sinus

L.V. R.V.

Posterior I.V. Vein

IV. The Relation of the Coronary Sinus to the Coronary Arteries

The inferior view of the heart: The veins are colored green in the drawings; their roofs have been removed to show their size and course.

Specimen A: 1 through 3: The coronary sinus and the great vein merge at the site of attachment of the left atrial oblique vein or, if the latter is absent, at the site of the valve of Vieussens (V.V.). The coronary sinus is located 10 mm above the attachment of the left atrium. In this specimen, a well-developed **small cardiac vein** (V.P.) runs, well above the right coronary artery, over the wall of the right atrium to terminate in the coronary sinus.

3: Observe: (a) The L.V. branch of the right coronary artery is unbent as it crosses the floor of the crux. (b) The coronary sinus orifice and its transilluminated valve (valve of Thebesius) are at the junction of the medial and inferior walls of the right atrium.

Specimen B: 4 and **5**: As in most specimens, the small cardiac vein is absent. Note the valve of Vieussens and the diaphanous coronary sinus valve. The left posterior vein, which enters the coronary sinus near its terminus, is large and the left marginal vein is small. Ordinarily the veins do not run adjacent to the arteries and cannot be used as a guide for the identification of the latter. **The right coronary artery is, with very rare exceptions, inferior to the coronary sinus.** This location is to be anticipated, as the inferior portion of the tricuspid ostium is inferior to the mitral portion of the left ventricular ostium and the coronary sinus is above the latter and the right coronary artery is related to the former before passing to the left.

Most often, the posterior interventricular vein is found on the left of the posterior descending artery—this, too, is not surprising. The coronary sinus terminates at the left margin of the posterior superior process of the left ventricle—well to the left of the posterior I.V. groove. The posterior descending coronary artery runs in relation to the latter, and the posterior interventricular vein terminates in the coronary sinus; it may be reduplicated; it is always superficial to an underlying coronary artery.

Specimen C: 6: On page 206, this specimen illustrates the high location on the atrium of the left coronary artery prior to its termination as the posterior branch to the left ventricle. Unlike the right coronary artery, which is inferior to, and separate from the coronary sinus, the left coronary artery may be deep to, and very exceptionally, superior to the sinus. Usually the vein and the artery are in contact at the obtuse margin. Here, the great vein passes from the ventricular to the atrial wall, and an artery directed to the obtuse margin frequently passes from the atrial to the ventricular wall. When the posterior division terminates as a posterior branch to the left ventricle or continues to the crux, it will usually be in contact with the coronary sinus.

V. The Relations of the Anterior Veins

The Anterior Interventricular Vein

1: L.A.O. view: Here we see the ventricles of the specimen which will be featured on the next five pages. Commencing 3 cm above the apex, two veins run on each side of the artery; they soon unite and form the anterior interventricular vein which ascends along the left side of the artery. It would be anticipated that the anterior interventricular artery, arising from the medially located aorta, should lie, as it usually does, to the right of its related vein, which merges with the great vein which courses over the summit of the left ventricle.

2: A.P. view: Observe: (a) Much less often, the vein is found on the right of the anterior interventricular artery, as seen in this specimen. (b) Small venous branches may be anterior to the anterior interventricular artery. Unless handled meticulously, the veins will cause annoying bleeding when the artery is being exposed at operation. (c) The posterior interventricular vein, not infrequently, originates from branches located on the anterior aspect of the apex. (d) A large preventricular arterial branch (P.V.B.) of the right coronary artery passes obliquely across the anterior wall of the right ventricle and recurs onto the inferior wall.

The Anterior Cardiac Veins

3: Nonattitudinal R.A.O. view: A large conus artery (orange) is accompanied by a large venous branch, which receives most of the venous return from the anterior wall of the right ventricle, including a marginal venous branch inferiorly. On the left it communicates with the anterior interventricular vein. Its terminus is located in the right atrium below the appendage (R.A.A.). It is connected to the coronary sinus by the small cardiac vein. The anterior cardiac veins pass superficially or deep to the right coronary artery. **The presence of a large conus vein is of interest,** because the related conus artery or a conus branch are important avenues for collateral development in the presence of occlusive disease. Collaterals are often seen at the time when the veins are also filled with contrast material, and this large conus vein might obscure, and possibly be misinterpreted as, an arterial branch serving a collateral role. James stresses the importance of the conal vein as a source of intersystemic collateral (between the coronary and anterior venous systems) and a beautiful demonstration of a vein fulfilling this role is seen on pages 199 and 200 of his monograph.

4: A superior view summarizing the main venous branches of the heart: (1) The coronary sinus has been retracted from the posterior superior process of the left ventricle: The small cardiac vein (vena parva) and the posterior interventricular vein (the middle vein) empty into its terminal centimeter. The coronary sinus is the most constant feature of the cardiac veins. Little variation exists in its termination and location. Although variations in its length and diameter are reported, one can state that, as a rule, in an 80-kilo man, the sinus is 40 mm in length and 10 mm in diameter. It is a good guide to the

posterior part of the ostium of the left ventricle in radiographic studies. The valve of Vieussens is usually present, though incompetent. **(2) The posterior vein of the left ventricle** is present in 75% of hearts and empties into the coronary sinus in 95% of these instances (Baroldi). (3) **The left atrial oblique vein** terminates at the junction of the great vein and the coronary sinus. (4) **The left marginal vein** usually enters the great vein; it may be replaced by the posterior left ventricular vein. (5) **The great vein** connects the anterior I.V. vein and the coronary sinus. It has been divided into the ascending portion (which is called here the anterior I.V. vein) and the horizontal portion (which is called here the great vein). Between it and the anterior system are communicating veins—so-called intersystemic veins—these pass on both aspects of the aorta. (6) **The anterior and the posterior interventricular veins** are rough indicators of their respective grooves; at the apex, important communications are found between these and the posterior left ventricular, the obtuse marginal, and the marginal vein (of the anterior system). (7) **The anterior venous sys-**

tem consists of three to six veins which drain the right two-thirds of the anterior wall of the right ventricle. Each vein crosses the anterior right A.V. sulcus and may empty by a separate ostium into the right atrium. They may merge into a reduced number, often one which empties into the upper or lower part of the right atrium. Often the veins empty into a venous lake which terminates in the anterior aspect of the atrium. It may be connected to the coronary sinus by the small cardiac vein. The conus and marginal veins are usually prominent.

Comment: In the monograph of Baroldi the wide variations in the termination of the obtuse marginal, posterior L.V., and posterior I.V. veins are described in detail. The relation of these terminations to the sampling site (of a catheter in the coronary sinus) is critical in metabolic studies. What part of L.V. is reflected by the sample? Should not these terminations be established by contrast studies before pathophysiologic inferences be drawn? Hyperselective sampling may also be valuable.

1. Coronary Sinus	5. Great Vein	9. Right Marginal
2. Posterior L.V.	6. Ant. Interventricular	10. Conus
3. Oblique L. Atrial	7. Small Cardiac	11. Anterior R.V.
4. Left Marginal	8. Post. Interventricular	12. Communicating

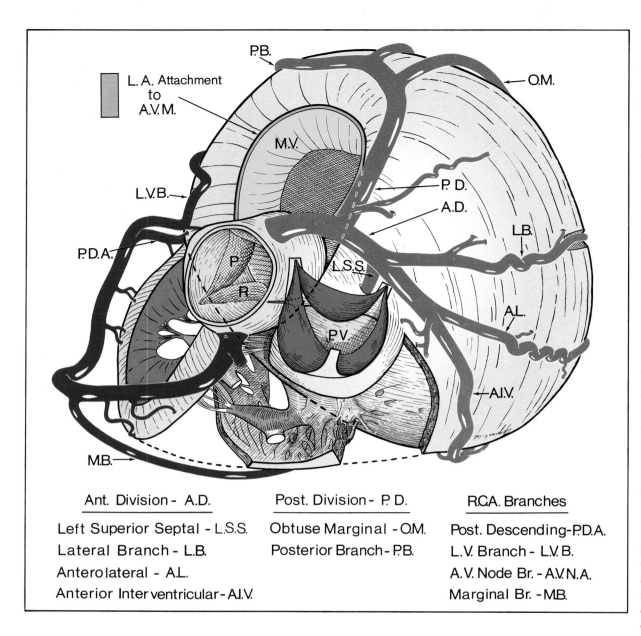

L. A. Attachment to A.V.M.

P.B.

M.V.

L.V.B.

P.D.

A.D.

O.M.

L.B.

P.D.A.

P

R

L.S.S.

A.L.

PV

A.I.V.

M.B.

Ant. Division - A.D.	Post. Division - P. D.	R.C.A. Branches
Left Superior Septal - L.S.S.	Obtuse Marginal - O.M.	Post. Descending-P.D.A.
Lateral Branch - L.B.	Posterior Branch- P.B.	L.V. Branch - L.V.B.
Anterolateral - A.L.		A.V. Node Br. - A.V.N.A.
Anterior Interventricular- A.I.V.		Marginal Br. -M.B.

C. The Course of the Coronary Arteries in Relation to the Major Landmarks of the Heart

I. The Horizontal Plane

As an introduction to this section see pages 122 and 179. The quality of our interpretation of an arteriogram is dependent on the state of our knowledge of these great landmarks in the three dimensions. In each of the four classical radiographic views (found on pages 193–196), two of these dimensions can be studied; the third is added when we observe the direction and relations of structures in the horizontal plane shown on this page; its basic importance is implied by the enlargement of the scale of this drawing. First study each anatomic feature here, then predict its disposition in the four radiographic views; finally examine pages 193, 195, and 196. For this purpose, we will use a single specimen (A). which has just been seen (**189—1–6** and **191—1**). Observe: (a) **The aortic sinuses:** As seen on the next page, they are indicated by the aortic annuli; they

occupy the aortic part of the ostium of the left ventricle. (b) The **ostium of the left ventricle** in its entirety is identified by the (yellow) A.V. membrane in the views where the ostium is visible, and stripes oriented in its axis when it is not visible; it faces to the right, posteriorly and superiorly, as does the tricuspid to a lesser degree. Together the ostia are disposed in an R.A.O.-L.P.O. axis. The lateral part of the mitral portion of the ostium extends to the left, posteriorly and inferiorly; hence, the lateral portion of the posterior division passes in these directions. (c) The **tricuspid ostium** is indicated by the purple of the leaflets of its valve and by the stipple in the views where these are not seen. (1) The superior segment (this includes the proximal segment) of the right coronary artery is related to the posterolateral wall of the right ventricle. (2) The right anterior and right inferior segments of the artery circle the ostium. (3) As the tricuspid ostium is anterior to the mitral division of the ostium of L.V., the left ventricular segment of the right coronary artery passes, not only to the left, but posteriorly. (d) The major part of the **pulmonary**

ostium is both anterior and to the left of the aorta. The left main branch and its bifurcation are posterior to it; the retropulmonary segment of the anterior division extends anteriorly and to the left at a 45° angle: The inclination of the segment in a vertical plane varies with the shape of L.V. and the length and axis of the left main branch—it may be horizontal. (e) In its descent to the acute margin, the **anterior interventricular groove** and its related arterial branch extends anteriorly and to the left of (1) the pulmonary ostium and (2) the mitral portion of the ostium of L.V. (to which the lateral portion of the posterior division is related). (f) The **walls of L.V.:** (1) The **septal wall,** except for its upper portion, is disposed in the L.A.O.-R.P.O. plane and is fully displayed in the R.A.O. view (see page 119). The septal arteries of this specimen are seen in the A.P. and both oblique views on pages 172 and 173. (2) The **posterior wall** (seen only in part here) is examined best in the A.P. plane (see page 193 and page 165, where its right angle examination is described). (3) The **lateral wall** is seen best in the lateral view. In this specimen, the anterolateral and the lateral branch of the anterior division identify the 60° and 90° sectors of this wall. The lateral branch divides the lateral wall into a larger anterior and a smaller posterior portion; in the L.A.O. view, the anterior portion is almost perpendicular and the posterior portion is parallel to this plane of examination. The reverse is true in the R.A.O. view. In the A.P. view, both halves are viewed tangentially.

Now systematically examine the component segments and branches listed below of the left coronary artery, then the right. In each, visualize its location in the four traditional radiographic views. Optimal examination of a vessel is carried out at a right angle to it. Hence, it is essential to be constantly aware of the direction of the vessel which is determined by its course, which must be established in relationship to the great anatomic landmarks and to the contour of the left ventricle. This exercise will be followed in the following pages, where reference to this horizontal plane in each instance is recommended.

The Left Coronary Artery: 1. The left main branch. 2. The retropulmonary, and 3. the anterior interventricular segments of the anterior division. 4. The branches of this division to the lateral wall. 5. The septal branches. 6. The lateral and posterior portions of the posterior division are related to the corresponding parts of the mitral portion of the ostium of L.V. 7. The branches of the posterior division.

The Right Coronary Artery: 1. The superior segment. 2. The right anterior segment (in relation to the anterior right A.V. sulcus). 3. The right inferior segment (in relation to the posterior right A.V. sulcus). 4. Posterior descending branch. 5. The left ventricular segment and its branches, including the A.V. node artery.

In the following pages, the most commonly used view of each plane of examination appears on the right side of the horizontal row—the opposite view is placed on the left; to facilitate the study of the former, the mirror image of the latter is placed between the two.

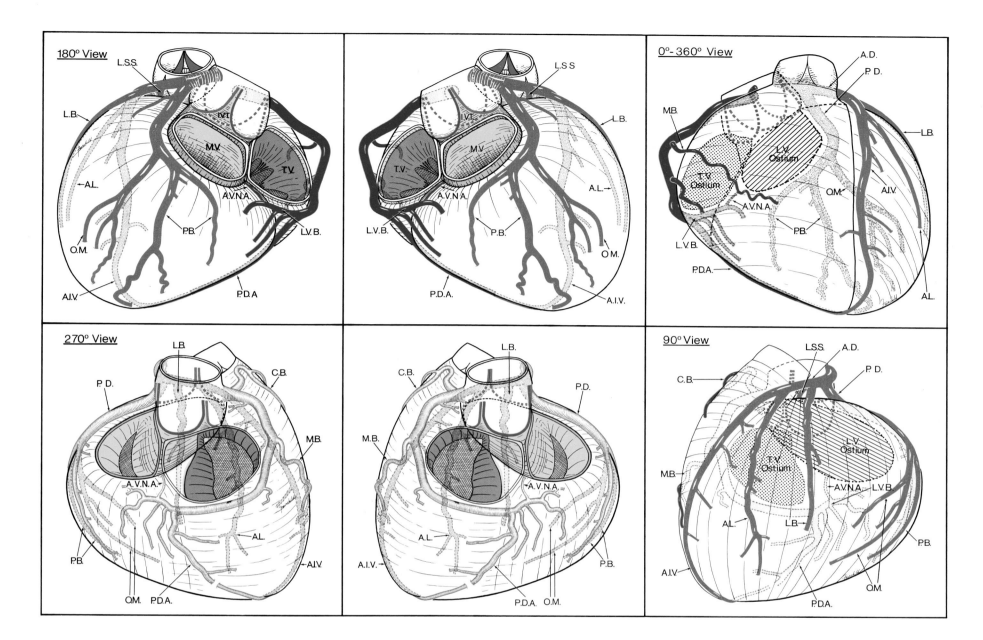

II. The A.P.-P.A. Plane of Examination

Specimen A: 1–6: For numerical designations see **4–6**. In the lateral plane, the right coronary artery is viewed clinically at 270° and the left at 90° if distortion is to be minimized (page 8).

The Left Coronary Artery: (a) **The left main branch** is seen best in this view when a transverse axis is present. (b) **The pulmonary ostium** (and the related retropulmonary portion of the anterior division) is superior and to the left of the ostium of L.V. (c) **The left lateral margin of the ostium of L.V.** (and a related lateral part of the posterior division) is (1) lateral to the aorta and (2) medial to the anterior interventricular groove and artery and (3) directly above the posterior part of the lateral wall of L.V. (4) It is directed to the left and posteroinferiorly; hence, its related artery is seen obliquely and relatively end-on in this view. (d) **The posterior part of the ostium of L.V.** is above the posterior wall of L.V. and is related to the corresponding part of the posterior division. (e) The branches to **the posterior wall of L.V.** are best seen in this view. (f) The 60° anterolateral (A.L.) and the 90° lateral branches (L.B.) identify the location of these sectors of **the lateral wall of L.V.** in this view: The lateral branch of the anterior division runs along the left radiographic border in this view.

The Right Coronary Artery: The four segments appear: (a) The superior—essentially end on; (b) Right anterior—essential perpendicular; (c) Right inferior—oblique; (d) Left ventricular—extends posteriorly and to the left (see superior view) and superiorly (the tricuspid ostium extends below the ostium of L.V.). **The posterior descending branch** runs at an unusually lew level.

III. The Lateral Plane of Examination

The Left Coronary Artery: (a) The **left main branch** is seen end-on. (b) The **retropulmonary segment** of the anterior division is seen obliquely. (c) The **lateral portion of the posterior division** is relatively well seen (see the angle formed by it and the plane of examination in **192—1**). (d) This view is essential in the recognition of the division of origin and in the study of the **branches** of the lateral wall. It provides an additional view of the anterior interventricular artery. (e) The two posterior wall branches overlap each other and the obtuse marginal branch.

The Right Coronary Artery: Observe: (a) When located in the midline of the sinus, the orifice will be seen better here than in the L.A.O. view. (b) Note the relationship of the four segments to the tricuspid and left ventricular ostia. The L.V. segment (small in this specimen) courses posteriorly and superiorly and to the left. The posterior descending branch follows its groove. (c) Overlap is present between the right coronary artery and the anterior I.V. and lateral wall branches of the left coronary artery. This is not, therefore, a good view for studying an anterior division being filled by intercoronary collateral circulation. (d) This view is valuable in the study of this artery, in particular the parts at and beyond the crux. (e) The A.V. node artery should be studied in all views. Apart from its inherent interest it provides a landmark: It terminates at the hub of the heart—the attachment of the junctions of A.V. membrane to the ostium of L.V.

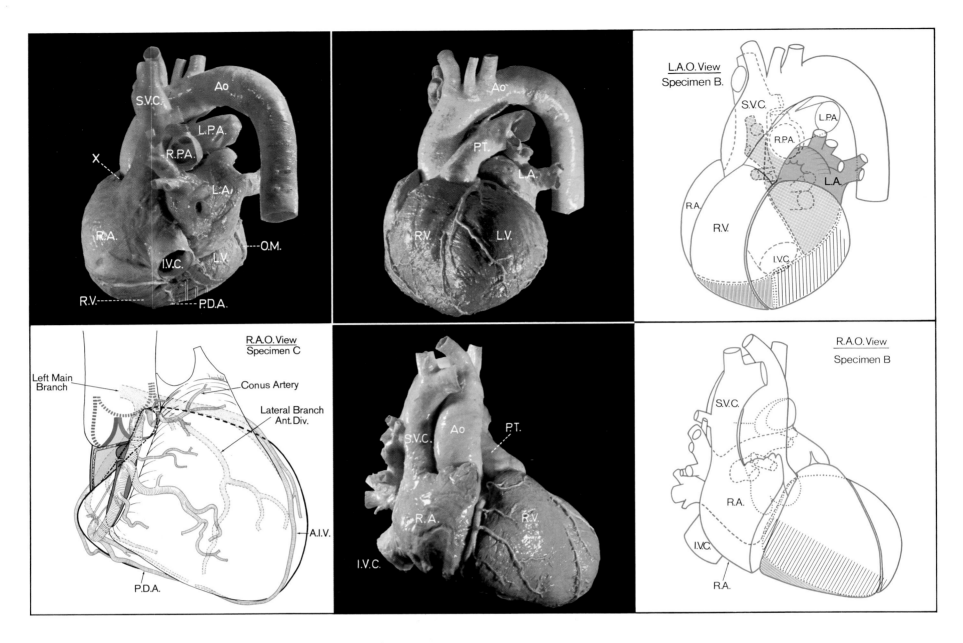

IV. Major Landmarks and Borders of the Heart in the Oblique Planes

Specimen B (1, 2, 3, 5, and **6)** has been seen in the lateral plane on page 7 (**1–6**) and the A.P. plane on page 31 (**4–6**). In **194**—**3** and **6** the lines indicate the direction and extent of the inferior wall of the right ventricle and the posterior wall of L.V., the left upper border of which marks the obtuse margin. The left atrium is red. Note: Dots=ventricles, dashes=atria. The letter A is assigned on these opposing pages to the specimen featured in this section.

L.A.O.-R.P.O. Plane
Views: 1: Mirror image R.P.O. **2** and **3**: L.A.O. Observe: (a) In this horizontal heart, the posterior A.V. sulcus is depressed. It is usually angled 45° above the horizontal. (b) The posterior wall is foreshortened. Its surface is projected posteriorly at a 45° angle in the R.A.O.-L.P.O. and at a 45° angle above the horizontal in the A.P. plane. Hence, its double obliquity is seen here. Arteries on the posterior wall are seen end-on and obliq-

uely, particularly in a horizontal heart. (c) The obtuse marginal artery (O.M.) runs near the **left border** of the heart. (d) The superior cavo-atrial junction (X) and the superior vena cava are behind the aorta (see **1** and **5**). (e) The left atrium is projected posteriorly; it is largely superimposed on the left ventricle. (f) The posterior interatrial sulcus is staggered to the left of the posterior interventricular.

R.A.O. view
Specimen C: 4: Note the location of the large lateral branch of the anterior division in the lateral plane on page 108 and the L.A.O.-R.P.O. plane on page 119. In the R.A.O. view, the upper half of the lateral branch is near the anterosuperior border of the left ventricle; the anterior half of the lateral wall of L.V. is between the two; the posterior half is between the artery and the obtuse margin. On pages 110–113, review the interrelationship of the axes of the left ventricle and its ostium and the axes of the right ventricle and its ostia. The axes of the nearly closed tricuspid ostium and the ostium of L.V. intersect at an angle of approximately 25°.

The axes are not sufficiently dissimilar, however, to prevent superimposition of the related posterior division of the left coronary artery and the right coronary artery. This feature is demonstrated in this specimen.

Specimen B: 5: R.A.O. view **6:** An R.A.O. composite drawing made in the same manner as **3**. (The mirror image L.P.O. is not shown).

Observe: (a) In this horizontal heart the obtuse margin is depressed below its usual location which is midway between the upper and lower borders of the left ventricle. (b) The posterior walls extend superiorly and to the left, oblique to the examining plane. (c) Note the relationship of the anterior interventricular groove to the upper cardiac border—the variation in this relationship is important in determining the degree of overlap of the related arterial branches. (d) The lateral wall is between the groove and the obtuse margin. (e) The superior cavo-atrial junction lies to the side of the aorta in this view and posterior to the aorta in the L.A.O.-R.P.O. plane. (f) The short right heart is seen.

V. The L.A.O.-R.P.O. Plane of Examination

Specimen A: 1–4: For the photograph of **1**, see **13—1**. **2:** Mirror image R.P.O. **4:** The isolated A.V. unit. **5:** A selective right coronary arteriogram. **6:** The late phase of a selective left coronary arteriogram in a patient with occlusion of the proximal right coronary artery.

The Left Coronary Artery: (a) **The left main branch** is overlapped by the proximal parts of the divisions—see **2**. (b) **The anterior division:** (1) The retropulmonary segment is seen end-on. (2) The upper portions of the anterior interventricular segment and anterolateral branches are directed antero-inferiorly (page 192), hence, are seen relatively end-on; however, this view is useful in separating the two as they may be superimposed, specially in the R.A.O. view. (3) Proximally the anterolateral and lateral branches of the anterior division are superimposed on the posterior division—see **2** and **3**. (c) **The posterior division:** (1) The lateral segment (X) runs almost at a right angle to this plane (**2**); in **6** the contrast medium

has passed through it.* (2) The posterior segment (Y) (seen in **6**) is set obliquely; it is best seen in the A.P. view. As seen in **119—5** and **6**, the posterior half of the lateral wall parallels the L.A.O.-R.P.O. plane. The lateral and the obtuse marginal branches course along the anterior and posterior aspects of **the left border of the ventricle** in this view.

Note: When we view page 192 and this page, it is evident that a horizontal plane examination is not optimal in the examination of the proximal 5.0 cm of the divisions of the left coronary artery; elevation of 45° or more of the plane of examination is needed.

The Right Coronary Artery: (a) The orifice is located to the right in the sinus as it usually is; hence, the **proximal segment** is optimally visualized in this view. (b) Always visualize the segments in relation to the superior, anterior, and inferior parts of the tricuspid ostium. (They are seen in **1–3** and marked A, B, and C in **5**.) They, like the tricuspid ostium, are set at a right angle to this

plane, therefore, are usually optimally visualized here. The plane of the ostium is deflected posteriorly 20° (page 115). (c) In **6**, note (1) the left conal branch (C.B.) filling a collateral role and (2) the left ventricular segment of the right (L.V.B.) filled by collateral. This view is important in identifying patency of the right coronary artery beyond a proximal occlusion. (d) The A.V. node artery is directed superiorly in a nearly vertical axis (see **3**). (e) The arteries in the two interventricular grooves, particularly the posterior, are foreshortened as they are directed anteriorly in this plane of examination; they have a variable relationship to each other, dependent on the situs of the heart. They may be superimposed. (d) The septal branches (see **3** and **4**) between the two grooves and the septal margin on their right are superimposed on one another; their motion is an indicator of the function of their wall.

---

* The lateral part of the posterior division is visualized best at 60° although it may be obscured by lateral wall branches.

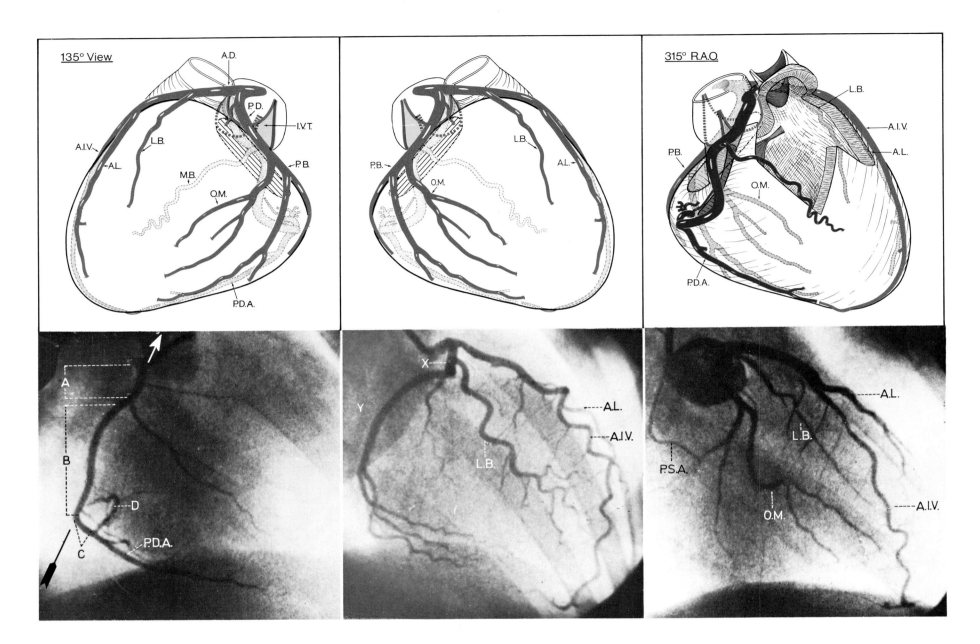

VI. The R.A.O.-L.P.O. Plane of Examination

Specimen A (seen on pages 192, 193, and 195) is shown here in the following three views: **1**: L.P.O.; **2**: mirror image L.P.O.; **3**: R.A.O.

4: A selective right and **5** and **6**: Two selective left coronary arteriograms. The views are R.A.O.

Left Coronary Artery: First re-examine the superior view of this specimen, 192—1. (a) The **left main branch** is well viewed only when its axis is directed anteriorly. (b) In this view, note the nearly horizontal course of the **retropulmonary segment of the anterior division;** it and the **interventricular segment of the anterior division** are optimally visualized, as is the posterior descending branch. Note that (a) an anterolateral branch may overlap the anterior interventricular branch and (b) branches to the posterior wall of L.V. may overlap branches in the posterior interventricular sulcus. In **1–3**, this overlap is seen in relation to the anterior interventricular sulcus; in **5** and particularly

in **6**, the anterolateral branch is above and better separated from the interventricular branch. (c) The **septal arteries** are best seen in this view. Recall however that the upper portion of the septum faces anteriorly and superiorly, hence, is oblique to this plane (see pages 165 and 173). (d) **The posterior division**: (1) **It terminates** as the obtuse marginal branch in **6**, the posterior branch in **1–3**, and the posterior descending branch in **5**. (2) **Its segments**: The upper end of the obtuse margin (Y in **5**) roughly demarcates **the left lateral** and **the posterior. The right lateral** division of the ostium of L.V. is marked by the A.V. node artery. (3) A short proximal segment (X in **5**) descends vertically to the ostium of L.V. (see 141—4). (4) From the latter segment, the lateral branch arises in **5**. (e) The L.V. branches to the posterior wall overlap one another. (f) The height of the **obtuse marginal artery** varies (see **3** and **6**). The specimen presents a poor example of an obtuse marginal artery; usually the artery extends midway between the upper and lower borders of L.V. in this view—in a horizontal heart it runs below this level. (g) Note the relationship of the anterosuperior

border of L.V. to **the lateral branch** of the posterior division (L.B.) in **5** and **6**. (h) **The posterior sinus node** arteries arise far posteriorly from a minor atrial circumflex branch in **6**.

Right Coronary Artery: Observe: (a) In the L.A.O.-R.P.O. plane, **its axis** (shown by the arrow) is directed anteriorly as well as superiorly (see page 110). It often overlaps the posterior division of the left coronary artery. (b) The proximal segment is seen end-on. (c) Review the spatial disposition of **the four segments** of the artery marked A, B, C in **195—5**—only segment B, which runs in the anterior right A.V. sulcus, is reasonably well seen. The view is useful, however, in studying the posterior descending branch and, in particular, in recognizing its **circummarginal variations**. (d) The tricuspid ostium extends below the crux, and, the right inferior segment C is seen relatively end-on in this view and overlap occurs between it and the origin of the posterior descending. The left ventricular segment D is also seen foreshortened.

Chapter 14:
The Five Modes of Termination
of the Posterior Division
of the Left Coronary Artery

Introduction

This chapter will focus on what is perhaps the most difficult aspect of coronary artery anatomy, the posterior division of the left coronary artery. We will examine 12 specimens **primarily demonstrating its mode of termination** and relation to the ostium of L.V. In addition, we will observe the general features of the specimens, e.g., the mode of branching and the course of both the right and left coronary arteries in relation to the A.V. sulci and the myocardium.

In the study of the mode of branching, the following determinations should be made: (a) the relative size of the right and left coronary arteries; (b) the relative size of the divisions of the left coronary artery; (c) the relative size of the branches to each wall of the left ventricle; (d) the relative size of branches of (1) each division and (2) the right coronary artery, e.g., the size of the posterior descending and the left ventricular branches of the right coronary artery or the posterior division of the left.

On the last two pages, 208–209, two specimens displaying **a dominant left pattern** appear. In the first, the diameters of the proximal part of the two divisions of the left coronary artery are approximately equal in size. In the second, the larger posterior division supplies not only the posterior wall, but a large part of the lateral wall and, as the posterior descending branch is larger than the anterior interventricular branch, probably a larger area of the septal wall than usual—in total, approximately 60–70% of the entire left ventricle—truly **a dominant posterior division**.

On the first two pages, 198–199, **a large dominant right coronary artery (Type III)** is seen in three specimens. In each, a large left ventricular branch, 2.5 mm in diameter accompanies a small non-graftable posterior descending branch, demonstrating the necessity of assessing **the relative size of the branches of the right coronary artery to the posterior and septal walls of the left ventricle.**

In relation to the ostium of the left ventricle, the posterior division or a branch thereof which reaches the posterior wall may be: (1) on the atrial wall usually 10 mm above its attachment—this course will be termed the major atrial circumflex; (2) deep in the A.V. sulcus—the last specimen to be studied (on page 209) exemplifies this rare course; (3) widely separated from the ostium throughout, the posterolateral radial artery passes radially or diagonally around the obtuse margin to the posterior wall; (4) from an obtuse marginal artery (Type I), branches pass transversely or obliquely across and supply the posterior wall of the left ventricle. These branches bear no relation to the ostium of the left ventricle.

The **major atrial circumflex course** warrants attention. This course is defined as one wherein the posterior division courses on the left atrium high (approximately 10 mm) above its attachment and reaches the posterior surface of the heart. This course may be followed from the origin in the left coronary fossa to the crux; in other specimens, the lateral segment of the posterior division is uninvolved. An artery pursuing this course will be deep to and occasionally above the level of the coronary sinus, which is normally 10 mm above the left atrial attachment; the course should be recognized in an arteriogram if the relation of the posterior division to the coronary sinus in the R.A.O. view is always observed. The location of a major artery in relation to the left atrium is relevant in all operations within the atrium and of particular importance in some—e.g., the creation of a baffle for the correction of transposition of the great vessels. Authors have alluded to the course over the atrium when the posterior division terminates as the posterior descending artery. However, it will be seen in three specimens (on pages 206 and 207) which, in turn, exemplify a dominant right, a balanced, and a dominant left pattern. This artery should be differentiated from a minor atrial circumflex, which is a small branch originating from the left lateral portion of a posterior division which terminates either as (a) a posterolateral radial branch or (b) an obtuse marginal branch.

In the two specimens seen on pages 200–203, the posterior division terminates as the **posterolateral radial artery** which is never close to the ostium of the left ventricle as it passes from its origin to its termination at the posterior I.V. sulcus; it does, however, give off a small branch, the minor atrial circumflex, which roughly follows the left A.V. sulcus to the crux. In the second of these specimens, at midpoint of the anterior right A.V.

sulcus, the right coronary artery gives off a small branch which follows the sulcus to the crux; the parent trunk then emerges from the sulcus, crosses the anterior and inferior walls of the right ventricle, and forms the posterior descending artery. These interrelationships are shown in **167—5**.

The **collateral circulation** has been studied using injection and corrosion as well as microradiographic techniques. The monography of James (1961), Fulton (1965) and Baroldi (1967) are good sources of information on these methods. Using gross techniques, we can demonstrate the branches which are available for the development of collateral circulation. **Four major sites are present**: (1) the apex, (2) the septal wall, (3) the anterior surface of the right ventricle, (4) the atria. Collateral circulation may be divided into **five types**: (1) intercoronary—between the right and left coronary arteries, (2) interdivisional—between the divisions of the left coronary artery, (3) intradivisional—between branches of a division, (4) right intracoronary—between branches of the right coronary artery, (5) intraradicular—between two parts of a branch—this has been called "bridge collateral". In the presence of a dominant left coronary artery, the potential for the development of collateral is reduced and the subject will be examined in this connection on pages 208 and 209.

The incidence of the different types of termination of the posterior division was noted in 100 specimens:

Termination of Posterior Division

	No. of specimens
1. Diminutive	7
2. Posterolateral radial	6
3. Obtuse marginal	
Type I	9
Type II	43
4. Posterior branch	23
5. Posterior descending branch	12

When the posterior branch to the left ventricle is the mode of termination, it may be found in a balanced (17%) or a dominant right pattern (6%).

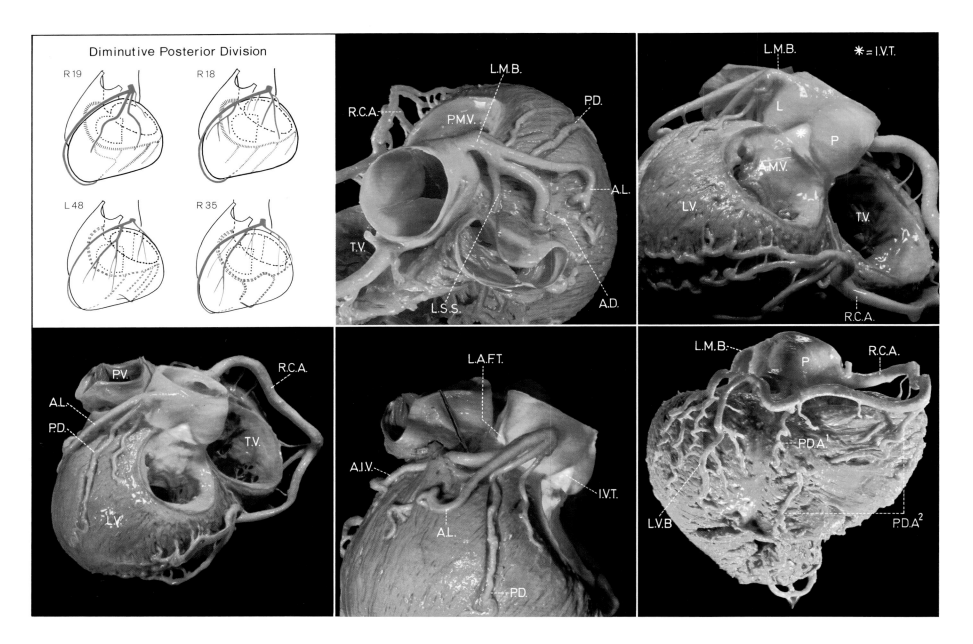

Mode of Termination I—
The Diminutive Posterior Division

The posterior division of the left coronary artery may frequently supply only a small area of the left ventricular wall and have only a fleeting or no relationship to the ostium of L.V. and the lateral left A.V. sulcus.

1: The left lateral arteriographic simulation of four specimens, two of which will be seen (R 19 on this page and R 18 in **1** through **3** on the next page).

Specimen A (R 19): 2–6

2: The superior view: This specimen is seen in its entirety in the superior view in **145—3**. Observe: (a) The left main coronary branch (L.M.B.), 5 mm in length and in diameter, demonstrates a posterior axis in the presence of a very dominant right coronary artery. (b) The pulmonary valve is reflected anteriorly, displaying a 2-mm, left superior septal artery (L.S.S.) entering the septal wall behind the right third of the posterior pulmonary sinus. (c) As seen in the majority of specimens, lateral to the pulmonary ostium, the anterior interventri-

cular branch courses intramurally. (d) The smaller high anterolateral branch and the major component of the diminutive posterior division (P.D.) also run intramurally.

3: P.A. view: In the frontal plane, the axis of the left main branch is 20° above the horizontal; it meets the aorta at an angle of 80°. The axis of the aortic bulb and the horizontal form an angle of 60°.

4: An elevated L.P.O. view and **5**, a more lateral, still nonattitudinal view are both seen with interior lighting. The longer (P.D.) of the two branches, representing the posterior division, measures 1.8 mm in diameter; the area of the left ventricle supplied by it can be seen. A high anterolateral branch (A.L.) and the anterior I.V. branch measure 2.2 and 3.2 mm in diameter, respectively. In passing, note (a) the extensive (16 mm) attachment of the left aortic annulus to the ostium and the absence of the left fibrous trigone. (b) The left aortic annulus is defined between the left anterior fibrous trigone (L.A.F.T.) and the intervalvular trigone (I.V.T.)—the left coronary artery orifice is below its usual loca-

tion, the line joining the upper extremities of the annulus.

6: The inferior view: Observe: (a) The posterior descending branch is represented by an upper vessel (P.D.A.[1]) in the posterior I.V. sulcus, and a second branch (P.D.A.[2]), which arises at the acute margin, extends at a right angle along the margin, then again turning at right angles to cross the posterior wall of the right ventricle. This specimen is diagrammed in **167—4C** as a variant in the retroventricular course of the posterior descending branch. (b) A large, 2.5-mm left ventricular branch (L.V.B.) descends vertically on the posterior wall of L.V. This vessel can be used for the anastomosis of a vein graft in the presence of disease in the proximal right coronary artery.

Note: (a) the scale in **2**, **3**, and **5** is 1:1. (b) Examine **161—3** and **4**, the posterosuperior view. (c) in **2**, the continuation of the retropulmonary segment (A.D.) becomes the anterior interventricular branch at the upper end of the anterior I.V. sulcus.

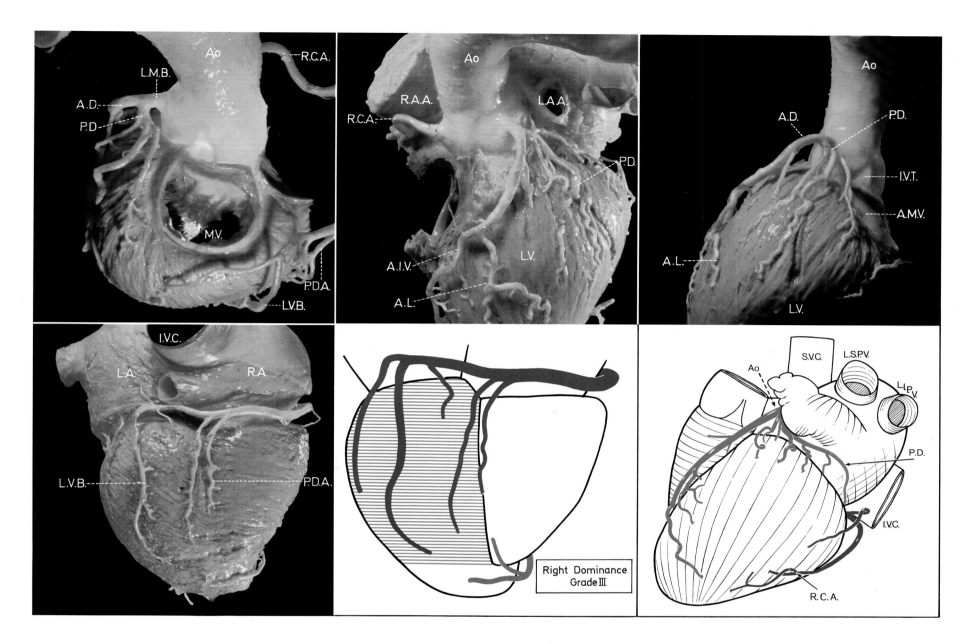

Specimen B (R 18): 1–3: First, on page 165, examine the left ventricular segment of the dominant right coronary artery; then in **145—4**, note the arteries on the anterior aspect of this specimen.

1: A superior P.A. view of the aorta and left ventricle: The left main branch bifurcates at a right angle. From the posterior division (P.D.), one major and two minor branches arise.

2: A nonattitudinal superior L.A.O. view: The right ventricle, pulmonary trunk, and left atrial appendage have been removed. (a) A small branch crosses the left atrial wall and supplies a small area of the ventricle at the obtuse margin. (b) The major branch (P.D.) passes posterolaterally onto the lateral wall of the ventricle. A large intermediate anterolateral branch (A.L.) is present.

3: L.P.O. view: Only a relatively small portion of the left ventricular wall is supplied by the posterior division. **The main element of the posterior division is well separated from the ostium of L.V.**

Specimen C: 4–6: An A.P. view of this specimen, showing the large right coronary artery and the slender anterior interventricular branch, is seen in **36—1**: The superior and L.A.O. views are seen in **59—3** and **4**. It is diagrammed—R 60 in **164—1** and **166—3**.

4 and 5: Observe: (a) The posterior descending branch, like the anterior interventricular branch, is small. The intermediate of the three left ventricular branches is the predominant termination of the right coronary artery. (b) Note the linear, superficial, elevated course of the right coronary artery in relation to both the posterior right and posterior left A.V. sulci and the crux. The artery is only rarely elevated above the left ventricle to this degree. (c) In this specimen, as in most perfusion-fixed hearts, a posterior interventricular groove is not identifiable.

6: Left lateral view: The right coronary artery reaches the lateral aspect of the left ventricle. The branches of the posterior division are short and under 1 mm in diameter. A striking lack of graftable branches to the entire lateral wall of the ventricle is apparent.

In these three specimens, note the following: (1) **The posterior division:** (a) It supplies only a small area of the lateral wall of the ventricle; (b) it ends proximal to the obtuse margin; (c) it does not bend around the heart (L. circum—around; flexus—flectere—to bend); (d) its course is separate from the ostium of the left ventricle in all three of the specimens and from the A.V. sulcus in two. (2) **The posterior descending artery** may be small and fragmented—the left ventricular branch is the mode of termination of the right coronary artery—the reverse may occur. (3) One would anticipate a relationship between **the axis of the left main branch** and the relative dominance of its divisions; none appears to exist. In these three specimens with pronounced dominance of the anterior division, the axes in the horizontal plane are: In A=posterior; in B=transverse; in C=anterior (see page 59).

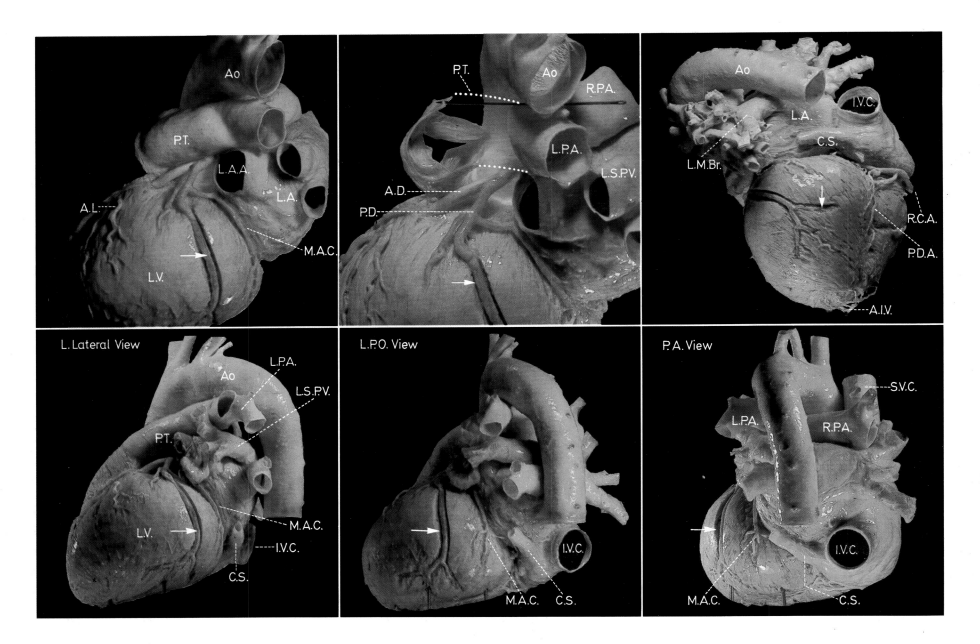

Mode of Termination II—
The Posterolateral Radial Artery

Note: This mode of termination will be seen in two specimens—the first on these two pages and the second on the following two pages.

Specimen A: Pages 200–201. This specimen is also seen in Chapter 8, in the study of the right heart in the four classical radiographic views and is diagrammed, R.50, in **164—1.**

1 and **2:** L.P.O. views before and after removal of the pulmonary trunk and sinuses: The long, left main branch divides into anterior and posterior divisions as it emerges from the left coronary fossa. Below the orifice of the left atrial appendage (L.A.A.), the posterior division gives off a small branch, the minor atrial circumflex (M.A.C.) which runs along the lower portion of the lateral and posterior walls of the left atrium, terminating on the uppermost portion of the posterior wall of the left ventricle. **The posterior division terminates as a pos-**

terolateral radial artery, which is marked by an arrow in all views. Prior to entering the muscle, it displays the characteristic U-shaped bend. During the remainder of its course, it continues in an intramural location. The anterior division is covered by muscle in the proximal 3 cm of the anterior I.V. groove. The anterolateral branch, originating from this intramural segment, might be injured during the dissection of the artery of origin.
3: The obtuse margin view: The posterolateral artery passes radially around the obtuse margin and extends transversely towards the interventricular groove. It crosses and supplies the posterior wall of the left ventricle.

Its spatial disposition and intramural location are seen in **4, 5,** and **6,** the left lateral, the L.P.O., and the P.A. views. In **4** and **5,** note the posterolateral direction of the termination of the posterior division—the posterolateral radial artery. In passing, note that: (a) The inferior vena cava is largely medial to the axis of the superior vena cava and is close to the aorta. (b) The coronary sinus is directed superiorly and to the left, indicating the location

of the posterior portion of the left ventricular ostium in the A.P.-P.A. plane of examination. Note the relationship of the two structures in the lateral and L.P.O. views. (c) Note the small minor atrial circumflex and its relation to the A.V. sulcus in these views: (d) The left atrium is the posterior chamber of the heart.

Comment: Does it not seem reasonable to consider the minuscule minor atrial circumflex with its limited area of supply of the L.V. as the branch, and the artery marked by the arrow with its major role in supply of L.V. as the mode of termination of the posterior division? The key to the arteriographic identification of this vessel is found in the R.A.O. view, viz., its vertical course from its origin to its termination at the posterior I.V. groove. It contributes a branch to the apex and it may be confused with an obtuse marginal artery, particularly in the views other than R.A.O. However its separation from the ostium of L.V. in the lateral view and **its radial course around the axis of the ventricle** should be noted in the A.P. and L.A.O. views.

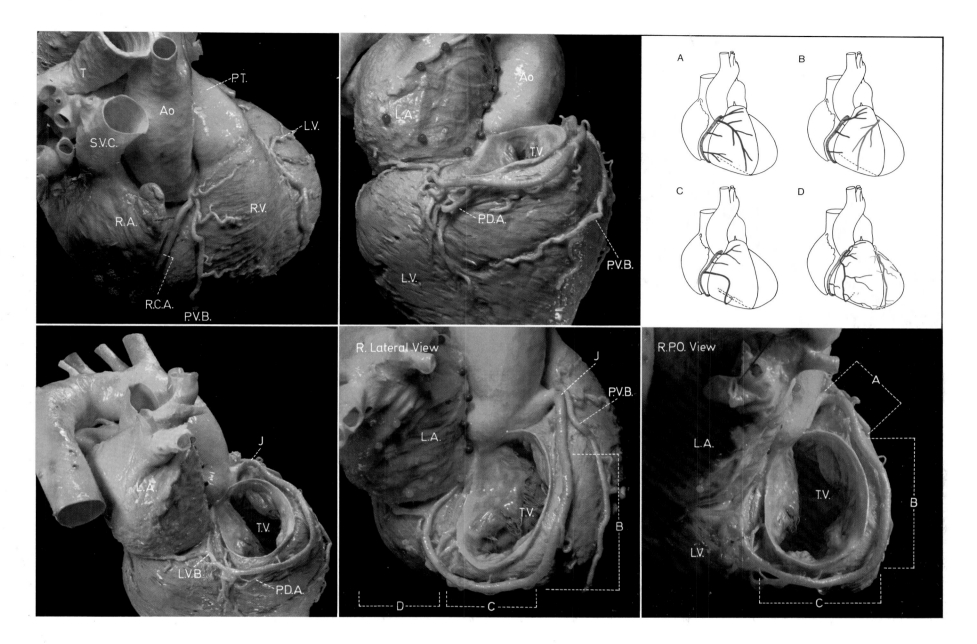

The Preventricular Branch of the Right Coronary Artery

After giving off a small minor atrial circumflex (M.A.C.) branch which runs in relation to the A.V. sulcus, the posterior division of the left coronary artery passes around the obtuse margin en route to the posterior I.V. sulcus. The right coronary artery gives off a smaller lower branch (the preventricular) which passes radially around the acute margin on its course to the posterior I.V. sulcus. The major element continues in the right A.V. sulcus to the crux and supplies the posterior descending and L.V. branches. This is seen diagrammed, R 50, in **167—5**.

1: Superior R.A.O. view: From the right aortic sinus, the right coronary artery emerges; from its proximal segment, the **preventricular branch** (P.V.B.) arises and supplies the right two-thirds of the anterior wall of the right ventricle. This vessel could be divided by the right extremity of a transverse right ventriculotomy.

2: After removal of the right atrium, the specimen is rotated and seen from a right inferior view: The preven-

tricular artery passes around the acute margin, supplying a large part of the inferior wall of the right ventricle before reaching the posterior interventricular sulcus.

3: Four patterns of preventricular branches: In D the A.P. view of this specimen is shown. In C, the pattern exhibited by the specimen on the next two pages is seen—a large vessel circumnavigates the acute margin to become the "posterior descending branch".

The Subdivisions of the Right Coronary Artery

4: Nonattitudinal R.P.O. view: The junction (J) between the proximal and continuing segments of the right coronary artery can be seen.

5: The right lateral view, and **6:** the R.P.O. view: Observe: (a) The proximal segment extends from the right aortic sinus at a right angle, meeting the continuing segment at an obtuse angle. In this specimen, the former is best seen in the L.A.O.-R.P.O. plane (**6**). (b) In **5** and **6** the four segments of the right coronary

artery are seen. The right superior segment (A) includes the proximal segment as it has been just described; it is related to the posterolateral wall of the right ventricle and is above the superior part of the tricuspid ostium. The right anterior segment (B) and the right inferior segment (C) are related to their respective parts of the tricuspid ostium. The left ventricular segment (D) is small in this specimen.

In the 270° view segment B and segment A (with the exception of the proximal segment) demonstrate an essentially vertical course (see **5**). In the R.A.O. view, the entirety of A and B forms a straight line which is deflected posteriorly on its vertex, as seen in this and another specimen in **111—3** and **5** and in an arteriogram, **196—4**. After examining **6** and the arteriogram **195—5**, the foreshortening of segment A in the 270° and 315° views is apparent.

Comment: This spatial division of the right coronary artery is intended to direct careful attention to the direction of each segment in the study of arteriograms.

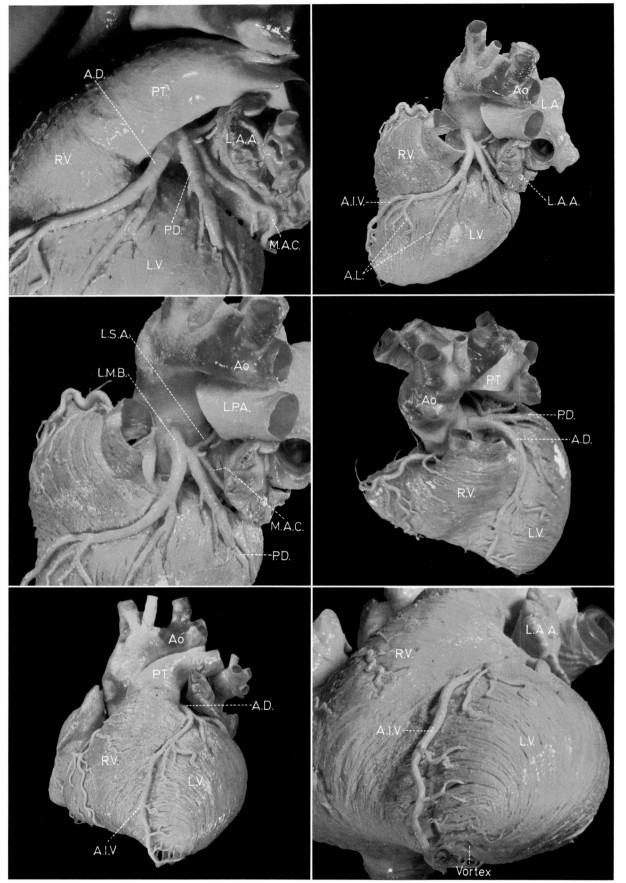

Mode of Termination II —
The Posterolateral Radial Artery

In order to attract attention to this previously unde-scribed artery, and because of its inherent interest the specimen occupying pages 202–203 will be examined.

1, 2, and **3** are superior left lateral views: In **2**, a segment of the pulmonary trunk has been excised. In **3**, the poste-rior pulmonary sinus is inverted. The 12-mm-long left main branch (L.M.B.) is directed transversely and hori-zontally. The divisions form an angle of 35° as they are directed towards their entrance into the myocardium. The anterior division (A.D.) is in contact with the pos-terior pulmonary sinus. The posterior division is well separated from the left ventricular ostium. The anterior division commences its intramural course on reaching the upper interventricular groove. The anterior division has two large anterolateral branches (A.L.), one high and one intermediate. All branches but the latter run intramurally at least in some part of their course. The posterior division gives off, first, the left sinus node artery, then a **minor atrial circumflex** (M.A.C.), from which an appendageal branch which has been ruptured arises. It then continues on to enter the myocardium and terminate as a posterolateral radial artery.

4: Superior A.P. view: The left main branch is posterior to the pulmonary trunk. The retropulmonary portion of the anterior division measures 3 cm between its origin and its termination in the anterior interventricular groove, where it becomes the anterior interventricular branch.

5: L.A.O. view: **The reverse-S configuration of the ante-rior division** of the left coronary artery, described by James results from its relationship to the pulmonary trunk (seen in **2**, **3**, and **4**) and the anterior and posterior interventricular grooves (seen in **5** and **6**)—the latter in turn reflect the shape of the left ventricle and the fact that the right wraps around the left ventricle. This 1961 observation is valuable in the examination of coronary arteriograms. This specimen was photographed some years ago and lighting produced heat injury to the aorta.

6: The apex is seen after the specimen has been tilted posteriorly. The small arterial branches, passing between the muscle bundles as they enter the myocardium, will be compressed in systole.

Comment: The variation in the contour, shape, and axis of L.V. should be noted when hearts are examined. In this heart, the left ventricle is long and somewhat oval—a shape resembling the one seen in animals. The axis of the left atrium is directed posterosuperiorly, roughly continuing the axis of L.V.; note its relation to a line drawn between the venae cavae. These features are best seen in **2** and **203**—**1**.

Note: This specimen is L-6 in **164**—**3** and **167**—**5**.

1: L.P.O. view: Observe: The posterolateral radial artery (P.D.) is seen commencing its intramural course; it passes almost radially around the left ventricle towards the posterior I.V. sulcus.

2: A left oblique view of the inferior surface: The posterior wall of L.V. receives an upper radial and a lower oblique branch from the upper product of the bifurcation of the posterolateral radial artery. These provide its major supply. A minor atrial circumflex is present (c.f. **200—1**).

The Circum-Marginal Course of the Posterior Descending Branch of the Right Coronary Artery

3 and its drawing **5** are the superior R.A.O. view: A large number of branches originate from the right coronary artery in the depth of the right coronary fossa. Knowledge of the walls and their relationships affords the prediction of the branches which may be found. (a) The posterolateral wall of the right ventricle receives branches anteriorly. (b) Inferiorly at the attachment of this wall to the unit, a right superior septal branch may enter the septum. (c) The anteromedial wall of the right atrium receives a low right anterior atrial branch. (d) Branches pass to the anterior wall of the infundibulum, one in an intramural location. (e) Adventitial branches supply the great vessels (the great arteries). The main artery bifurcates—the larger branch first passes anteriorly, then inferiorly across the anterior wall of the right ventricle, coursing around the acute margin to terminate as the posterior descending artery, as is shown in the drawing in **6**.

4: R.A.O. view: Observe: (a) In the midportion of the anterior right A.V. sulcus, the bifurcation of the right coronary artery is seen. The larger branch supplies a large area of the right ventricle and the septum, and could be injured by a right ventriculotomy. (b) An intermediate right atrial artery, marked by an arrow, ascends in the notch between the inferolateral appendage (I.L.F.) (which is better seen in **2**) and the prominent appendage (R.A.A.). An artery arising in this site in dogs characteristically becomes the sinus node artery; this is a rarity in human material. Apart from our present topic, observe. (a) The azygos vein terminates at the junction of the shorter postero-inferiorly directed upper segment (X) and the longer antero-inferiorly directed lower segment (Y). The azygos vein is seen in **1**. (b) The infundibulum or conus is well developed.

6: The inferior view: The terminations of both the right and the left coronary arteries pass, not in the A.V. sulci, but radially around the acute and obtuse margins, and reach the posterior interventricular groove. On the left, the minor atrial circumflex (related to the A.V. sulcus) divides to supply branches to the posterior wall of the left atrium and a small area of the left ventricle. On the right, the smaller branch continues in the right A.V. sulcus, dividing into a ventricular and an atrial branch, the latter terminating as the A.V. node artery. This specimen demonstrates the importance of noting the precise origin, course, and termination of both the right and left coronary arteries; the simplistic relegation of the vessels to the A.V. sulci is misleading and imprecise.

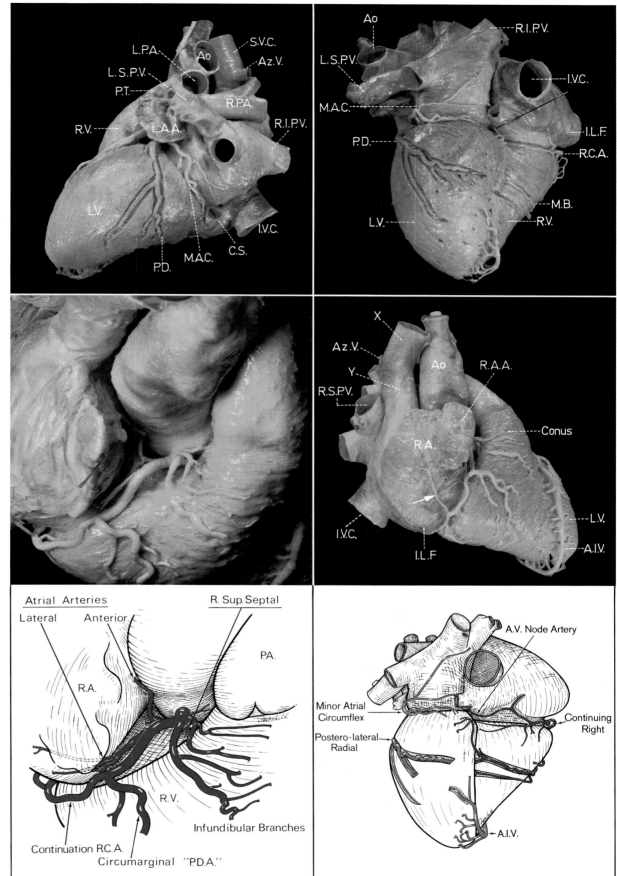

203

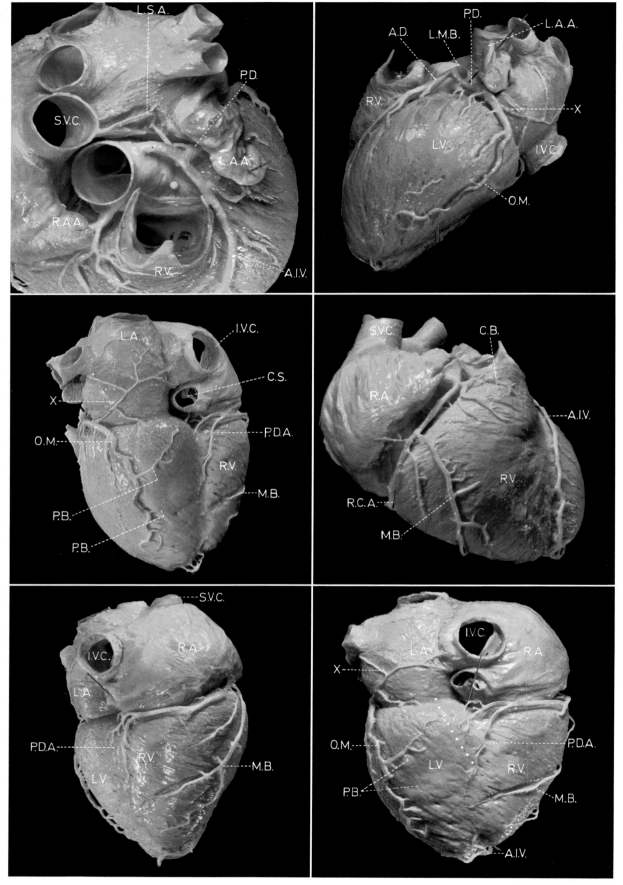

Mode of Termination III— The Obtuse Marginal Artery

Type I

The suggested classification of obtuse marginal arteries appears on page 164. On this page an example of Type I appears. On the next page, two specimens are examples of Type II; additionally, they pose a problem in the terminology of a branch to the lateral wall of L.V.

Specimen A: 1 through 6

1: Superior view: Observe: (a) In the horizontal plane, the axis of the 16-mm-long left main branch is directed anteriorly 12°. (b) The left sinus node artery (L.S.A.) is given off from the posterior division, 6 mm beyond its origin. It passes to the anterior wall of the left atrium, where it not only penetrates the interatrial muscle bundle, but lies in direct contact with the left atrial endocardium. At what anatomic plane of dissection is a large atrial thrombus removed coincident to an operation on the mitral valve? Could this 2-mm artery be divided, resulting in an arterio-cameral fistula? I have, not infrequently, removed the endocardium along with the thrombus in order to leave a clean, healthy albeit muscular surface. An artery with this course is in jeopardy. If the procedure is carried out with a clamped aorta, recognition of the bleeding vessel would be unlikely.

2: Left lateral view: (a) The left main branch and the divisions (of this specimen) are seen and discussed on page 148. (b) When a posterior division terminates as an obtuse marginal artery, **the following courses between the origin and the margin may be seen:** (1) tightly applied to the surface of the ventricle and close to the ostium—e.g. **149—2** and **3**; (2) on the wall of the left atrium high above the ostium—e.g., **205—5**; (3) in a superficial or aerial course which may be marked—e.g., **184—3** or moderate as in this specimen. (c) Note the origin of the posterior left atrial branch (X)—its further course may be seen in **3** and **6**. This artery is discussed on page 151.

3: The obtuse margin is examined: (a) The obtuse marginal artery courses over the margin to the apex. Two branches (P.B.) extend obliquely and superiorly over the posterior wall of L.V.—this is an example of Type I.

(b) Often the posterior I.V. sulcus is not recognizable: In this specimen, the adjacent walls of the ventricles protrude, and a junction rather than a sulcus results.

(c) Note the slender posterior descending branch which terminates above the middle of the "sulcus".

4: R.A.O. view: The wall of the right ventricle is supplied by a large conus branch (C.B.) above and a large circum-marginal artery (M.B.) below. See the diagram of this specimen, L 52, in **167—5**.

5: The acute margin: The circum-marginal branch crosses the acute margin and contributes to the supply of the inferior wall of the right ventricle.

6: Observe: (a) The large circum-marginal reaches the junction of the middle and lower third of the interventricular groove. (b) The supply of the posterior wall of L.V.: (1) The essentially triangular area above the dotted line is supplied by the right coronary artery; this pattern is common. (2) A small area at the apex is supplied by the anterior interventricular branch. (3) The posterior atrial branch (X) contributes a small branch to the left upper corner.

Specimen B: 1 through 4

1: A superior R.A.O. view: The prominent proximal segment of the right coronary artery is 8 mm in diameter. The right and left coronary arteries and their branches are large.

2: Left lateral view: The posterior division descends to the obtuse margin, terminating as the obtuse marginal artery, which follows that margin to the apex. A second, higher, parallel branch (X) is present.

3: The obtuse margin is viewed: The obtuse marginal artery provides no branches to the posterior wall of L.V., which is supplied by the right coronary artery. A prominent minor atrial circumflex branch (M.A.C.) curves around the atrial wall to reach the atrial septum.

4: The inferior view: (a) The posterior descending branch arises at the midpoint of the posterior right A.V. sulcus. In the posterior interventricular groove, it descends intramurally; such a course is displayed by this branch in approximately 5% of specimens. (e) Two large left ventricular branches of the right coronary artery descend vertically. Only minor branches from the minor atrial circumflex and the obtuse marginal branch reach the posterior wall of the left ventricle which is supplied essentially by the right coronary artery—an obtuse marginal artery, Type II, is present.

Specimen C: 5: Left lateral view: Observe: (a) The posterior division is superficial in the left coronary fossa. After a 2-cm course, it bifurcates into an upper and a lower branch. (b) The "upper" branch is destined to become the obtuse marginal artery (O.M.); before it reaches the margin, it runs high above the ostium of L.V. (which is marked by the blue beads). This "irrational" and indirect route demonstrates the unpredictability of the course of this artery. (c) The "lower" branch (X) passes to the apex midway between the upper and lower borders of L.V. The branch marked (X) in **2** has a similar course; these branches may be termed the lateral axial branch of the posterior division. (d) The posterior wall is supplied by the right coronary artery, a branch of which (R.C.A.) is seen winding over the inferior border of the left ventricle. This is the second example of an obtuse marginal artery, Type II.

Specimen D: 6: The posterior division of the left coronary artery bifurcates. Again one branch may be classified as a lateral axial branch of the posterior division (X). It replaces an obtuse marginal branch. The second passes to the posterior wall of the left ventricle as a small posterolateral radial branch (Y).

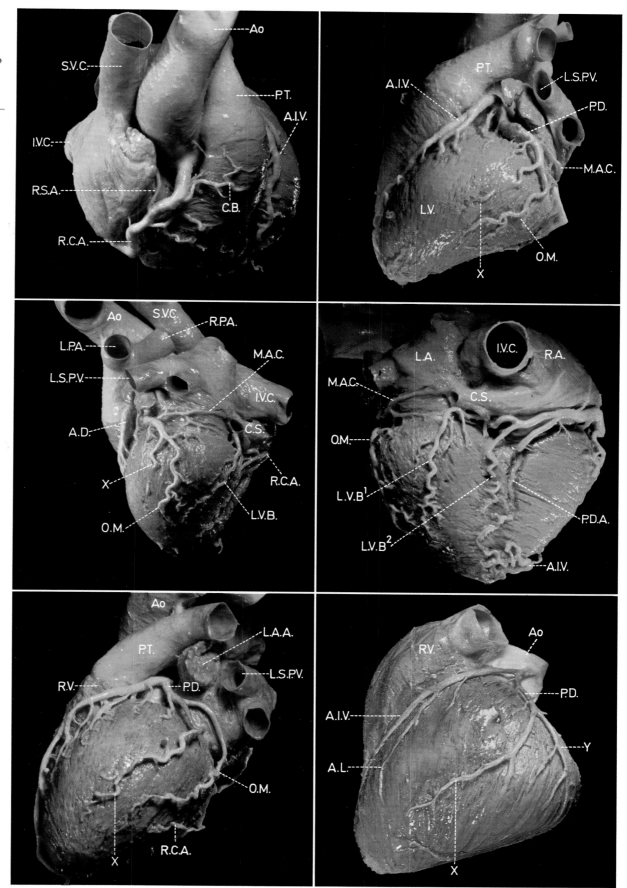

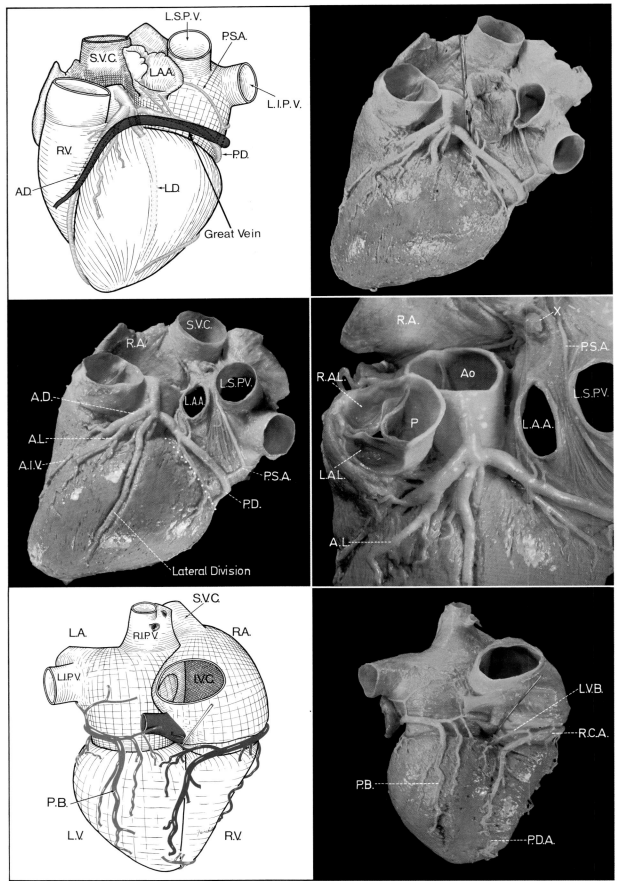

Mode of Termination IV—The Posterior Branch

Specimen A: 1–6: The superior left lateral view is seen in **1–4**.

1 and **2:** The great vein is superficial to the posterior division; it has been removed in **2**. Observe: (a) **The left main branch trifurcates.** (b) **The lateral division:** (1) A gentle convexity is above its entrance into the muscle; (2) during its intramural course, it is not discernible—like a snake under the sand, a telltale ridge may be present.

3: The left atrial appendage and the myocardium covering the lateral division have been removed. Observe: (a) **A lateral division,** like a lateral branch of a division, will (1) run intramurally throughout its course and (2) will initially be directed vertically. (3) In its final course, it will run either to the posterior I.V. groove or toward the apex—the latter is seen here. (b) **The posterior division** is 10 mm above the ostium of L.V. which is marked by the white dots. (c) Only a slender (1 mm) branch passes to the upper obtuse margin; in the presence of a large lateral division and a large posterior branch of the posterior division this is not surprising but not predictable. (d) Below the inferior pulmonary vein, the posterior sinus node artery arises.

4: 1:1 scale: (a) The axes of the anterior and posterior divisions form an angle of 110°. (b) The anterior division passes intramurally in the proximal inch of the interventricular groove. (c) A high anterolateral branch is present. (d) The atrial appendage (characteristically) receives two branches. (e) A diverticulum (X) of the left atrium (seen in no other specimen) protrudes through the fibers of the interatrial muscle. (f) The axis of the left main branch is transverse and sharply inferior—as a result, a prominent incisura is present in the orifice.

Note: The left lateral view is seen diagrammed, P2, in **164—4**.

5 and **6:** Inferior view: Observe: (a) **The posterior division:** (1) It terminates as a 3-mm artery which descends vertically to the "collateral area" at the apex. A smaller transverse branch continues medially towards, but fails to reach, the crux. (2) It courses high on the atrial wall—an example of **the major circumflex course in the presence of a dominant right coronary artery.** Its relation to the coronary sinus appears in **190—6**.
(b) **The right coronary artery:** (1) It terminates as a large (3.2 mm) posterior descending artery which reaches the apex; (2) the branch to the left ventricle (L.V.B.) is slender. After supplying a 2.1-mm main septal artery in the proximal anterior I.V. sulcus, the anterior interventricular branch continues, only 1.8 mm in diameter. Note the importance of assessing the size of the arteries in the I.V. sulci. This specimen presents an example of a dominant posterior descending branch—its importance in the perfusion of the left ventricle is belied when its parent artery is classified as a dominant right coronary artery—type I (the slender L.V. branch supplies less than 20% of the posterior wall—see page 163). The specimen on page 186 has a similar posterior descending branch.

The Major Atrial Circumflex Course in a Balanced Pattern of Circulation

Specimen B: 1 and **2**: First, examine the left main branch and the divisions of this specimen and their relations to the great vein on page **188—4, 5,** and **6**.

1: Left lateral view: (a) The lateral branch of the posterior division characteristically descends almost vertically in an intramural course. (b) The posterior division is above the great vein, high on the atrial wall.

2: Inferior view: (a) The posterior division: (1) It courses 1.2 cm above the atrial attachment which is indicated by the red beads. This, the major atrial circumflex course, is seen on both the lateral and posterior surfaces of the left atrium. (2) It terminates as the posterior branch (P.B.) to L.V. A smaller transverse branch passes to the posterior superior process of L.V. and supplies the A.V. node. (b) The right coronary artery terminates as the posterior descending branch. We see a balanced pattern of circulation.

The Intramural and Major Atrial Circumflex Course in a Dominant Left Pattern of Circulation

Specimen C: 3–6: Incisions have separated this specimen into anterior and posterior segments: The posterior is seen here.

3: Left lateral view: The large main trunk bifurcates into anterior and posterior divisions, which are 4 and 6 mm in external diameter. The posterior division courses superficially to a point 1 cm behind the attachment of the left atrial appendage, where it bifurcates into a 4-mm obtuse marginal branch and a second branch which passes into the left atrial wall 1.5 cm above its attachment to the A.V. membrane (this attachment is indicated by red beads). In **4**, the artery is seen to reach the crux and terminate as the posterior descending branch. The muscle covering the artery is best seen in **5** and **6**, which are shown in a 1:1 scale; however, it may be recognized between the arrows in all three photographs. While under its muscle cover, the artery was also under the great vein and coronary sinus. The coronary sinus is not a vein but a muscle-walled tube, and in its dissection, "left atrial" muscle fibers frequently require division. The coronary sinus, to exaggerate a point, may be located intramurally. This muscle duality will not be deemed singular if one recalls the origin of the coronary sinus from the left horn of the sinus venosus. The intramural location of a high-lying posterior division—the intramural major atrial circumflex course—is not uncommon. These combination of factors necessitate special care if the surgeon ever finds it necessary to expose this segment of the artery.

Note: (1) The posterior division may terminate as a posterior branch in association with a dominant right (Specimen A) or a balanced pattern (Specimen B). (2) The major atrial circumflex course occurs in a dominant right (Specimen A), a balanced pattern (Specimen B), or a dominant left pattern (Specimen C).

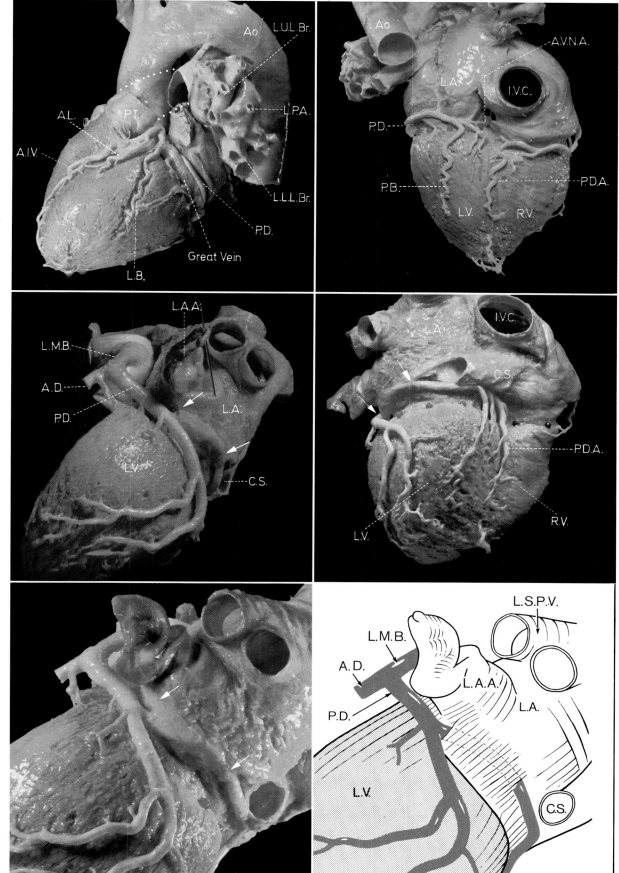

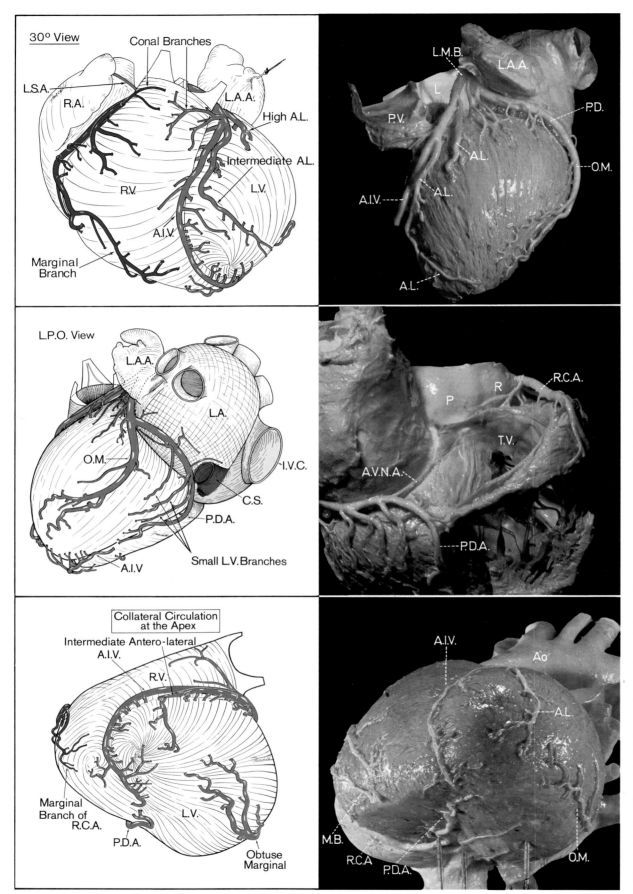

Mode of Termination V —
The Posterior Descending Branch

The "dominant left" pattern, a canine characteristic, is seen in approximately 10% of human hearts. On these two pages, we will note (1) the relative size of the two divisions, (2) the relative size of the arteries in the interventricular grooves, (3) the course of the posterior division, (4) the decreased potential for the development of collateral circulation imposed by the presence of a dominant left coronary artery: The **four major areas** (enumerated on page 197) for its development will be examined. The diameter of the branches, in millimetres will he noted.

Specimen A: 1–5
1: Observe: (a) A left sinus node artery (L.S.A.) is present—the left coronary artery also supplies the atria! No relationship exists between arterial dominance and the origin of the sinus node arteries. (b) The large right conal and marginal branches provide the only avenue for intercoronary collateral.

2: A nonattitudinal L.A.O. view. (a) Silhouetted against the transilluminated aorta are the left main branch and the two divisions. **The posterior is slightly larger in diameter** (4.5:4.0mm). (b) The lateral part of the posterior division is just above the ostium of the left ventricle (red beads); nevertheless it impinges on the atrial appendage which is attached at a low level. (c) The anterior division and its branches are large. From the retropulmonary segment, a 2.0-mm, high anterolateral branch and a 2.2-mm, left superior septal branch arise. From the 3.0 mm anterior interventricular branch a 2.0 mm intermediate anterolateral branch arises.

3: L.P.O. view: (a) An obtuse marginal branch (O.M.) is commonly seen in a dominant left pattern; it passes midway between the borders of L.V. in this specimen. (b) at the obtuse margin the posterior part of the posterior division ascends onto the left atrial wall, where it remains until it reaches the crux.

4: A nonattitudinal R.P.O. view: The right atrium and the anterior and inferior walls of the right ventricle have been removed. The posterior descending and the L.V. branches of the posterior division are small in comparison with branches of the anterior division. The A.V. node artery of this specimen (seen more clearly in **160—1**) is tightly applied to the attachment of the left atrium.

5: The potential for the development of **collateral circulation at the apex** in the presence of this dominant left coronary artery:
Intercoronary—the right is represented only by its marginal branch.
Interdivisional—(1) the arteries in the I.V. grooves. (2) the anterolateral and obtuse marginal branches.
Intradivisional—the anterior interventricular and the anterolateral branches of the anterior division.

Specimen B: 6: The apex view: This heart, with a dominant right coronary artery, is presented for comparison. The important difference is the potential for intercoronary collateral circulation between the arteries in the interventricular grooves.

Specimen C: **1**: A.P. view: A segment of the pulmonary trunk has been removed. In contrast to specimen A, the anterior interventricular (2.0 mm) and the intermediate anterolateral branches are small.

2: Superior A.P. view: Note the transverse axis of the left main branch.

3: Superior left lateral view: Note the relative inaccessibility of the left main branch in the left coronary fossa.

4: Same view: The length of the left main branch is 5 mm. It courses almost in contact with the aortic sinus wall. The anterior and posterior divisions measure 3 and 5 mm in diameter, demonstrating dominance of the latter.

5: Left lateral view: The 3.5-mm obtuse marginal and the lateral axial branch (X) supply the major part of the lateral wall of the ventricle; the anterior division supplies only a small intermediate anterolateral and an even smaller lateral branch.

6: Inferior view: Observe: (a) In contrast to specimen A, the posterior descending and L.V. branches (both 2.5 mm in diameter) are suitable recipients for a vein graft. (b) The artery courses at a low level in the A.V. sulcus. Much more commonly, the major atrial circumflex course is associated with this mode of termination of the posterior division.

Note the contrast in these two examples of a dominant left coronary artery.

(I) **The Dominance of the Divisions**: As the posterior wall will be supplied by the posterior division, the determinative variations occur in the mode of supply of the septal and lateral walls. In specimen C, **the dominance of the posterior division** is attributable to the following: (a) The anterolateral branch is small; the obtuse marginal and lateral axial are large and dominate in the supply of the lateral wall. (b) The posterior descending is larger than the anterior interventricular, suggesting a greater role of the former in the perfusion of the septal wall. A bypass operation into these arteries is often required in the presence of proximal occlusive disease. If one is normal, its size may provide some indication of the size of the other. This information is needed, particularly when the diseased artery is poorly or not visualized in the arteriogram.

In specimen A, the divisions are nearly equal in size.
(a) The two anterolateral branches supply a larger area of the lateral wall. (b) The anterior interventricular artery is larger than the posterior descending. As seen on **31—4-7**, the reverse occurs in Specimen B.

(II.) **The Course of the Posterior Division**: In specimen A, the posterior part of the posterior division is high above the ostium of L.V.—its usual site. In specimen C, it is unusually low.

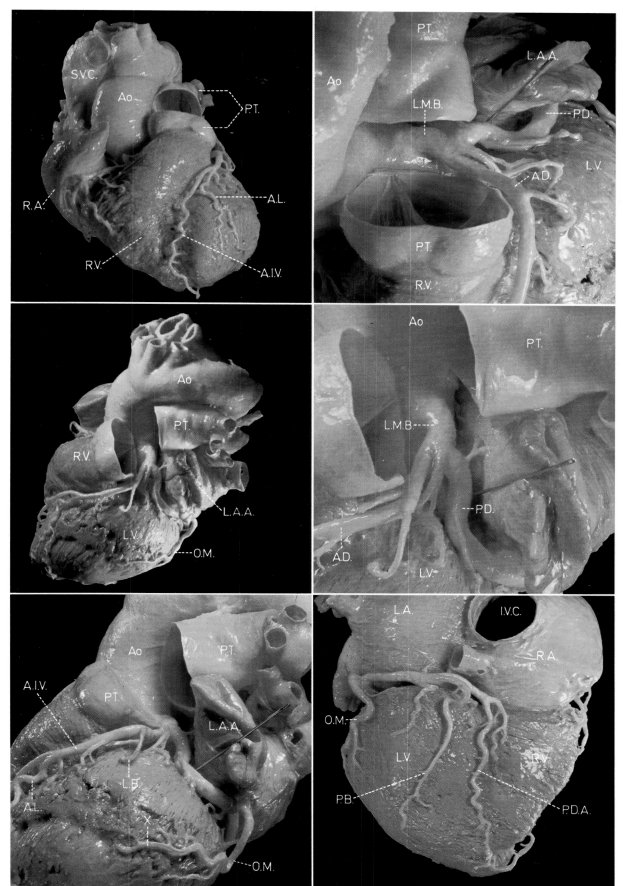

References

A

Abrahams, D.G., Barton, C.J., Cockshott, W.P., Edington, G.M., Weaver, E.J.: Annular subvalvular left ventricular aneurysms. Quart. Med., N. S. **31**, 345 (1962).

Abrikossoff, A.: Aneurysma des linken Herzventrikels mit abnormer Abgangstelle der linken Koronararterie von der Pulmonalis bei einem fünfmonatlichen Kinde. Virchows Arch. Path. Anat. **203**, 413 (1911).

Alavi, S.M., Keats, T.E., O'Brien, W.M.: The angle of tracheal bifurcation: its normal mensuration. Amer. J. Roentgenol. **108**, 546 (1970).

Amer. Heart Assn. Committee Report: A reporting system on patients evaluated for coronary artery disease. Circulation **51**, 7 (April 1975).

Amplatz, K., Anderson, R.: Angiographic appearance of myocardial bridging of the coronary artery. Invest. Radiol. **3**, 213 (1968).

Amplatz, K., Formanek, G., Stanger, P., Wilson, W.: Mechanics of selective coronary artery catheterization via femoral approach. Radiology **89**, 1040 (1967).

Arnold, J.R., Ghahramani, A.R., Hernandez, F.A., Sommer, L.S.: Calcification of annulus of tricuspid valve (observation in two patients with congenital pulmonary stenosis). Chest **60**, 229 (1971).

B

Bachmann, G.: Interauricular time interval. Amer. J. Physiol. **41**, 309 (1916).

Baltaxe, H.A., Amplatz, K., Levin, D.C.: Coronary Angiography. Springfield, Ill.: Charles C. Thomas, 1973.

Baroldi, G., Scomazzoni, G.: Coronary circulation in the normal and the pathologic heart. Washington: Armed Forces Institute of Pathology, 1965.

Baron, M.G., Wolf, B.S., Steinfeld, L.: Angiocardiographic diagnosis of subpulmonic ventricular septal defect. Amer. J. Roentgenol. **103**, 93 (1968).

Beck, W., Schrire, V.: Idiopathic mitral subannular left ventricular aneurysm in the Bantu. Amer. Heart. J. **78**, 28 (1969).

Becker, A.E., Becker, M.J.: Juxtaposition of atrial appendages associated with normally oriented ventricles and great arteries. Circulation **41**, 685 (1970).

Bellhouse, B.J., Bellhouse, F.H., Reid, K.G.: Fluid mechanics of the aortic root with application to coronary flow. Nature (Lond.) **219**, 1059 (1968).

Bishop, M.B., Free, S.L., Davies, J.N.P., Albert, R.P.: The coronary arterial pattern of deer in New York State with special reference to the third (posterior) coronary artery. Amer. Heart J. **80**, 785 (1970).

Björk, L.: Anastomoses between the coronary and bronchial arteries. Acta radiol. Diagnosis **4**, 93 (1966).

Björk, L.: Angiographic demonstration of extracardial anastomoses to the coronary ateries. Radiology **87**, 274 (1966).

Black, L.L., McComb, R.J., Silver, M.D.: Vascular injury following heart valve replacement. Ann. thorac. Surg. **16**, 19 (1973).

Brock, R.C.: The surgical and pathological anatomy of the mitral valve. Brit. Heart J. **14**, 489 (1952).

Brock, Sir Russel: Control mechanisms in the outflow tract of the right ventricle in health and disease. Guy's Hosp. Rep. **104**, 356 (1955).

C

Campeti, F.L., Ramsey, G.H., Gramiak, R., Watson, J.S. Jr.: Dynamics of the orifices of the venae cavae studies by cineangiocardiography. Circulation **19**, 55 (1959).

Cheitlin, M.D., De Castro, C.M., McAllister, H.A.: Sudden death as a complication of anomalous left coronary origin from the anterior sinus of Valsalva. A not-so-minor congenital anomaly. Circulation **50**, 780 (1974).

Cheitlin, M.D., McAllister, H.A., de Castro, C.M.: Myocardial infarction without atherosclerosis. J. Amer. med. Ass. **231**, 951 (1975).

Chesler, E., Joffe, N., Schamroth, L., Meyers, A.: Annular subvalvular left ventricular aneurysms in the South African Bantu. Circulation **32**, 43 (1965).

Chesler, E., Korns, M.E., Porter, G.E., Reyes, C.N., Edwards, J.E.: False aneurysm of the left ventricle secondary to bacterial endocarditis with perforation of the mitral-aortic intervalvular fibrosa. Circulation **37**, 518 (1968).

Chiari, H.: Ueber Netzbildungen im rechten Vorhofe des Herzens. Beitr. Path. Anat. **22**, 1 (1897).

Chiechi, M.A., Lees, W.M., Thompson, R.: Functional anatomy of the normal mitral valve. J. thorac. Surg. **32**, 378 (1956).

Chinn, J., Chinn, M.A.: Report of an accessory coronary artery arising from the pulmonary artery. Anat. Rec. **139**, 23 (1961).

Cockshott, W.P., Antia, A., Ikeme, A., Uzodike, V.O.: Annular subvalvar left ventricular aneurysms. Brit. J. Radiol. **40**, 424 (1967).

Crainicianu, A.: Anatomische Studien über die Coronararterien und experimentelle Untersuchungen über ihre Durchgängigkeit. Virchows Arch. Path. Anat. **238**, 1 (1922).

D

Danielson, G.K., Cooper, E., Tweeddale, D.N.: Circumflex coronary artery injury during mitral valve replacement. Ann. thorac. Surg. **4**, 53 (1967).

Davis, P.K.B., Kinmonth, J.B.: The movements of the annulus of the mitral valve. J. cardiovasc. Surg. **4**, 427 (1963).

DiDio, L.J.A.: The atrioventricular branches of the human coronary arteries. J. Morph. **123**, 397 (1967).

Dorland's Illustrated Medical Dictionary, 24th edit. Philadelphia, Pa.: W.B. Saunders, 1965.

E

Eckner, F.A.O., Brown, B.W., Overll, E., et al.: Alteration of the gross dimensions of the heart and its structures by formalin fixation: A quantitative study. Virchows Arch. (Path. Anat.) **346**, 318 (1969).

Eckner, F.A.O., Brown, B.W., Davidson, D.L., Glagov, S.: Dimensions of normal human hearts after standard fixation by controlled pressure coronary perfusion. Arch. Path. **88**, 497 (1969).

Editorial: The sick sinus. J. Amer. med. Ass. **225**, 632 (1973).

Edwards, J.C., Burnsides, C., Swarm, R.L., Lansing, A.I.: Arteriosclerosis in the intramural and extramural portions of coronary arteries in the human heart. Circulation **13**, 235 (1956).

Edwards, J.E.: An atlas of acquired diseases of the heart and great vessels. Philadelphia: W.B. Saunders, 1961.

Edwards, J.E., Burchell, H.B.: Effects of pulmonary hypertension of the tracheobroncial tree. Dis. Chest **38**, 272 (1960).

Edwards, J.E., Carey, L.S., Neufeld, H.N., Lester, R.G.: Congenital heart disease. Philadelphia: W.B. Saunders, 1965.

Esmond, W.G., Moulton, G.A., Cowley, R.A., Attar, S., Blair, E.: Peripheral ramification of the cardiac conducting system. Circulation **27**, 732 (1963).

Eustachi, B.: 'Opuscula anatomica' Venetiis. Vincentius Luchinus excudebat, 1563.

F

Farrer-Brown, G., Rowles, P.M.: Vascular supply of interventricular septum of human heart. Brit. Heart J. **31**, 727 (1969).

Fehn, P.A., Howe, B.B., Pensinger, R.R.: Comparative anatomical studies of the coronary arteries of canine and porcine heart. II. Interventricular septum. Acta anat. (Basel) **71**, 223 (1968).

Feldt, R.H., DuShane, J.W., Titus, J.L.: The anatomy of the atrioventricular conduction system in ventricular septal defect and tetralogy of Fallot: correlations with the electrocardiogram and vectorcardiogram. Circulation **34**, 774 (1966).

Ferrer, M.I.: Sick sinus syndrome in atrial disease. J. Amer. med. Ass. **206**, 645 (1968).

Franklin, K.J.: Cardiovascular studies. Springfield, Ill.: Charles C Thomas, 1948.

Friedman, S., Ash, R., Klein, D., Johnson, J.: Anomalous single coronary atery complicating ventriculotomy in a child with cyanotic congenital heart disease. Amer. Heart J. **59**, 140 (1960).

Fulton, W.F.M.: Coronary arteries. Springfield, Ill.: Charles C. Thomas, 1965.

G

Gadboys, H.L., Slonim, R., Litwak, R.S.: The treacherous anomalous coronary artery. Amer. J. Cardiol. **8**, 854 (1961).

Gasul, B.M., Arcilla, R.A., Lev, M.: Heart disease in children. Philadelphia: Lippincott 1966.

Geens, M., Gonzalez-Lavin, L., Dawbarn, C., Ross, D.N.: The surgical anatomy of the pulmonary artery root in relation to the pulmonary valve autograft and surgery of the right ventricular outflow tract. J. thorac. cardiovasc. Surg. **62**, 262 (1971).

Geiringer, E.: The mural coronary. Amer. Heart J. **41**, 359 (1951).

Glagov, S., Eckner, F.A.O., Lev, M.: Controlled pressure fixation apparatus for hearts. Arch. Path. **76**, 640 (1963).

Godwin, T.F., Auger, P., Key, J.A., Wigle, E.D.: Intrapericardial aneurysmal dilatation of the left atrial appendage. Circulation **37**, 397 (1968).

Goor, D., Lillehei, C.W., Edwards, J.E.: The "sigmoid septum". Amer. J. Roentgenol. **107**, 366 (1969).

Grant, R.P.: Architecture of the right ventricular outflow tract in man. Circulation **24**, 223 (1961).

Grant, R.P.: The embryology of ventricular flow pathways in man. Circulation **25**, 756 (1962).

Green, G.E., Bernstein, S., Reppert, E.H.: The length of the left main coronary artery. Surgery **62**, 1021 (1967).

211

Gross, L.: The blood supply to the heart in its anatomical and clinical aspects. New York: Paul B. Hoeber, 1921.

H

Hackensellner, H.A.: Koronaranomalien unter 1000 auslese-frei untersuchten Herzen. Anat. Anz. **101**, 123 (1955).

Healey, J.E., Jr., Gibbon, J.H., Jr.: Intrapericardial anatomy in relation to pneumonectomy for pulmonary carcinoma. J. thorac. Surg. **19**, 864 (1950).

Helwing, E.: Untersuchungen über die Variabilität der Länge der Arteria coronaria sinistra. Thoraxchirurgie und Vaskuläre Chirurgie **15**, 218 (1967).

Henle, J.: Handbuch der Gefäßlehre des Menschen. Braunschweig, 1876.

Hillestad, L., Eie, H.: Single coronary artery. Acta med. scand. **189**, 409 (1971).

Hudson, C.L., Moritz, A.R., Wearn, J.T.: The extracardiac anastomoses of the coronary arteries. J. exp. Med. **56**, 919 (1932).

Hudson, R.E.B.: Cardiovascular pathology. London: Edward Arnold 1965. Baltimore, Md.: Williams & Wilkins, 1965.

Hurwitz, L.E., Roberts, W.C.: Quadricuspid semilunar valve. Amer. J. Cardiol. **31**, 623 (1973).

Hutter, A.M., Jr., Page, D.L.: Atrial arrhythmias and lipomatous hypertrophy of the cardiac interatrial septum. Amer. Heart J. **82**, 16 (1971).

Hwang, W.S.: Single coronary artery with unusual intramural course in interventricular septum. Singapore med. J. **8**, 147 (1967).

J

James, T.N.: Anatomy of the coronary arteries. New York: Harper & Row, 1961.

James, T.N.: Anatomy of the human sinus node. Anat. Rec. **141**, 109 (1961).

James, T.N.: Morphology of the human atrioventricular node with remarks pertinent to its electrophysiology. Amer. Heart J. **62**, 756 (1961).

James, T.N.: Connecting pathways between the sinus node and A.V. node and between the right and the left atrium in the human heart. Amer. Heart J. **66**, 498 (1963).

James, T.N., Sherf, L., Fine, G., Morales, A.R.: Comparative ultrastructure of the sinus node in man and dog. Circulation **34**, 139 (1966).

Johnsson, K.A.: Collateral circulation between bronchial and coronary arteries—report on two cases verified by selective catheterization of the bronchial arteries. Acta radiol. (Stockh.) **8**, 393 (1969).

K

Kattan, K.R.: Angled view in pulmonary angiography: a new roentgen approach. Radiology **94**, 79 (1970).

Keith, A.: The anatomy of the valvular mechanism round the venous orifices of the right and left auricles, with some observations on the morphology of the heart. J. Anat. (Lond.) **37**, 2 (1903).

Keith, A.: The evolution and action of certain muscular structures of the heart. Lancet **1**, 555 (1904).

Keith, A.: An account of the structures concerned in the production of the jugular pulse. J. Anat. (Lond.) **42**, 1 (1907).

Keith, A., Flack, M.: Form and nature of the muscular connections between the primary divisions of the vertebrate heart. J.Anat. (Paris) **41**, 172 (1907).

Kennel, A.J., Titus, J.L.: The vasculature of the human sinus node. Proc. Mayo Clin. **47**, 556 (1972).

Killen, D.A., Gobbel, W.G., Jr., France, R.: Spontaneous aortic-cleft ventricular fistula associated with myxomatous transformation. Ann. thorac. Surg. **8**, 570 (1969).

Kirk, R.S., Russell, J.G.B.: Subvalvular calcification of mitral valve. Brit. Heart J. **31**, 684 (1969).

Kirklin, J.W., Ellis, F.H., McGoon, D.C., DuShane, J.W., Swan, H.J.C.: Surgical treatment for the tetralogy of Fallot by open intracardiac repair. J. thorac. Surg. **37**, 22 (1959).

Korn, D., DeSanctis, R.W., Sell, S.: Massive calcification of the mitral annulus. New Engl. J. Med. **267**, 900 (1962).

Kugel, M.A.: Anatomical studies on the coronary arteries and their branches. I. Arteria anastomotica auricularis magna. Amer. Heart J. **3**, 260 (1927).

Kyger, E.R. III, Chiariello, L., Hallman, G.L., Cooley, D.A.: Conduit reconstruction of right ventricular outflow tract. Ann. thorac. Surg. **19**, 277 (1975).

L

Lam, J.H.C., Ranganathan, N., Wigle, E.D., Silver, M.D.: Morphology of the human mitral valve. I. Chordae tendineae: a new classification. Circulation **41**, 449 (1970).

Lancisi, G.M.: Dissertatio de vena sine pari. In: Morgagni, J.B. (1765), Opera omnia. Patavil, sumptibus Josephi Remondini, Veniti **1**, 173.

Lane, E.J., Jr., Whalen, J.P.: A new sign of left atrial enlargement: posterior displacement of the left bronchial tree. Radiol. **93**, 279 (1969).

Lenegre, J.: The etiology and pathology of bilateral bundle branch block in relation to complete heart block. Progr. cardiovasc. Dis. **6**, 409 (1964).

LeRoux, B.T.: Anatomical abnormalities of the right upper bronchus. J. thorac. cardiovasc. Surg. **44**, 225 (1962).

LeRoux, B.T., Gotsman, M.S.: Giant left atrium. Thorax **25**, 190 (1970).

Lev, M.: The architecture of the conduction system in congenital heart disease: II. Tetralogy of Fallot. Arch. Path. **67**, 572 (1959).

Lev, M.: The anatomic basis for disturbances in conduction and cardiac arrhythmias. Progr. cardiovasc. Dis. **2**, 360 (1960).

Lev, M.: Conduction system. In pathology of the heart, 2nd edit. Springfield, Ill.: Charles C Thomas, 1960.

Lev, M.: Anatomic basis for atrioventricular block. Amer. J. Med. **37**, 742 (1964).

Longenecker, C.G., Reemtsma, K., Creech, O., Jr.: Surgical implications of single coronary artery, a review and two case reports. Amer. Herat. J. **61**, 382 (1961).

M

McAllister, H.A.: Personal communication. 1975.

MacVaugh, H., III, Joyner, C., Pierce, W.S., Johnson, J.: Repair of subvalvular left ventricular aneurysm occurring as a complication of mitral valve replacement. J. thorac. cardiovasc. Surg. **58**, 291 (1969).

MacVaugh, H. III, Joyner, C.R., Johnson, J.: Unusual complications during mitral valve replacement in the presence of calcification of the annulus. Ann. thorac. Surg. **11**, 336 (1972).

Magarey, F.R.: On the mode of formation of Lambl's excrescences and their relation to chronic thickening of the mitral valve. J. Path. Bact. **61**, 203 (1949).

Manninen, V., Rissanen, V.T., Halonen, P.I.: Coronary ostium outside the aortic sinus. A factor in the aetiology of ischaemic heart disease? Advanc. Cardiol. **4**, 94 (1970).

Marshall, J.: On development of the great anterior veins in man, etc. Phil. Trans. B **140**, 133 (1850).

Mathew, R., Replogle, R., Thilenius, O.G., Arcilla, R.A.: Right juxtaposition of the atrial appendages. Chest **67**, 483 (1975).

Merideth, J., Titus, J.L.: The anatomic atrial connections between sinus and a-v node. Circulation **37**, 566 (1968).

Meyer, B.W., Verska, J.J., Lindesmith, G.G., Jones, J.J.: Open repair of mitral valve lesions: the superior approach. Ann. thorac. Surg. **1**, 453 (1965).

Moberg, A.: Anastomoses between extracardial vessels and coronary arteries. Acta med. scand., Suppl. 485 (1968).

Morrow, A.G., Fisher, R.D., Fogarty, T.J.: Isolated hypertrophic obstruction to right ventricular outflow. Amer. Heart J. **77**, 814 (1969).

N

Nathan, H., Orda, R., Barkay, M.: The right bronchial artery. Anatomical considerations and surgical approach. Thorax **25**, 328 (1970).

O

Ogden, J.A.: Congenital anomalies of the coronary arteries. Amer. J. Cardiol. **25**, 474 (1970).

Onat, A., Ersanli, O., Kanuni, A., Aykan, T.: Congenital aortic sinus aneurysms with particular reference to dissection of the interventricular septum. Amer. Heart J. **72**, 158 (1966).

P

Petelenz, T.: Extracoronary arteries of the myocardium in man. Folia cardiol. (Milano) **22**, 223 (1963).

Petelenz, T.: Extracoronary shunts with coronary arteries in man. Cardiologia (Basel) **47**, 323 (1965).

Pocock, W.A., Cockshott, W.P., Ball, P.J.A., Steiner, R.E.: Left ventricular aneurysms of uncertain etiology. Brit. Heart J. **27**, 184 (1965).

Polacek, P., Kralove, H.: Relation of myocardial bridges and loops on the coronary arteries to coronary occlusions. Amer. Heart J. **61**, 44 (1961).

Powell, E.D.U., Mullaney, J.M.: The Chiari network and the valve of the inferior vena cava. Brit. Heart J. **22**, 579 (1960).

R

Ranganathan, N., Lam, J.H.C., Wigle, E.D.: Morphology of the human mitral valve. 2. The valve leaflets. Circulation **41**, 459 (1970).

Reeve, R., MacDonald, D.: Partial absence of the right ventricular musculature—partial parchment heart. Amer. J. Cardiol. **14**, 415 (1964).

Reid, K.: The anatomy of the sinus of Valsalva. Thorax **25**, 79 (1970).

Roberts, W.C., Morrow, A.G.: Causes of early postoperative death following cardiac valve replacement. J. thorac. cardiovasc. Surg. **54**, 422 (1967).

Roberts, W.C., Perloff, J.K.: Mitral valvular disease. Ann. intern. Med. **77**, 939 (1972).

Robinson, G., Attai, L., Kaplitt, M.J.: Clinical experience with superior approach to mitral valve. N.Y. St. J. Med., **71**, 2649 (1971).

Rodriguez, F.L., Robbins, S.L., Banasiewicz, M.: The descending septal artery in human, porcine, equine, ovine, bovine and canine hearts: a postmortem angiographic study. Amer. Heart J. **62**, 247 (1961).

Rosenbaum, M.B.: Hemiblocks: New concepts of intraventricular conduction based on human anatomical, physiological and clinical studies. Oldsmar, Fla.: Tampa Tracings, 1970.

Rusted, I.E., Scheifley, C.H., Edwards, J.E.: Studies of the mitral valve: I. Anatomic features of the normal mitral valve and associated structures. Circulation **6**, 825 (1952).

S

Saksena, D.S., Tucker, B.L., Lindesmith, G.G., Nelson, R.M., Stiles, Q.R., Meyer, B.W.: The superior approach to the mitral valve. A review of clinical experience. Ann. thorac. Surg. **12**, 146 (1971).

Schroeckenstein, R.F., Wasenda, G.J., Edwards, J.E.: Valvular competent patent foramen ovale in adults. Minn. Med. **55**, 11 (1972).

Shaher, R.M., Puddu, G.C.: Coronary arterial anatomy in complete transposition of the great vessels. Amer. J. Cardiol. **17**, 355 (1966).

Silverman, M.E., Hurst, J.W.: The mitral complex. Amer. Heart J. **76**, 399 (1968).

Simon, M.A., Liu, S.F.: Calcification of the mitral valve annulus and its relation to functional valvular disturbance. Amer. Heart J. **48**, 497 (1954).

Smith, J.C.: Review of single coronary artery with report of two cases. Circulation **1**, 1168 (1950).

Smol'iannikov, A., Naddachina, A.: Anomalies of the coronary arteries. Arkh. Pat. **25**, 3 (1963).

Sones, F.M., Jr., Shirey, E.K.: Cine coronary arteriography. Mod. Conc. cardiov. Dis. **31**, 735 (1962).

Sondergaard, T., Gotzsche, H., Ottosen, P., Schultz, J.: Surgical closure of interatrial septal defects by circumclusion. Acta chir. scand. **109**, 188 (1955).

Spalteholz, W.: Die Arterien der Herzwand. Leipzig: S. Hirzel, 1924.

Symbas, P.N., Walter, P.F., Hurst, J.W., Schlant, R.C.: Fenestration of aortic cusps causing aortic regurgitation. J. thorac cardiovasc. Surg. **57**, 464 (1969).

T

Taguchi, K., Sasaki, N., Matsuura, Y., Uemura, R: Surgical correction of aneurysm of the sinus of Valsalva. Amer. J. Cardiol. **23**, 180 (1969).

Tandler, J.: Anatomie des Herzens. Jena: G. Fischer, 1913.

Tenckhoff, L., Stamm, S.J., Beckwith, J.B.: Sudden death in idiopathic (congenital) right atrial enlargement. Circulation **40**, 227 (1969).

Thebesius, A.C.: Dissertatio de circulo sanguinis in corde. Lugdunum Batavorum, 1708.

Thomas, C.E.: The muscular architecture of the atria of hog and dog hearts. Amer. J. Anat. **104**, 207 (1959).

Titus, J.L.: Normal anatomy of the human cardiac conduction system. Proc. Mayo Clin. **48**, 24 (1973).

Titus, J.L., Daugherty, G.W., Edwards, J.E.: Anatomy of the normal human atrioventricular conduction system. Amer. J. Anat. **113**, 407 (1963).

U

Uhl, H.S.M.: A previously undescribed congenital malformation of the heart: Almost total absence of the myocardium of the right ventricle. Bull. Johns Hopk. Hosp. **91**, 197 (1952).

V

Vieussens, R.: Nouvelles decouvertes sur le coeur. Paris 1706.

Voboril, Z.B.: Todaro's tendon in the heart. I. Todaro's tendon in the normal human heart. Folia morph. **15**, 187 (1967).

W

Waldhausen, J.A., Petry, E.L., Kurlander, G.J.: Successful repair of subvalvular annular aneurysm of the left ventricle. New Engl. J. Med. **275**, 984 1966.

Wallach, J.D., Howcroft, T.: Variable number of coronary os in the aorta of the Zululand wildebeeste. Veterinary Medicine/Small Animal Clinician, **62**, 21 (1967).

Walmsley, R.: Orientation of the heart and appearance of its chambers in the adult cadaver. Brit. Heart J. **20**, 441 (1958).

Walmsley, R.: Gross anatomy of the heart. Anat. Rec. **136**, 298 (1960).

Walmsley, R., Watson, H.: The medial wall of the right atrium. Circulation **34**, 400 (1966).

Walmsley, R., Watson, H.: The outflow tract of the left ventricle. Brit. Heart J. **28**, 435 (1966).

Walmsley, R., Watson, H.: Clinical Anatomy of the heart. In: Watson, H.: Pediatric cardiology. St. Louis: C.V. Mosby, 1968.

Walmsley, T.: The heart. In: Quain's elements of anatomy, 11th edit., vol. 4. London: Longmans Green, 1929.

Waterston, D.J.: Treatment of Fallot's tetralogy in infants under the age of one year. Rozhl. Chir. **41**, 181 (1962).

Widran, J., Lev, M.: The dissection of the atrioventricular node, bundle and bundle branches in the human heart. Circulation **IV**, 863 (1951).

Wright, R.R., Anson, B.J., Cleveland, H.C.: The vestigial valves and the interatrial foramen of the adult human heart. Anat. Rec. **100**, 331 (1948).

Y

Yater, W.M.: Heart block due to calcareous lesions of the His bundle. Ann. intern. Med. **8**, 777 (1935).

Yates, J.D., Kirsh, M.M., Sodeman, T.M., Walton, J.A., Jr., Brymer, J.F.: Coronary ostial stenosis. A complication of aortic valve replacement. Circulation **49**, 530 (1974).

Z

Zimmerman, J.: A new look at cardiac anatomy. J. A. Einstein med. Cent. **7**, 77 (1959).

Zimmerman, J., Bailey, C.P.: The surgical significance of the fibrous skeleton of the heart. J. thorac. cardiovasc. Surg. **44**, 701 (1962).

Subject Index

218

Abbreviations

I. The Left Heart

A. The Aorto-Ventricular Unit _ _ _ _ _ A.V. Unit
   Aorta _ _ _ _ _ _ _ _ _ _ Ao
   Aortic Sinuses, Leaflets and Annuli
      Right (Anterior) _ _ _ _ _ _ _ R
      Left (Left Posterior) _ _ _ _ _ L
      Posterior (Right Posterior) _ _ _ P
   Aorto-Ventricular Membrane _ _ _ _ A.V.M.
      Junction of Divisions _ _ _ _ J or R.F.T
   Membranous Septum _ _ _ _ _ _ M.S.
      Atrial or Atrioventricular Portion _ _ A.M.S.
      Ventricular Portion _ _ _ _ _ V.M.S.
   Mitral Valve _ _ _ _ _ _ _ M.V.
      Anterior Leaflet _ _ _ _ _ _ A.M.V.
      Posterior Leaflet _ _ _ _ _ _ P.M.V.
      Superior Commissure _ _ _ _ _ S.C.
      Inferior Commissure _ _ _ _ _ I.C.
   Fibrous Trigones
      Right Anterior _ _ _ _ _ _ R.A.F.T.
      Left Anterior _ _ _ _ _ _ _ L.A.F.T.
      Left _ _ _ _ _ _ _ _ _ L.F.T.
      Right _ _ _ _ _ _ _ _ R.F.T.
      Intervalvular _ _ _ _ _ _ _ I.V.T.
   Left Ventricle _ _ _ _ _ _ _ L.V.
   Papillary Muscles
      Lateral _ _ _ _ _ _ _ _ L.P.M.
      Posterior _ _ _ _ _ _ _ _ P.P.M.

B. Left Atrium _ _ _ _ _ _ _ _ L.A.
   Left Atrial Appendage _ _ _ _ _ L.A.A.
   Pulmonary Veins e.g., Right Superior _ _ R.S.P.V.

II. The Right Heart

A. Right Atrium _ _ _ _ _ _ _ _ R.A.
   Superior Vena Cava _ _ _ _ _ _ S.V.C.
   Inferior Vena Cava _ _ _ _ _ _ I.V.C.
   Coronary Sinus _ _ _ _ _ _ _ C.S.
   Appendages and Fossae:
      Superior _ _ _ _ _ _ _ _ R.A.A.
      Inferomedial _ _ _ _ _ _ _ I.M.F.
      Inferolateral _ _ _ _ _ _ _ I.L.F.
   Muscle Bundles:
      Terminal _ _ _ _ _ _ _ _ T.B.
      Sagittal _ _ _ _ _ _ _ _ S.B.
      Precaval _ _ _ _ _ _ _ _ P.C.B.
      Posterior Limbic _ _ _ _ _ _ P.L.B.
      Anterior Limbic _ _ _ _ _ _ A.L.B.
      Lower _ _ _ _ _ _ _ _ _ L.B.
   Valves:
      Inferior Vena Cava (Eustachius) _ _ _ V.E.
      Coronary Sinus (Thebesius) _ _ _ _ V.T.
   Supravalvular Lamina _ _ _ _ _ S.V.L.
   Fossa Ovalis _ _ _ _ _ _ _ F.O.

B. Right Ventricle _ _ _ _ _ _ _ R.V.
   Infundibular Muscle Band
      Parietal _ _ _ _ _ _ _ _ P.B.
      Septal _ _ _ _ _ _ _ _ _ S.B.
      Moderator _ _ _ _ _ _ _ M.B.
   Valves:
      Tricuspid _ _ _ _ _ _ _ _ T.V.
      Pulmonary _ _ _ _ _ _ _ P.V.
   Pulmonary Leaflets:
      Posterior _ _ _ _ _ _ _ _ P
      Right Anterolateral _ _ _ _ _ R.A.L.
      Left Anterolateral _ _ _ _ _ _ L.A.L.

Papillary Muscles:
   Superior (Luschka or Lancisi) _ _ _ _ S.P.M.
   Anterior _ _ _ _ _ _ _ _ A.P.M.
   Inferior _ _ _ _ _ _ _ _ I.P.M.

C. Pulmonary Trunk _ _ _ _ _ _ _ P.T.
   Right Pulmonary Artery _ _ _ _ _ R.P.A.
   Left Pulmonary Artery _ _ _ _ _ L.P.A.

III. The Coronary Arteries

A. Left Coronary Artery _ _ _ _ _ _ L.C.A.
   Left Main Branch _ _ _ _ _ _ L.M.B.
   Anterior Division _ _ _ _ _ _ A.D.
      Anterior Interventricular Branch _ _ _ A.I.V.
      Anterolateral Branch _ _ _ _ _ A.L.
      Lateral Branch _ _ _ _ _ _ L.B.
      Septal Branches:
         Left Superior Septal _ _ _ _ L.S.S.
      Lateral Division _ _ _ _ _ _ L.D.
      Posterior Division _ _ _ _ _ P.D.
         Lateral Branch _ _ _ _ _ _ L.B.
         Obtuse Marginal _ _ _ _ _ O.M.
         Posterior Branch _ _ _ _ _ P.B.
         Posterior Descending _ _ _ _ P.D.A.
B. Right Coronary Artery _ _ _ _ _ R.C.A.
   Conus Branch _ _ _ _ _ _ _ C.B.
   Marginal Branch _ _ _ _ _ _ M.B.
   Preventricular Branch _ _ _ _ _ P.V.B.
   Posterior Descending _ _ _ _ _ P.D.A.
   Left Ventricular Branch _ _ _ _ _ L.V.B.
   A.V. Node Branch _ _ _ _ _ _ A.V.N.A.
C. Atrial Branches
   Right Sinus Node Artery _ _ _ _ _ R.S.A.
   Left Sinus Node Artery _ _ _ _ _ L.S.A.
   Posterior Sinus Node
   Artery _ _ _ _ _ _ _ _ P.S.A.

IV. Miscellaneous

Pericardium
   Aortocaval Recess _ _ _ _ _ _ A.C.R.
   Retrocaval Recess _ _ _ _ _ _ R.C.R.
Trachea _ _ _ _ _ _ _ _ _ T
Left Main Bronchus _ _ _ _ _ _ L.M.Br.

List of Abbreviations in Alphabetical Order

A.C.R. _ _ Aortocaval Recess
A.D. _ _ Anterior Division of the Left Coronary Artery
A.I.V. _ _ Anterior Interventricular Branch of the
   Left Coronary Artery
A.L. _ _ Anterolateral Branch of the Left Coronary Artery
A.L.B. _ _ Anterior Limbic Band (of the Right Atrium)
A.M.V. _ _ Anterior Leaflet of the Mitral Valve
Ao _ _ Aorta
A.P.M. _ _ Anterior Papillary Muscle (of the Right Ventricle)
A.V. Unit _ _ Aorto-Ventricular Unit
A.V.N.A. _ _ A.V. Node Artery
C.B. _ _ _ Conus Branch
C.S. _ _ Coronary Sinus
F.O. _ _ Fossa Ovalis
I.A.B. _ _ Interatrial Muscle Bundle
I.C. _ _ _ Inferior Commissure of the Mitral Valve
I.L.F. _ _ Inferolateral Fossa (of the Right Atrium)
I.M.F. _ _ Inferomedial Fossa (of the Right Atrium)
I.P.M. _ _ Inferior Papillary Muscle (of the Right Ventricle)
I.V.C. _ _ Inferior Vena Cava
I.V.T. _ _ Intervalvular Trigone

J _ _ _ Junction of Divisions of the
   Aorto-Ventricular Membrane
L _ _ _ Left (Left Posterior) Aortic Sinus, Leaflet
   or Annulus
L.A. _ _ Left Atrium
L.A.A. _ Left Atrial Appendage
L.A.F.T. _ Left Anterior Fibrous Trigone
L.A.L. _ Left Anterolateral Pulmonary Sinus,
   Leaflet or Annulus
L.B. _ _ Lateral Branch of the Left Coronary Artery
L.C.A. _ Left Coronary Artery
L.D. _ _ Lateral Division of the Left Coronary Artery
L.F.T. _ Left Fibrous Trigone
L.M.B. _ Left Main Branch of the Left Coronary Artery
L.M.Br. _ Left Main Bronchus
L.P.A. _ Left Pulmonary Artery
L.P.M. _ Lateral Papillary Muscle
L.S.A. _ Left Sinus Node Artery
L.S.S. _ Left Superior Septal Artery
L.V. _ Left Ventricle
L.V.B. _ Left Ventricular Branch of the Right Coronary Artery
M.A.C. _ Minor Atrial Circumflex Branch of the
   Left Coronary Artery
M.B. _ _ Moderator Bundle or Band (in Right Ventricle)
M.S. _ _ Membranous Septum
M.V. _ Mitral Valve
O.M. _ _ Obtuse Marginal Artery
P _ _ Posterior (Right Posterior) Aortic Sinus,
   Leaflet or Annulus
P _ _ Posterior Pulmonary Sinus, Leaflet or Annulus
P.B. _ _ Parietal Muscle Bundle of the Right Ventricle
P.B. _ _ Posterior Branch of the Left Coronary Artery
P.C.B. _ Precaval Muscle Bundle
P.D. _ _ Posterior Division of the Left Coronary Artery
P.D.A. _ Posterior Descending Artery
P.L.B. _ Posterior Limbic Band (of the Right Atrium)
P.M.V. _ Posterior Leaflet of the Mitral Valve
P.P.M. _ Posterior Papillary Muscle (Left Ventricle)
P.S.A. _ Posterior Sinus Node Artery
P.T. _ _ Pulmonary Trunk
P.V. _ _ Pulmonary Valve
P.V.B. _ Preventricular Branch
R _ _ _ Right (Anterior) Aortic Sinus, Leaflet or Annulus
R.A. _ _ Right Atrium
R.A.A. _ (Superior) Right Atrial Appendage
R.A.F.T. _ Right Anterior Fibrous Trigone
R.A.L. _ Right Anterolateral Pulmonary Sinus,
   Leaflet or Annulus
R.C.A. _ Right Coronary Artery
R.C.R. _ Retrocaval Recess
R.F.T. _ Right Fibrous Trigone
R.M.Br. _ Right Main Bronchus
R.P.A. _ Right Pulmonary Artery
R.S.A. _ Right Sinus Node Artery
R.S.P.V. _ Right Superior Pulmonary Vein
S.B. _ _ Septal Band of the Right Ventricle
S.C. _ _ Superior Commissure of the Mitral Valve
S.P.M. _ Superior Papillary Muscle (of the Right
   Ventricle) — Luschka or Lancisi
S.V.C. _ Superior Vena Cava
S.V.L. _ Supravalvular Lamina
T _ _ _ Trachea
T.B. _ _ Terminal Muscle Bundle of the Right Atrium
T.V. _ _ Triscuspid Valve
V.E. _ _ Inferior Vena Cava (Eustachius) Valve
V.T. _ _ Coronary Sinus (Thebesius) Valve